BIOCHEMISTRY RESEARCH TRENDS

CREATININE

PRODUCTION, DIAGNOSTIC USES AND ROLE IN RENAL DISEASE

BIOCHEMISTRY RESEARCH TRENDS

Additional books in this series can be found on Nova's website
under the Series tab.

Additional e-books in this series can be found on Nova's website
under the e-book tab.

NEPHROLOGY RESEARCH AND CLINICAL DEVELOPMENTS

Additional books in this series can be found on Nova's website
under the Series tab.

Additional e-books in this series can be found on Nova's website
under the e-book tab.

BIOCHEMISTRY RESEARCH TRENDS

CREATINE

PRODUCTION, DIAGNOSTIC USES AND ROLE IN RENAL DISEASE

IVAN H. PERKINS
AND
CATHERINE M. CHAPMAN
EDITORS

New York

Library of Congress Cataloging-in-Publication Data

ISBN: 978-1-62257-475-9
Library of Congress Control Number: 2012942810

Published by Nova Science Publishers, Inc. † New York

Contents

Preface

Creatinine, a muscle waste product, is widely interpreted as a measure of renal function. However, the serum level reflects not only renal excretion, but also the generation, intake, and metabolism of creatinine. In this book, the authors present current research in the study of the production, diagnostic uses and role in renal disease of creatinine. Topics include the diagnostic use of creatinine in preeclampsia; serum creatinine and its effect and management in renal and hepatic disease; evaluation of renal function in patients with cirrhosis; the role of creatinine in kidney disease in neonates, infants and children; and retinol X creatinine in kidney disease.

Chapter I – Preeclampsia is a major complication in pregnancy, occurring in 7-10% of all pregnant women. Hypertension in pregnancy is associated with fetal and maternal adverse outcomes: the risks are higher when significant proteinuria is associated. Proteinuria may be measured in single voided urine samples or in 24-hour pools, the latter considered as the gold standard test. Errors in pooling may occur, especially in outpatient tests and without the control with creatininuria levels. Moreover, a quick diagnostic test may be needed due to the severity of clinical manifestations: an alternative solution is assessing protein in single urine voided samples.

Despite the fact that the reagent stick is the most commonly used proteinuria screening test for preeclampsia after the assessment of blood pressure, its use has been challenged by several authors. The urine protein-to-creatinine ratio proved to be an accurate method for the diagnosis of preeclampsia when correlated with the 24-hour proteinuria. It is a more reliable means of assessing protein in single voided urine specimens. This rate is an efficient, quick and easy test for the diagnosis of preeclampsia.

The predictive diagnosis of preeclampsia and a differential diagnosis from other forms of hypertension can be difficult to accomplish at first clinical presentation, especially in the presence of proteinuria. The identification of markers has been the objective of many researchers.

Many investigators have written about hypocalciuria in preeclampsia compared with normotensive pregnant women. It could be the result of reduced glomerular filtration rate, which appears at the same time as proteinuria, but the mechanism of hypocalciuria is still unclear. Studies using measurements of 24-hour urinary calcium excretion have documented decreased excretion in women with preeclampsia or who developed a disease some time after the collection of urine.

Twenty-four hour calciuria has been used as an indicator of disease, but sometimes a prompt examination or a rapid test is required for monitoring high-risk pregnancies: the calcium-to-creatinine ratio seems to be a good candidate for use in both cases.

This chapter was based on a case-control study that evaluated the relationship between hypocalciuria and preeclampsia by comparing pregnant women with severe and mild preeclampsia, and hypertensive and normotensive cases, analyzing the calcium-to-creatinine ratio and the correlation with 24-hour calciuria as a diagnostic test for preeclampsia.

There were statistically significant differences between the groups when comparing severe preeclampsia and chronic hypertension, severe preeclampsia and normal pregnancy, and mild and severe preeclampsia ($p<0.0001$). The Spearman index between the calcium-to-creatinine ratio and 24-hour calciuria was 0.65 (high correlation). The best cutoff point was 0.053 mg/mg, showing a sensitivity of 70% and a specificity of 85%, with positive and negative predictive values of 80% and 74%, respectively.

The calcium-to-creatinine ratio can reliably estimate 24-hour calciuria, differentiating severe preeclampsia from mild preeclampsia, chronic hypertension and normal pregnancy, helping to diagnose hypertension diseases during the pregnancy.

Chapter II - Plasma creatinine is one of the most frequently prescribed blood tests in clinical practice. Indeed, although it has used for many decades, it remains the reference marker to assess renal function. In this chapter, the authors propose to detail the physiological aspects that explain that creatinine is a relatively good marker of endogenous glomerular filtration. The authors will review the determinants of plasma creatinine independent of GFR, in terms of muscle production, non-renal clearance and tubular secretion. The value and limitations of the urinary clearance of creatinine will be discussed. The authors will present the formulas derived from serum creatinine to estimate GFR.

Chapter III - Chronic kidney disease (CKD) comprises a spectrum of pathology with significant medical and financial burden, affecting at least 26 million individuals in the United States. The staging of CKD has implications upon the utilization of medical therapeutics and procedural interventions, including renal replacement therapies such as hemodialysis and transplantation. The ability to measure CKD is based upon many parameters, an important one being the glomerular filtration rate (GFR). The assessment of GFR, despite numerous iterations, still for practical reasons, relies heavily upon the serum creatinine level, a suboptimal marker. Creatinine exists within a complex biology wherein its serum level is affected by intrinsic factors such as age and nutritional status, and extrinsic factors such as medications and other forms of iatrogenic intervention. Furthermore, the nature of the creatinine assays themselves are non-standardized, and their ability to sense true creatinine concentrations are affected at times quite severely by non-creatinine chromogens. Unfortunately many clinical decisions are made with the simple assumption that the reported serum creatinine level truly represents an *in vivo* level and that by extension the severity of CKD. Beyond the immediate consequences of this assumption, the long-term consequences can be quite significant. Medical surveillance, specific pharmacologic and procedural replacement therapies, including transplantation of a kidney and simultaneous liver-kidney transplantation rest in large measure upon the serum creatinine level and its expression of kidney function. Implementation of therapy can be life-extending, however, unfortunately in other cases, medically-deserving patients are denied treatment given the limitations and/or mis-allocation of these resources based upon the same creatinine measurement. In this review, the complexities of creatinine analysis, it's evolving role in assessing kidney function, and it's ultimate effect upon renal and liver replacement therapies will be discussed.

Chapter IV - Renal function in patients with cirrhosis is an important prognostic factor, both before and following liver transplantation (LT). The importance of renal function is reflected by serum creatinine (Cr) being in the model for end stage liver disease (MELD) score, which predicts the likelihood of death within 3 months for patients on liver transplant waiting lists and is used for prioritization of recipients ("sickest first"). Creatinine is also part of the UKELD score which predicts waiting list mortality over 1 year. Cr is a routine laboratory test and is part of the definitions of acute kidney injury, and hepatorenal syndrome in patients with progressive liver disease. However, it is only an indirect marker of renal function, i.e. of glomerular filtration rate (GFR). Unfortunately, all methods currently in use for assessment of renal function have several limitations and also do not have a good correlation with true GFR. Creatinine estimations are readily available but affected by changes in creatinine generation rate, volume of distribution and assay interference that can affect their interpretation. For example, serum creatinine is dependent upon other factors, including dietary meat, the conversion rate of creatine to creatinine, renal tubular secretion of creatinine, urinary flow rate, hydration status, as well as the total pool of body creatine (total muscle mass). The latter can lead to different Cr concentration between individuals with the same renal function but of different age, race and sex.

Creatinine assays are also subject to interference by chromogens: bilirubin (both conjugated and unconjugated) which typically reduces the creatinine numerical value. In patients with cirrhosis the interference of bilirubin with Cr measurement is a major problem leading to differences in MELD scores up to 7 points, particularly in patients with the highest priority for LT. Modifications to reduce bilirubin interference are used, including enzymatic methods, but these are mostly more expensive and still underestimate creatinine at high bilirubin concentrations..It is important to recognise that there is no universal reference standard for creatinine, and hence, laboratory standardisation of techniques and 'normal' values would be necessary for all liver transplant units to avoid systematic biases in UKELD and MELD-based allocation systems, or others which incorporate Cr values.

Unfortunately, other renal biomarkers, such as cystatin C also have limitations, as cystatin C production is not constant and varies with inflammation. Inulin clearances are impractical in clinical practice. Single bolus isotopic and iodinated radiocontrast methods tend to over estimate "true" GFR in volume expanded patients with ascites, and further inaccuracy is added when attempts are made to correct for body surface area. A recently published modified Tikhonov method may improve isotopic estimation. Further studies are needed in large series of cirrhotic patients to correlate "true" GFR with potential serum or urinary markers, which could result in the creation and validation of more specific mathematical formulae for GFR in patients with cirrhosis.

Chapter V- Glomerular filtration rate (GFR) is an accepted parameter for assessing kidney function. Measurement of clearance of external substances that are freely filtered in the glomerulus but not reabsorbed or excreted in the tubules (inulin or some isotopic agents) is the "gold standard" for GFR, but this method is cumbersome for critical practice and so GFR is usually based in the clearance of endogenous substances, i.e. serum creatinine (Crs).

So, for the critically ill patient, 24 hours creatinine clearance (or shorter intervals) is the method of reference for the estimation of the GFR, although this is often not measured but estimated by equations based on anthropometric data and isolated valued of Crs (i.e.

Cockroft-Gault or MDRD equations), event though these were not designed for ICU patients and perform poorly in this setting.

Whatever the method employed, renal evaluation rests in Crs but this is subjected to wide variations dependent on multiple factors, among which we should highlight race, sex, nutritional status, proteins intake and, specially significant in critical care, the over-hydration and the loss of muscle mass. Also the laboratory method used, either the Jaffe or the more recently introduced enzymatic one, introduce variations in Crs.

It is significant that in subjects with normal kidney function, when the Crs amounts to 2 mg/dL, over a fifty per cent of the kidney reserve has been lost. Also it has been proven that small increases in Crs, either absolute or as relative changes over the basal value, has serious repercussion on the prognosis of patients.

But even when it is well accepted that acute kidney injury (AKI) is common in patients in ICU and it conditions a longer stay and an increase on cost, as well as an increase in associated mortality, it has not been until the last decade that really serious efforts have been undertook by the professionals directly involved in AKI management (nephrologists and intensivists) in order to unify diagnostic criteria and to stratify risk.

In this sense, since the beginning of this century, various approaches such as the SHARF or SIRE initiatives initiated what eventually crystallized in the RIFLE and later in the AKIN systems. Both are based on the evaluation of sequential changes in GFR (estimated either through clearance or Crs) or urine flow.

The experience accumulated with these systems has made evident their usefulness but also some potential problems and areas for improvement.

For one side RIFLE or AKIN have provided a common definition of AKI for those who treat ICU patients and because their sensitivity for detecting AKI have meant a considerable advantage for the clinician (previously we had more than 25 definitions of renal failure) but, on the other side this same fact is a drawback for clinical research because potentially overestimating AKI incidence if we count on the early stages of these systems (R or 1) as kidney failure. Other significant problem is the unavoidable delay before a patient is classified that is perhaps the one to be overcome in the near future.

Chapter VI - Kidney disease has become a global pandemic in the last decade and it is estimated that more than 2 million people in the United States will require transplantation or dialysis for kidney failure by the year 2030. Chronic kidney disease is defined as an estimated glomerular filtration rate (GFR) of less than 60ml/min/1.73m2 or the presence of kidney damage (detected by abnormalities in urinalysis, imaging or pathology) for 3 months or more. Several studies have shown that kidney disease is an independent predictor for cardiovascular and all-cause mortality. There is also ample evidence to show that early detection and effective treatment may halt or retard the progression of kidney disease. This highlights the importance of raising awareness among health care providers and increases their familiarity with the most commonly used methods of evaluating kidney function.

Serum creatinine is the most commonly used measure for estimating kidney function. It is an amino acid derived from the non-enzymatic breakdown of creatine and creatine phosphate in skeletal muscle. Several factors affect its generation including age, gender, race or ethnic group, body habitus, diet, and malnutrition. It is freely filtered across the glomerulus and is neither metabolized nor reabsorbed by the kidney. It is however secreted by the organic cation secretory pathways in the proximal tubules: thus, the creatinine clearance exceeds the actual GFR. Creatinine is measured in most laboratories in the US using the colorimetric alkaline picrate (Jaffe) method which is prone to analytical errors because it also detects non-creatinine chromogens like acetoacetate. Enzymatic methods for measuring creatinine have been reported to have less interference than the Jaffe method.

Elevations in serum creatinine (SCr) almost always reflects decreased glomerular filtration rate (GFR) especially in the absence of drugs that interfere with its tubular secretion (like cimetidine or trimethoprim) or rhabdomyolysis where there is increased creatinine generation. However the relationship between SCr and GFR is not linear, hence small increases in SCr signify marked reduction in GFR. Because of these limitations of SCr as an index of GFR, several prediction equations are in use for estimating GFR and appear to provide a substantial improvement over the measurement of SCr alone in the clinical assessment of kidney function. The commonly used prediction equations are the Cockcroft-Gault (CG) and Modification of Diet in Renal Disease (MDRD) equations. More recently, the Chronic Kidney Disease Epidemiology Collaboration (CKD-EPI) equation is being increasingly used, particularly in many clinical trials. However, these equations have their own limitations, not least because they also depend on SCr measurements. In addition, these equations were derived in specific populations, so it may be inaccurate when used in different subpopulations.

In conclusion, although measurement of SCr and the GFR estimation equations are imperfect methods for evaluating kidney function (especially in populations without kidney disease); they facilitate early detection, evaluation and management of the renal disease.

Chapter VII - Creatinine, a muscle waste product, is widely interpreted as a measure of renal function. However, the serum level reflects not only renal excretion, but also the generation, intake, and metabolism of creatinine. In stable normal or reduced renal function they are determined by the rate of creatinine production and the endogenous creatinine clearance, and, during changing renal function, also by the apparent volume of distribution of creatinine. The rate of creatinine production is proportional to body weight, and it decreases with age and is slower in females than in males. Elevated creatinine levels suggest the differential diagnosis of renal failure. History and a complete physical examination are important. An ultrasound scan is particularly useful for eliminating an obstructive cause while complementary blood tests and imaging studies might be useful. The authors reviewed the principles of physiology, metabolism of creatinine, and its diagnostic uses and role in renal disease.

Chapter VIII - The renal excretion of creatinine is very similar to that of inulin and creatinine has been extensively used for estimation of the glomerular function rate (GFR) in adults and children by calculating the clearance of creatinine. GFR is considered the best index of renal function and while it can be measured directly by clearance studies of exogenous markers, such as inulin, these procedures are costly and time consuming. GFR estimation based on endogenous creatinine correlates well with inulin clearance, but necessitates precise urine collection which is not feasible in infants and young children. Estimated GFR, based on plasma creatinine level (PCr) and body length, is a key method for estimating renal function and identifying patients with chronic kidney disease (CKD). Several formulas have been used for estimating GFR, using mainly PCr, body length or height, and a constant. The new Schwartz formula (2009) is in current use, but others have been recently studied.

Serial measurement of PCr is also a useful bedside index of kidney function, especially during the neonatal period. PCr is high at birth, reflecting maternal levels, decreases during the first weeks of life in parallel with an increase in GFR, reaches trough values by the end of the first month, then increases gradually during childhood. Its level is inversely correlated with both gestational age and postnatal age. PCr is estimated using several methods, including modified Jaffe methods, enzymatic methods, high-performance liquid chromatography, isotope dilution mass spectrometry (IDMS) and gas chromatography. Commercially available methods for creatinine measurement have limitations and there are differences in results among methods due to lack of assay standardization and the non specificity of the alkaline picrate method used in most laboratories. Recent international efforts have been made to improve creatinine standardization by assuring traceability to a reference system.

Chapter IX - Chronic kidney disease (CKD) is an important public health problem. CKD is defined as kidney damage or glomerular filtration rate (GFR) less than 60 ml/min/1.73m^2 for 3 months or more, irrespective of cause. CKD is classified into stages according to the level of GFR. Therefore, estimation of the GFR is essential for the evaluation of patients with CKD. GFR allows us to detect early impairment of renal function, prevent further deterioration and complications, to correct the dosage of drugs cleared by the kidney so as to avoid potential drug toxicity and to help us to manage CKD patients.

Over the last decades several different markers for estimation of GFR have been proposed. The ideal marker of GFR should be an endogenous molecule, which, being produced at a constant rate, is cleared solely by the kidneys via free glomerulari filtration, without being either secreted by tubular cells or reabsorbed into peritubular circulation. The "gold standard" for estimation of GFR is clearance of exogenous substances such as inulin, iohexol, ^{51}CrEDTA, ^{99m}TcDTPA or ^{125}I-iothalamate. These techniques are time-consuming, labour-intensive, expensive and require administration of substances, that make them incompatible with routine monitoring.

During the last decades, in clinical practice as in most studies, serum creatinine concentration has become the most commonly used marker to estimate GFR. Creatinine is completely filtered across the glomerular membrane and is neither reabsorbed nor metabolized in kidneys and is partially secreted into proximal tubule. Tubular secretion causes the increase of creatinine clearance by 10 – 20%. Creatinine is usually measured by the Jaffé reaction (the kinetic method without deproteinisation- isotope dilution mass spectrometry traceable creatinine assay), based on a complex formation between alkaline picrate and creatinine. According to this method, other non-creatinine cromogens are present in serum, which are not found in urine. Thus creatinine concentration is overestimated in serum and the calculated clearance is underestimated (by 10 to 20%). In individuals with normal renal function both irregularities are abolished and creatinine clearance is very close to the inulin clearance. Other factors, including age, gender, race, body size, muscle mass and food intake (meat in diet), also affect the serum creatinine concentration. Creatinine clearance gives a better estimation of GFR than serum creatinine concentration, but it requires the inconvenience of urine collections. The current Kidney Disease Outcomes Quality Initiative (K/DOQI) guidelines emphasize the need to assess kidney function using predictive equations rather than just serum creatinine. Various creatinine-based equations have been developed in an attempt to improve the estimation of GFR from serum creatinine. Recently, serum cystatin C and cystatin C-based formulas were proposed as a new endogenous marker of GFR.

All the above-mentioned topics will be closely analyzed and described in the details in the chapter.

Chapter X - Creatinine is a guanidino metabolic product of muscular creatine phosphate, produced in constant level relative to body muscular mass, thus its renal clearance is used as a marker of kidney function. Renal creatinine handling includes glomerular filtration and active proximal tubular secretion. Pathological conditions as severe renal failure cause reduction in glomerular filtration of creatinine, such that total creatinine excreted is dependent on active tubular secretion. The latter involves proximal tubule directional transport by basolateral uptake via organic cation transporter (OCT) 2, followed by apical efflux into the urine via multidrug and toxin extrusion (MATE) 1 and MATE2-k transporter proteins. Other transporters, as OCT3, have been suggested to contribute to creatinine active renal secretion. A number of factors may alter creatinine renal secretion. Genetic polymorphisms of transporters involved in active renal efflux of creatinine may impair its secretion. Furthermore, drugs as cimetidine, trimethoprim and levofloxacin may affect renal creatinine excretion. Gender-based differences in creatinine transport have also been implicated. Extra-renal transport of creatinine, as its cerebral clearance via OCT3 efflux protein in the blood-cerebrospinal fluid barrier, contributes to creatinine tissue distribution. Translational research faces difficulty in interpreting mechanisms of creatinine renal handling from animal experiments due to inter-species variation. Still, human pharmacogenomic and molecular studies may provide insights that can be applied to clinical situations.

Chapter XI - Acute kidney injury (AKI) is characterized by a rapid decline in glomerular filtration rate (GFR) over hours to days that results in the retention of urea and other nitrogenous waste products normally cleared by the kidneys. It is associated with a 25% to 80% risk of in-hospital death and has been rising in the incidence over the past several decades. The RIFLE and AKIN criteria have greatest utility in epidemiologic studies. However, these definitions may be problematic when applied to patients at bedside because the baseline creatinine may be unknown. The creatinine (Cr) level may not perfectly reflect the severity of kidney injury because serum Cr is altered by age, sex, muscle mass, nutritional status, and medications. The novel biomarkers, such as Kidney injury molecule-1 (KIM-1) and Neutrophil gelatinase associated lipocalin (NGAL), are promising in the diagnosis of intrinsic AKI and may permit development of a new paradigm for classifying AKI in the future.

Chapter XII - Chronic kidney disease is renal injury in progressive and irreversible loss of renal glomerular, tubular and endocrine functions. Its most advanced stage is called chronic renal failure (CRF) and it is the final common pathway for a variety of renal disorders. According to a recent consensus of the National Kidney Foundation, the IRC is characterized by a glomerular filtration rate (GFR) below 60 ml/min/1, 73m^2 body surface. The degree of CKD varies according to the glomerular filtration rate and values below 15 ml/min/1, 73 m^2 already indicate kidney failure. In clinical practice, GFR is assessed by measuring creatinine in serum or plasma or by determining the creatinine clearance, being that the creatinine clearance remains one of markers most used in evaluation of renal function, despite of overestimating the GFR and depend on muscle mass. Retinol is the major circulating form of vitamin A and it plays an essential role in maintaining the health of mammals. After absorption, vitamin A is transported from the hepatic tissue to peripherals sites; for such transport to happen, retinol needs be connected to complex retinol-binding protein 4 (RBP4) - transthyretin. In order to allow excretion of retinol, catabolism of protein of the complex (RBP4) must occur, which takes place in the kidney, the main catabolic site of this protein; for this reason the homeostasis of circulating vitamin A depends on the renal function. Patients who have renal diseases present elevated levels of retinol because in this pathology the renal function decreases, as well as its catabolic activity will also be reduced, causing a reduction of the catabolism of RBP4 and consequently of excretion of retinol. In fact, there is a strong positive direct correlation between the concentrations of vitamin A and serum creatinine. Thus, according to the increase of the severity degree, chronic renal insufficiency suffers a decrease of renal function reflected by the augment of serum creatinine as well as of retinol levels. The determination of vitamin A in patients with renal disease has great importance because high concentrations of this vitamin have a pro-oxidant proven by the relation with biomarkers of oxidative stress such as malondialdehyde and antioxidant enzymes (glutathione peroxidase, catalase and superoxide dismutase). However, the determination of vitamin A in the laboratory routine has limitations mainly due to its high cost and for requiring more complex methodologies. Since there is a direct relation between serum retinol and creatinine, it can estimate the levels of retinol from the levels of creatinine. On the other hand, creatinine is considered a low cost methodology, standardized and accessible to all clinical laboratories, and the relation between retinol and creatinine consists an additional tool for clinical monitoring and treatment of patients with kidney disease.

In: Creatinine
Editors: I. H. Perkins and C. M. Chapman
ISBN: 978-1-62257-475-9

Chapter I

Creatinine: Diagnostic Uses in Preeclampsia

Rose Gasnier, Edimárlei Gonsales Valério and José Geraldo Lopes Ramos
Universidade Federal do Rio Grande do Sul,
Hospital de Clínicas de Porto Alegre, Brazil

Abstract

Preeclampsia is a major complication in pregnancy, occurring in 7-10% of all pregnant women. Hypertension in pregnancy is associated with fetal and maternal adverse outcomes: the risks are higher when significant proteinuria is associated. Proteinuria may be measured in single voided urine samples or in 24-hour pools, the latter considered as the gold standard test. Errors in pooling may occur, especially in outpatient tests and without the control with creatininuria levels. Moreover, a quick diagnostic test may be needed due to the severity of clinical manifestations: an alternative solution is assessing protein in single urine voided samples.

Despite the fact that the reagent stick is the most commonly used proteinuria screening test for preeclampsia after the assessment of blood pressure, its use has been challenged by several authors. The urine protein-to-creatinine ratio proved to be an accurate method for the diagnosis of preeclampsia when correlated with the 24-hour proteinuria. It is a more reliable means of assessing protein in single voided urine specimens. This rate is an efficient, quick and easy test for the diagnosis of preeclampsia.

The predictive diagnosis of preeclampsia and a differential diagnosis from other forms of hypertension can be difficult to accomplish at first clinical presentation, especially in the presence of proteinuria. The identification of markers has been the objective of many researchers.

Many investigators have written about hypocalciuria in preeclampsia compared with normotensive pregnant women. It could be the result of reduced glomerular filtration rate, which appears at the same time as proteinuria, but the mechanism of hypocalciuria is still unclear. Studies using measurements of 24-hour urinary calcium excretion have documented decreased excretion in women with preeclampsia or who developed a disease some time after the collection of urine.

Twenty-four hour calciuria has been used as an indicator of disease, but sometimes a prompt examination or a rapid test is required for monitoring high-risk pregnancies: the calcium-to-creatinine ratio seems to be a good candidate for use in both cases.

This chapter was based on a case-control study that evaluated the relationship between hypocalciuria and preeclampsia by comparing pregnant women with severe and mild preeclampsia, and hypertensive and normotensive cases, analyzing the calcium-to-creatinine ratio and the correlation with 24-hour calciuria as a diagnostic test for preeclampsia.

There were statistically significant differences between the groups when comparing severe preeclampsia and chronic hypertension, severe preeclampsia and normal pregnancy, and mild and severe preeclampsia ($p<0.0001$). The Spearman index between the calcium-to-creatinine ratio and 24-hour calciuria was 0.65 (high correlation). The best cutoff point was 0.053 mg/mg, showing a sensitivity of 70% and a specificity of 85%, with positive and negative predictive values of 80% and 74%, respectively.

The calcium-to-creatinine ratio can reliably estimate 24-hour calciuria, differentiating severe preeclampsia from mild preeclampsia, chronic hypertension and normal pregnancy, helping to diagnose hypertension diseases during the pregnancy.

Hypertension in Pregnancy

Preeclampsia was described for the first time in 1894 by William Smith with the name of pregnancy toxicosis. The American College of Obstetrics and Gynecology Classification, proposed in 1972, and reviewed in 2000, it is of good clinical application: preeclampsia/eclampsia, arterial chronic hypertension (of any etiology), arterial chronic hypertension with superposed preeclampsia, gestational arterial hypertension.

In 2000, o USA National High Blood Pressure Education Program Working Group (NHBPEP), as Brown (Brown 2000), revised the classification systems, and your recommendations were adopted by the International Society for the Study of Hypertension in Pregnancy during the 12° Mundial Congress in 2000 and by the Australasian Society Consensus Statement [1,2,3].

Preeclampsia, a pregnancy specific syndrome of reduced organ perfusion secondary to vasospasm and endothelial activation, is a major complication in pregnancy, occurring in 7–10% of all pregnant women [4], and is one of the major causes of maternal morbidity and mortality, preterm birth, intrauterine growth restriction, and perinatal mortality [5,6]. Hypertension in pregnancy is associated with fetal and maternal adverse outcomes [7]. Maternal and fetal risks are higher when significant proteinuria ($\geq$ 300 mg / 24 hour) is associated [8,9], justifying the correct diagnosis of significant proteinuria. Pregnant women with mild chronic hypertension, without proteinuria, have demonstrated outcomes comparables to non-hypertensive pregnant women [10].

North and cols, comparing pregnant women with preeclampsia and those with transient gestational hypertension, found an odds ratio of 4.8 (95% CI: 2.4-9.5) for severe maternal disease.

Premature labor and infants born small for gestational age were more frequent in the group with preeclampsia (OR 14.6 95% CI: 5.8-37.8 and OR 2.6 95% CI: 1.2-5.3) than in the group of normotensive women. Among pregnant women classified as having transient hypertension, severe maternal disease was more frequent in those with "+" urine protein (41.7%) than in the ones with no proteinuria detected (15.9%) with OR of 3.8 95% CI: 1.5-98

[8]. These findings support the idea that pregnant women with hypertension and proteinuria have a poorer prognosis: its correct diagnosis being thus mandatory.

The diagnosis of arterial hypertension is made when systolic arterial pressure ≥ 140 mmHg and/or diastolic arterial pressure ≥ 90 mmHg, in at least 2 occasions, measured at intervals greater than 6 hours. Blood pressure is measured with calibrated conventional sphygmanometers, in the right arm; diastolic pressure is considered in the Korotkoff phase V, with the patients in sitting position. It can be chronic (known before 20 weeks of pregnancy) or pregnancy-specific.

The latter begins after the week 20 (exception for the cases of mole disease and hydropsia), and can be associated to significative proteinuria (≥ 300mg in 24-hour), characterizing preeclampsia disease (or eclampsia, in the presence of convulsion).

In the cases whose proteinuria is not significative, is classified as gestational arterial hypertension (Report of National High Blood Pressure Education Program Working Group on High Blood Pressure in Pregnancy, 2000; North, 1999) [1,8].

Preeclampsia is recognized as hypertension that begins after week 20 of pregnancy with significative proteinuria that disappears until 12 weeks after the labor. Some criteria help to diagnose and make the disease more severe (NHBPEP 2000) (1): 24-hour proteinuria > 2g (begins in pregnancy and disappears in the post labor period), diastolic arterial pressure ≥ 110 mmHg or systolic arterial pressure ≥ 160 mmHg, hepatic dysfunction, microangiopatic hemolysis, low platelets, imminent eclamptic signs, persistent epigastric pain, progressive renal function loss, cardiac insufficiency, pulmonary edema, retina hemorrhagy, exsudatos, papilar edema, fetal restriction weight, oligodramnio.

Chronic hypertension is diagnosed before week 20 or in a late pregnancy period, not disappearing after the labor. In cases of preeclampsia superposed to chronic hypertension, occur proteinuria ≥ 300 mg after a week 20 or, in cases of patients with hypertension and previous proteinuria, occur proteinuria rising, arterial pressure levels rising in previous controlled patients, laboratorial abnormalities – platelets, transaminases, hiperuricemia – or premonitory signs.

In cases of gestational arterial hypertension, the hypertension is detected after the week 20, without significative proteinuria. If the levels return to the normal pattern until 12 weeks after the labor, is denominated transient gestational hypertension.

The Australasian Society for the Study of Hypertension in Pregnancy (ASSHP) has suggested that in the preeclampsia diagnostic criteria not be included proteinuria, since that was present renal insufficiency and/or hepatic dysfunction and/or neurological problems and/or hematological abnormalities and/or fetal restriction weight.

This classification recognizes the multisystemic aspect of the disease, with a more sensitive diagnostic. However, concerned with the scientific methodology, recommend, as definition for research, the obligatory presence of proteinuria, despite of reducing the sensitivity for diagnose. For the USA National High Blood Pressure Education Program (NHBPEP), a more restrictive criterion is necessary, including proteinuria, but establishes suspected criteria in the ausence of proteinuria: always suspect of preeclampsia in the presence of headache, visual abnormalities, abdominal pain or abnormal laboratorial exams, as low platelets and hepatic enzymes elevation.

Proteinuria

In pregnant women with preeclampsia, glomerular filtration rate and renal plasmatic circulation decrease in relation to normal pregnant women, because of vasospasm, and proteinuria appears as consequence of glomerular membrane damage [11]. Proteinuria level is a parameter of renal vasospasm severity and fibrinoid deposition in endotelial cells. Glomerular capillary endoteliosis is the preeclampsia characteristic lesion, observed by renal biopsy [12]. Proteinuria is formed by molecular high weigh proteins, as albumin, but also hemoglobin, globulins and transferrin, besides other proteins of little height [13].

Health individuals show protein urinary excretion of 30-150 mg in 24 hours, most related to albumin. In pregnant women, because of physiological rise in glomerular filtration rate and renal plasmatic circulation, it can be accepted 300 mg in 24 hours as superior level [14]. Fever and exercise can raise urinary protein excretion. Position alterations in advanced pregnancy can cause physiological modifications in renal function (renal metabolism of sodium, water and uric acid can be altered) and in arterial pressure, but do not modify the proteinuria [15]. Proteinuria can be reflex of renal or systemic diseases, not related to pregnancy. Systemic diseases that can raise glomerular capillary permeability (cardiac insufficiency, viral infection, fever) cause urinary protein loss. Renal disease can be primary (membranous glomerulopathy or focal glomerulosclerosis) or secondary to systemic disease with local repercussion (diabetic nephropathy, lupic nephropathy or hypertensive nefrosclerosis).

Proteinuria measurement in pregnant women with hypertension establishes the diagnosis and it is one of the severity criteria of this disease. The International Society for the Study of Hypertension in Pregnanacy – ISSHP has defined significative proteinuria as urinary excretion ≥ 300mg in 24 hours or protein-to-creatinine ratio (PCR) in randomly specimens > 30 mg/mmol (> 0.26 mg/mg) [3]. The NHBPEP accepts, as severity disease criteria, 24-hour proteinuria > 2g (1), and The American College of Obstetrics and Gynecology – ACOG classifies preeclampsia as severe when proteinuria is more than 5g in 24 hours (2002). Other groups considered proteinuria as severe ≥ 2g or even 3g.

24-Hour Proteinuria

The gold standard test for significative proteinuria, more accepted in the world and more reliable, is 24-hour proteinuria. Significant proteinuria is defined by the International Society for the Study of Hypertension in Pregnancy as excretion of ≥ 300 mg of protein in a 24-hour urine specimen [3]. These is usually correlated to proteins ≥ 30mg/dl in urinary samples (or "+"in dipsticks) in patients without urinary infection [1,16], but can occur errors, especially in outpatient exams.

Outside pregnancy the 24-hour urine collection has well documented problems with completeness, timeliness, and ease of performance. In pregnancy, however, problems are increased by the physiological dilatation of the ureters (which can hold up to 200 ml of urine) and incomplete bladder emptying as a result of the enlarging uterus, both of which may cause significant collection errors. These errors can be avoided by adequate hydration to maintain urine flow (500 ml fluid to generate a urine flow of > 6 ml/min) and standardization of the technique at the beginning (urine discard) and end of the collection (lying in left lateral recumbency for 45 minutes to remove any partial obstruction of the ureters related to supine or upright posture). Ideally a urinary catheter would be placed, which is impractical, relatively invasive, and may lead to infection. It follows from these limitations that it should not be the standard against which new measures are evaluated.

Lindheimer et al suggest a more physiological approach to assessment of proteinuria: if clinicians and investigators looked at proteinuria in terms of how the kidney handles protein in health and disease it would lead to a more rational and evidence-based approach to proteinuria in pregnancy. The current cutoff for abnormal proteinuria should be used to diagnose preeclampsia, but the level of proteinuria should not guide management. Other variables, such as status of blood pressure control, evidence of increasing organ damage in the liver and hematological systems, evidence of falling glomerular filtration rate, and signs of neurological involvement, are more reliable indicators of severity of preeclampsia [17].

The cutoff usually used to classify significative proteinuria in pregnant women of 300 mg/24 hour had done based on healthful pregnant populations, in small surveys, accepting as "abnormal population" that with proteinuria above percentil 95 [18,19,20]. There is no study that presents this cutoff as clinical outcomes prediction. Studies that had correlated proteinuria levels to maternal and fetal outcomes demonstrated discordant findings [21-27]. A Cochrane revision (2009) concluded that proteinuria tests can't predict maternal and fetal complications in preeclampsia [28]. Lindheimer concluded that clinical decisions can't be based on proteinuria, even massive, that is not a good marker for severity disease: other signs more reliable should be used to guide management.

It might be best for individual hospital laboratories to establish their own population norms as well as upper limits of their 95% confidence levels. It appears that better designed studies are required in defining both abnormal protein excretion and when to designate a patient who develops new onset hypertension in late pregnancy as preeclamptic. Proteinuria seems to be greater in the second compared with the first half of pregnancy: either filtrance or tubular reabsorption of proteins may change in late pregnancy [17].

Proteinuria in Voided Urine Samples

Proteinuria may be measured in single voided urine samples or in 24-hour pools, the latter considered as the gold-standard test and the main quantitative assessment of the amount of proteinuria in pregnant women (Report of the National High Blood Pressure Education Program Working Group on High Blood Pressure in Pregnancy – NHBPEP – 2000). Errors in pooling may occur, especially in outpatient tests, as urine losses and non-observance of the necessary rest during the period, and it would not be of cost benefit to undertake the test routinely on admission. Moreover, a quick diagnostic test may be needed due to the severity of clinical manifestations, when 24 hours is an unduly long time, as in active labor phase. Late diagnosis of proteinuria in the labor phase delays the more timely decision to use magnesium sulphate for seizure prophylaxis. An alternative solution is assessing protein in single voided urine samples.

Reagent Sticks

Reagent stick tests are a simple and rapid test for proteinuria diagnosis (29,30]: 1+ is related to 30 mg/dl, 2+ is related to 100 mg/dl, 3+ is related to 500 mg/dl and 4+ is related to more than 500 mg/dl. Despite the fact that the reagent stick is the most commonly used proteinuria screening test for preeclampsia, after the assessment of blood pressure, its use has been challenged by several authors [31-34]. The dipstick is inexpensive, easy to use, and provides a rapid result but has been shown to have low sensitivity and specificity for urinary protein excretion over 24 hours. Meyer and cols, in 1994, reported that a cutoff point of "+"or greater had positive predictive value of 92%, with negative predictive value of only 34% [31]. Phelan and cols, by using "+"as significant proteinuria, have encountered 71% of false-positive and 9% of false-negative results (14% with traces amounts and 7% with no protein). Reagent sticks led to the incorrect diagnosis of preeclampsia in 50% of the cases, especially when ketonuria was present. Assuming no protein and trace amounts as true-negative tests, they have failed to identify 1 in every 11 cases [32]. Other studies have analyzed the factors causing errors in reagent stick test results, such as urine concentration, urine ph, examiner error (in non-automated reading), radiocontrast and glicosuria [30,32,33]. Cochrane revision (2004) concluded that the accuracy of dipstick is of limited value to diagnose presence or ausence of proteinuria in preeclampsia, considering 1 + in the exam. The accuracy could be better for more elevated values [35].

Protein measurement in single voided urine specimen done by dipping reagent sticks, detect total urine protein concentration and do not necessarily, increased excretions. Patients with low urinary output may test positive with the dipsticks, even when protein excretion is normal, the opposite being true in patients with increased protein excretion and high urine output [29,30,31,36,37]. Dipsticks detect protein concentration of 30 mg/dl: less than this value, they are negative or with traces. A patient with protein excretion of 300 mg/24-hour in a total of 1500 ml of urine, with a concentration of 20 mg/dl, has a negative test. Dipstick should not be used as the sole method for screening preeclampsia and, in obstetrical emergencies, clinical presentation of the patient should be given priority over the dipstick. Other methods of screening of proteinuria should also be assessed with the objective of reducing false-negative results.

Roy and cols compared reagent dipsticks for protein-to-creatinine ratio (PCR) to conventional sticks measurements, considering laboratorial PCR as gold-standard test: found 1 case (in 102 pregnant women) of incorrect diagnosis with RPC sticks compared to 20 cases with conventional sticks [38].

Protein-to-Creatinine Ratio (PCR)

Côté et al, in 2006, presented a paper in the " 15th World Congress of the International Society for the Study of Hypertension in Pregnancy", carried out with 199 patients, demonstrating less than 50% of accuracy of 24-hour proteinuria, with creatininuria for complete collection measurement. The group suggested that alternative methods, as PCR, should be considered [39].

The urine protein-to-creatinine ratio is an efficient, quick and easy test for preeclampsia diagnosis, with excellent correlation to 24-hour collection [40-46] and has shown excellent correlations with 24-hour proteinuria. Relevant Australasian and international guidelines advocate use of the spot protein-to-creatinine ratio [2,3].The test is available from any laboratory that determines protein and creatinine concentrations on 24-hour urine collections. This ratio was used in the beginning for non-pregnant patients and has been used for more than 20 years in pregnancy. 24-hour proteinuria and/or PCR are essentials to evaluate pregnancies complicated by hypertension, but some controversies persisted about the more adequate test.

The urine protein-to-creatinine ratio proved to be an accurate method for the diagnosis of preeclampsia when correlated with the 24-hour proteinuria (used as gold-standard). It has some advantages compared to the 24-hour proteinuria: it can be measured in a single voided urine sample, bypassing the 24 hour waiting time, what is particularly important when a quick diagnosis is needed; significant errors may occur in 24 hour pooling, such as loss of part of the urine by the patients [40]. Single-voided PCR is preferable to random spot urine protein because the ratio of two stables excretion rates (creatinine and protein) would cancel out the time factor and thus provide a better estimation of 24-hour protein excretion [41]. The PCR would be assessable in all trimesters of pregnancy: the association of gestational age with PCR and 24-hour proteinuria seems to be not significant [42].

In a previous study in our group (Hospital de Clínicas de Porto Alegre, Brazil) we have detected loss of 30% of the 24-hour proteinuria pools, considering as standard the presence of at least 600 mg of creatinine in 24 hour urine pools. In the study of Valerio and cols, 10 of 85 patients had trouble pooling, although hospitalized [47]. In 1999, a study by Ramos disclosed a 0.94 correlation coefficient ($p < 0.05$) between the urine PCR and the 24-hour proteinuria [40]. Neithard and cols, in 2002, had found r 0.93 ($p<0.01$) [42], and Yamasmit and cols, in 2003, found r 0.929 ($p<0.001$) [48]. Côte has reviewed 11 studies (1987-2003) in which the PCR was evaluated as the detection method for significant proteinuria, and concluded that it it has reasonable accuracy, reminding it should locally validated before used, due to the great variation in cutoff points and laboratorial tests employed [49].

Blackburn, in a cohort study with 208 hypertensive pregnant women, has found a negative predictive value of 100% using PCR ≤ 0.1 (mg/dl) as the cutoff point and a positive predictive value of 100% at PCR ≥ 0.4 [44]. Rodriguez-Thompson et al found Pearson correlation of 0.80 ($p<0.001$) and area under the ROC curve of 0.91 (CI 95% 0.87-0.96). They tried to elevate the sensitivity because of the risk to lose patients with preeclampsia. They concluded that a PCR < 0.14 excluded significative proteinuria, but the specificity was of only 51%. In order to have a better specificity, with a sensitivity $> 90\%$, a PCR ≥ 0.19 demonstrated sensitivity of 70%. The negative predictive value was 87%, in a population with a prevalence of 50% of significative proteinuria. Most of the cases of false-positive and negative values were identified in the interval of 50 mg of difference from the cutoff point of 300 mg in 24-hour. All false negative cases had mild proteinuria, not more than 380 mg/24 hour. It was not clear if the cases of false-negative are related to the clinic course of the disease, because of the mild severity. The false-positive cases, on the other hand, could be not really false-positive cases, since 24-hour proteinuria is more susceptible to underestimation because of incomplete collection [41].

Leanõs-Miranda, in a cross-sectional study with 927 hospitalized pregnant-women and a second cohort of 161 pregnant women, found high correlation between PCR and 24-hour proteinuria (r 0.98 $p < 0.001$). The PCR as an indicator of protein excretion ≥ 300 mg/24 hour was ≥ 0.3: sensitivity of 98.2%, specificity of 98.8%, positive and negative predictive values of 97.2% and 99.2%, positive and negative likelihood ratios of 79.2 and 0.02 [46]. Ramos et al found significative correlation coefficient between PCR in voided urine samples and 24-hour proteinuria of 0.94. Specificity and positive predictive value were 100% for PCR ≥ 0.8, and a PCR ≥ 0.3 is related to significative proteinuria in 92% of the cases. The best values of sensitivity, specificity, positive and negative predicitive values for preeclampsia diagnosis were with PCR of 0.5 (0.96, 0.96, 0.96, 0.96) [40].

Table 1. PCR in different papers

Author	Correlation coefficient
Ramos, 1999	r 0.94
Rodriguez-Thompson, 2001	r 0.80
Neithardt, 2002	r 0.93
Yamasmit, 2003	r 0.95
Nisell, 2006	r 0.95
Leanos-Miranda, 2007	r 0.95
Wheeler, 2007	r 0.98
Kyle, 2008	r 0.99
Dwyer, 2008	r 0.83

The PCR is a more reliable means of assessing protein in single voided urine specimens. Some studies have placed some doubts about the test due to PCR variation throughout the day [36,37,50]. Another concern refers to whether the sample obtained when the patient arrives at the clinic is a reliable one, since she is not at rest and it is known that exercise may increase proteinuria. The error to which the spot urine sample is maybe susceptible – the potential mild diurnal variation in protein excretion – is likely to be far outweighed by the error associated with 24 hour urine collection. Despite of this, the PCR has not been widely adopted in obstetric practice. Reasons may include the different cutoff points in four units, the fact that only the International and Australasian Societies for the study of hypertension in pregnancy have published a cutoff point of 30 mg/mmol for diagnosis of significant proteinuria, and the conservative perspective of obstetric care providers who must not miss a diagnosis of preeclampsia, and will be resistant to abandoning the traditional comparator [51]. The diagnostic performance of the urine PCR should be validated locally by each laboratory because of the variability in laboratory methods used to measure proteinuria and the criteria to establish cutoff points.

It has been questioned whether a random voided urine sample to determine the PCR is adequate or there is a period in the day it would be more reliable (correlated with the 24-hour proteinuria). In 1983, Allen has studied non-pregnant patients with proteinuria and normal controls and observed that the urine PCR of samples obtained in the morning period was less sensitive than, but equally specific, to the ratio of randomly obtained samples [37]. They suggested it could be due to positional variables. Ginsberg and cols (1983) have found better correlation between the ratio and the gold standard test during the day. Their study was done in non-pregnant patients with impaired renal function and a control group with normal renal function [52]. In 1991, Misiani has demonstrated that non-pregnant and puerperal women had greater albumin excretion during the day. Variation was significantly smaller in normotensive primiparous and, in women with preeclampsia, although in small number, there was no varying excretion (daytime increase) compared to the normotensive pregnant women. These finding suggest that urine protein excretion in pregnant women, normotensive or with hypertension, does not vary along 24 hour the way it happens in non-pregnant women [50].

Lindheimer and Kanter believe that 24-hour proteinuria is inadequate: obstetricians are using the PCR more frequently. The cutoff points have varied between 0.19-1.14. This rate seems to be stable in the same patient during 24 hours period [17]. Despite of the fact that was contested in the beginning, the importance of PCR has been progressively recognized [53].

Based on these data, a cross-sectional study was performed in our Service, in which the factor evaluated was the variation of the PCR in single voided urine specimens obtained at different periods of the day and the outcome was the 24-hour proteinuria. After arterial hypertension was diagnosed, a urine specimen for PCR determination was obtained, which was repeated at every 6 hours thereafter (4 samples in a 24 hour period) and, simultaneously, pooled 24-hour urine was collected for protein quantification. All patients were admitted to the hospital and were at rest throughout the sampling period. The PCR was calculated by dividing urine protein (mg/dl) by urine creatinine (mg/dl), in single voided urine samples, in different periods of the day. A significant correlation (0.8 or greater) of the 24 hour-proteinuria with the urine PCR, at every one of the four day periods ($p<0.001$), as well as with that in the first sample at arrival, irrespectively of the period of the day (p 0.003), was found. The area under the curve (ROC Curve) ranged between 0.935 and 0.962 in the four periods of the day and was 0.930 in the first voided urine sample. Based on these finding, have concluded that the single voided urine sample PCR does not vary significantly throughout the day and may be determined at any period, with strong correlation with the 24-hour proteinuria [47].

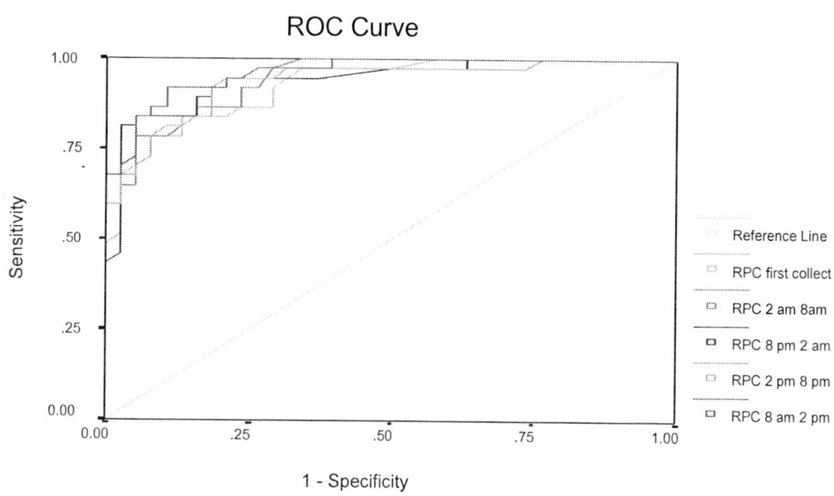

Figure 1. ROC Curve for the analysis of the relationship of the 24-hour proteinuria and the urine protein/creatinine ratio at different periods of the day.

The National Kidney Foundation has recommended that an increase in protein excretion be used as a screening tool in patients at risk of developing renal disease [54] and recommend the spot protein-to-creatinine and albumin-to-creatinine ratio (instead of 24-hour urine collection) to diagnose proteinuria in most situations, without specific mention of pregnancy [55]. For some authors, PCR seems to be correlated to 24-hour proteinuria for different levels of renal function. Morales et al, analyzing patients with primary glomerulonephrities, observed high correlation coefficients (r 0.91, 0.95 and 0.98) in patients with normal, reduced and severely reduced renal function: differences and variability between 24-hour proteinuria and PCR tended to increase with higher proteinuria levels, and this trend was observed for the three renal function levels. The best cutoff points to detect abnormal and nephrotic proteinuria were 0.3 and 2.6, respectively [56]. Price and cols. in a systematic review concluded that the PCR on a random specimen provides evidence to "rule out" the presence of significant proteinuria as defined by a 24-hour urine excretion measurement. This rate could avaliate proteinura, but methodological limitations exist [57].

Côté and cols (2006) carried out a systematic review of diagnostic accuracy of PCR for proteinuria in hypertensive pregnant women: 13 studies with 8 different cutoff points and different populations (1987-2003) [39]. In a new systematic review in 2008, the same group demonstrated that the sensitivities and specificities in the studies of the spot PCR varied, as expected. The diagnostic accuracy results using a cutoff point of 30 mg/mmol for the spot PCR, as recommended in published guidelines, showed no sensitivity to the range for proteinuria or method of urine collection: the positive likelihood was poor to fair. The negative likelihood ratio was fair to good, suggesting that a spot protein-to-creatinine ratio of less than 30 mg/mmol is a reasonable "rule out" test for proteinuria of 300 mg/day or more. The spot PCR has not been reliable for quantifying proteinuria either outside or during pregnancy [58].

Albumin specific assays are used extensively outside pregnancy for detection of "microalbuminuria", since albumin assays are more specific than total urinary protein for kidney disease as a result of diabetes mellitus or hypertension. The authors identified two studies that examined use of the spot albumin-to-creatinine ratio in pregnancy (ACR): the test was excellent at diagnosing proteinuria or albuminuria of 300 mg/day or more but data are too limited to advocate use of the test in pregnancy.

Wikström and cols concluded that, in women with preeclampsia, random albumin-to-creatinine ratio is not stable during the day and cannot predict 24-hour protein excretion accurately. ACR from the 24-hour collection, for otherwise, is an accurate predictor of total albumine amount and can be used to minimize errors from incomplete collection [59]. Hayashi et al evaluated, among other parameters, PCR and ACR in voided urine samples of not pregnant women (group 1), normotensive pregnant women (group 2) and pregnant women with preeclampsia (group 3). They found elevation of the two parameters in the group 2 in relation to group 1, and further elevation in group 3 in relation to group 2 (more notable in ACR than in PCR) [11]. In glomerular diseases, which include preeclampsia, increased urinary protein derives primarily from the circulating proteins presented to the glomerulus, and much of the increment is due to increased albumin excretion.

Boler al el (1987) found an excellent correlation between 24-hour proteinuria and PCR (r 0.99 $p<0.001$) among pregnant women in the third trimester (with or without hypertension) [60]. This correlation decreases when the protein loss is greater than 1g. Jaschevatzky et al (1990) related this fact with proteinuria greater than 2g [61]. More recently, Antunes et al observed a very good accuracy of PCR among patients with primary glomerulonephritis. The values under the ROC Curve were 0.99 (CI 95% 0.97-1) and 0.99 (CI 95% 0.99-1), both significatives, for 24-hour proteinuria of 0.2g and 3.5g [62].

Other Measurements for Proteinuria

Other concept for significative proteinuria is 1g or more per liter in 6 hours urine collection [63]. Few studies (and guidelines from the NHBPEP) have proposed using shorter timed urine collections (2, 4, 8 or 12 hours) to diagnose proteinuria in pregnancy [64 -68]. Shorter collections, however, share some of the limitations and concerns associated with 24-hour collection. Kieler et al concluded that 12-hour albuminuria collection could substitute 24-hour collection as gold-standard test in patients with preeclampsia, but the same not happened with voided urine samples [36]. Adelberg concluded that 8-hour proteinuria is related to 24-hour proteinuria ≥ 300 mg until 5g (r 0.82 $p<0.001$) and to proteinuria ≥ 5g (r 0.89 p 0.003). It was not relation between 8 and 24-hour collection among patients without significative proteinuria. 12-hour collection is related to 24-hour collection in cases without significative proteinuria, cases with significative proteinuria < 5g and cases with proteinuria > 5g (r 0.84 $p<0.001$ and r 0.95 p 0.003, respectively) [64].

Early Diagnosis of Preeclampsia

One way to reduce the impact of arterial hypertension on maternal mortality is to establish the correct diagnosis of preeclampsia, and to proceed with an early intervention when it is diagnosed. The predictive diagnosis of preeclampsia and the differential diagnosis with other forms of hypertension can be difficult, especially in the presence of proteinuria. Identification of markers has been the objective of many researchers. The clinical presentation appears in the late midtrimester, as an advanced disease and a late manifestation of a process that has continued since the beginning of pregnancy. The tests used for the early diagnosis of preeclampsia are, among others, Doppler ultrasound assessment of maternal and fetal circulation, uric acid concentration, and calciuria levels. Studies using measurements of 24-h urinary calcium excretion have documented decreased excretion in women with preeclampsia or who developed the disease some time after the collection of urine.

Calciuria in Preeclampsia

Several abnormalities of calcium metabolism have been described in women with this disease. Many investigators have written about hypocalciuria in preeclampsia compared with normotensive pregnant women [69-74]. Based on this evidence, the calciuria measurement has been suggested as a diagnostic test for preeclampsia. Calcium urinary excretion rise in all pregnant women, probably because of glomerular filtration rate. Calcium urinary excretion during pregnancy can reach 350-620 mg/day, compared to 100-250 mg/day in non-pregnant women.

The excretion usually rises each trimester, with the maximum level in the third one. Calcium homeostasis is altered in preeclampsia: is known an inverse correlation between eclampsia incidence and calcium intake. Several studies have shown hypocalciuria in pregnant women with preeclampsia.

Most of these studies were carried out with limited number of patients or had shown epidemiological deficiencies. Hypocalciuria seems to be important for differential diagnosis of hypertensive diseases in the pregnancy and indicator of gestational prognosis. As proteinuria, can be estimate by urine samples, analyzing calcium-to-creatinine ratio. Using hypocalciuria as predictor of preeclampsia has also conflicting results. It has been reported that hypocalciuria predicts preeclampsia long before the clinical manifestations exist.

Maternal calcium absorption from the gut increases significantly in the second and third trimesters, and maternal urinary calcium excretion is increased throughout pregnancy [75]. This combination of increased calcium absorption and excretion has resulted in the term "absorptive hypercalciuria" to describe the changes in calcium metabolism during pregnancy [76]. The etiology is unclear; it may only reflect renal compromise because of pregnancy-induced hypertension [77] or may be the result reductions in renal prostaglandins [78]. It could be the result of reduced glomerular filtration rate, which appears at the same time as proteinuria, but the mechanism of hypocalciuria is still unclear. It has been speculated that hypocalciuria may result from decreased dietary intake, decreased intestinal absorption, increased calcium uptake by the fetus and placenta [79], intrinsic renal tubular dysfunction [80], or high intracellular calcium [81].

Preeclampsia is associated with increased levels of intracellular calcium, decreased calcium dependent ATPase activity of erythrocytes and hypocalciuria [82]. Parathyreoid hormone (PTH) and dihydroxyvitamin D (1,25 OHD) alterations also could be related [83]. Halhali et al. suggested that 1,25-$(OH)_2$D and/or IGF-1 may be involved in the regulation of urinary calcium excretion [84].

Since there is no significant difference in creatinine clearance, but significant decrease in fractional excretion of calcium, hypocalciuria may be related to alteration of tubular reabsorption [81] or dissociation between calcium and sodium in the loop of Henle [63,85].

During pregnancy, an increase in calcium in endothelial cells stimulates the production of vasodilator substances such as nitric oxide and prostacyclin. Disruption in the balance between dietary, plasma and vascular cell calcium may be responsible for some of the manifestation of preeclampsia including procoagulation, decreased vasodilation, and increased vasoconstriction and vascular resistance [86].

Some investigators have evaluated the calcium-to-creatinine ratio (CCR) as a rapid method of measuring urinary calcium excretion. McGrowder et al. found a lower urinary calcium-to-creatinine ratio (0.17 ± 0.03) in preeclamptic women compared with normotensive women (0.45 ± 0.08) [87]. The value of this urinary ratio in preeclamptic women was different according to other authors [88,89]. This ratio is easy to measure, and has been used as a test to predict preeclampsia, although some investigators have found contradictory results [90,91].

Other workers showed that an increase in blood pressure was found after gestation week 30, but only among subjects who had a high excretion of calcium and magnesium at week 12, because of a functional deficit; this may be a risk indicator for gestational hypertension and preeclampsia [92].

Calcium-to-Creatinine Ratio for Preeclampsia Diagnosis

This chapter was based on a case-control study that evaluated the relationship between hypocalciuria and preeclampsia by comparing pregnant women with severe and mild preeclampsia, and hypertensive and normotensive cases, analyzing the calcium-to-creatinine ratio (CCR) and the correlation with 24-hour calciuria as a diagnostic test for preeclampsia. The patients selected were women between 20 and 37 weeks of gestation, in the period between March 2008 and November 2009. The subjects were separated into four groups: severe and mild preeclampsia, chronic hypertension, and normal pregnancies.

The preeclampsia subjects were taken from the obstetrics emergency service at the Hospital de Clinicas de Porto Alegre, Brazil, upon hospitalization. The groups of hypertensives were taken from the high-risk pregnancy outpatient clinic at the same hospital. The control group comprised normotensive patients with no history of preeclampsia or hypertension in previous pregnancies, from the basic health unit. The groups of chronic hypertension and normotensive controls collected a 24-hour urine pool at home. The preeclampsia group, who were hospitalized, had their urine collected at the hospital. All the patients collected a urine spot, for analysis of the calcium-to-creatinine ratio.

Patients who had an appointment at the Obstetric Center and at the Outpatient Clinic at the Hospital and that met the patient inclusion criteria, and patients who had an appointment at the Basic Health Unit and met the control inclusion criteria, and who wanted to participate, were included in the research. Patients who presented exclusion criteria during follow-up were excluded, as were patients who were lost to follow-up after the collection.

The exclusion criteria for cases and controls were malnutrition, previous or gestational diabetes, renal diseases, previous significant proteinuria, superimposed preeclampsia, continuous use of supplements with calcium or calcium channel blockers, major fetal malformations, intrauterine fetal death, or multiple pregnancies.

The criteria used to diagnose diabetes followed the ''Fourth International Workshop Conference on Gestational Diabetes Mellitus Recommendations'', based on routine screening with glucose fasting in prenatal care, and a 75-g diagnostic glucose-tolerance test when required [92]. The criteria adopted for preeclampsia diagnosis (systolic arterial blood pressure 140mmHg and/or diastolic arterial blood pressure 90mmHg with 300 mg/24-hour proteinuria) and for classification of preeclampsia as severe were those described by the National High Blood Pressure Education Program Working Group (NHBPEP), USA, in 2000 [1].

All the patients collected a 24-hour urine pool for analysis of protein, creatinine and calcium levels. In order to assure adequate 24-hour urine pooling, creatinine was assayed in the pool (24-hour urine pools with less than 600 mg creatinine were discarded) [93]. The creatinine control has been a routine in our Service, with the objective of possibility more reliable measurements: most of the papers whose had not found good correlation between 24-hour collection and voided urine samples for proteinuria or calciuria not controlled their patients for creatinine. The study was approved by the University Ethics Committee, and a written informed consent was obtained from each patient before she was admitted to the study protocol. Laboratory tests were performed at the Clinical Pathology Laboratories of the Hospital de Clinicas, Porto Alegre. To measure calcium levels in urine, automatic autoanalyzers Roche line (Hitachi 917 Roche) were used following the colorimetric method of cresolftalein reaction. Possible interference was eliminated through EDTA use.

To calculate the sample, the study by Ramos et al. was used, in which the preeclampsia group showed a calciuria of 82 ± 15.1 mg/24 h, and the control group showed a calciuria of 317 ± 86 mg/24 h [94], with 0.01 alpha and 0.90 beta risks. The number of patients in each group was 14. This previous study was done by the same research group, with the same population. The quantitative variables with asymmetrical distribution were described by the median, minimum and maximum, 25–75 percentile, and compared by the Kruskal–Wallis test. Next, one-way ANOVA with Ranking values and then a post hoc Tukey test were done. The results were analyzed by means of the Spearman correlation and ROC (Receiver Operating Characteristic) Curve. The adopted level of significance was 0.05. The database was constructed in Excel, and the analyses were performed with SPSS (Statistical Package for the Social Sciences) 16.0.

Results

The population characteristics at the time of inclusion in the study are presented in Table 2. Maternal age was statistically higher in the group with chronic hypertension than in the other groups. Fetal gestational age was significantly higher in patients with mild preeclampsia than in those with chronic hypertension. Arterial pressure means were significantly higher in the group with severe preeclampsia than in the other groups. The group with mild preeclampsia differed significantly from the other groups, except for those patients with chronic hypertension. More primigravidas were included in the preeclampsias groups than in the other groups. Preeclampsia history and BMI were not significantly different among the groups.

Table 2. Characteristics of the population

Characteristics	Severe PE (n 14)	Mild PE (n 14)	CH (n 14)	NP (n 14)	p
Maternal age	26.42 ± 6.03 ^{a}	26.23 ± 5.03 ^{b}	33.06 ± 6.44 ^{a,b,c}	26.71 ± 6.34 ^{c}	0.008
BMI (kg/m^2)	31.36 ± 6.80	31.07 ± 3.57	32.07 ± 3.55	29.49 ± 4.59	0.536(NS)
Fetal GA (weeks)	30.25 ± 3.43	32.54 ± 3.02 ^{a}	26.21 ± 6.40 ^{a}	29.05 ± 5.39	0.010
APM (mm Hg)	122.47 ± 15.18 $^{a, b, c}$	106.26 ± 10.51 $^{a, b}$	102.40 ± 8.77 $^{a, c}$	80.93 ± 11.86 $^{a, b, c}$	0.0001
Nullipara	9 (64.3%)	7 (53.8%)	2 (14.3%)	3 (21.42%)	0.01
PE history	3 (21.4%)	2 (15.4%)	4 (28.6%)	0 (0%)	0.709(NS)

Quantitative variables, for symmetrical distribution, were expressed as mean ± standard deviation, compared for ANOVA one way and posterior Tukey.

Categorical variables were expressed with n (%) and compared for Chi-square test, NS not significant, PE preeclampsia CH chronic hypertension NP normal pregnancy, BMI body mass index, GA gestational age at the urine collection, APM arterial pressure mean, APM was calculated as (SP + 2 x DP) / 3. The arterial pressure measurements were the highest in the first 24 h for preeclampsia and in the inclusion for the other groups, BMI was calculated as weight in kilograms divided by the square of the height in meters.

$^{a, b, c}$ To demonstrate which group is significant different from the other groups.

Calciuria levels showed a progressive decrease from normal pregnancy to severe preeclampsia. The differences in calciuria levels between women with severe preeclampsia and those with chronic hypertension, and between women with severe preeclampsia and those with normal pregnancies were statistically significant ($p < 0.0001$). Calciuria measurement could be used as a further test to differentiate between chronic arterial hypertensive disease and preeclampsia in pregnant patients, mainly in patients far from term, when attempting to maintain the pregnancy. Testing for hypocalciuria is not necessarily a means of diagnosis, but serves as an auxiliary examination to separate preeclampsia from chronic hypertension.

The CCR was lower in preeclamptic patients than in those with chronic hypertension and normal pregnancies. The CCR (but not the 24-hour measurement) differed between patients with severe and mild preeclampsia, as seen in Table 3.

Table 3. Twenty-four hour calciuria and calcium-to-creatinine ratio

	Severe PE (n 14)	Mild PE (n 14)	CH (n 14)	NP (n 14)	p
24-hour calciuria (mg)	81.5 (3-164) [a, b] P25 11.25 P75 155.5	118 (8-564) P25 80 P75 243	226 (50-612) [a] P25 168 P75 292	272 (60-489) [b] P25 128 P75 333	< 0.0001
Calcium-to-Creatinine Ratio (mg/mg)	0.0108 (0-0.14) [a,b,c,d] P25 0.0072 P75 0.0283	0.05 (0.01-0.36) [a,b] P25 0.02 P75 0.23	0.14 (0.02-0.38) [a,c] P25 0.065 P75 0.32	0.0995 (0.04-0.23) [a,d] P25 0.0703 P75 0.2025	0.0001

Data expressed as median, minimum-maximum and 25-75 percentile compared with Kruskall-Wallis test, ranking for Anova one way and posterior Tukey test, PE preeclampsia CH chronic hypertension NP normal pregnancy.

[a, b, c, d] To demonstrate which group is significant different from the other groups.

The correlation between 24-hour calciuria and the CCR showed a Spearman index of 0.65, which indicates a good correlation, as seen in Figure 2 ($p < 0.05$). The relationship between this ratio and the preeclampsia diagnosis, considering a 300 mg proteinuria, is shown in Figure 3. The ROC curve demonstrates the concordance of sensitivity and specificity of the ratio and the preeclampsia diagnosis, with an area under the curve of 0.792 ($p < 0.0001$). The best cutoff point was 0.053 mg/mg, showing a sensitivity of 70% and a specificity of 85%, with positive and negative predictive values of 80% and 74%, respectively. Although we did not have control for the gestational age, fetal gestational age upon inclusion in the study differed only between the groups of women with mild preeclampsia and chronic hypertension. Although literature reports indicate that there is a difference in calciuria with the progression of the pregnancy, higher throughout a normal pregnancy and lower throughout a pregnancy with preeclampsia, our data showed no correlation, perhaps because of the number of subjects.

The linear correlation between calciuria and gestational age with the entire patient population was not good (Spearman correlation -0.56), and the values in each group isolated were lower than in the entire group.

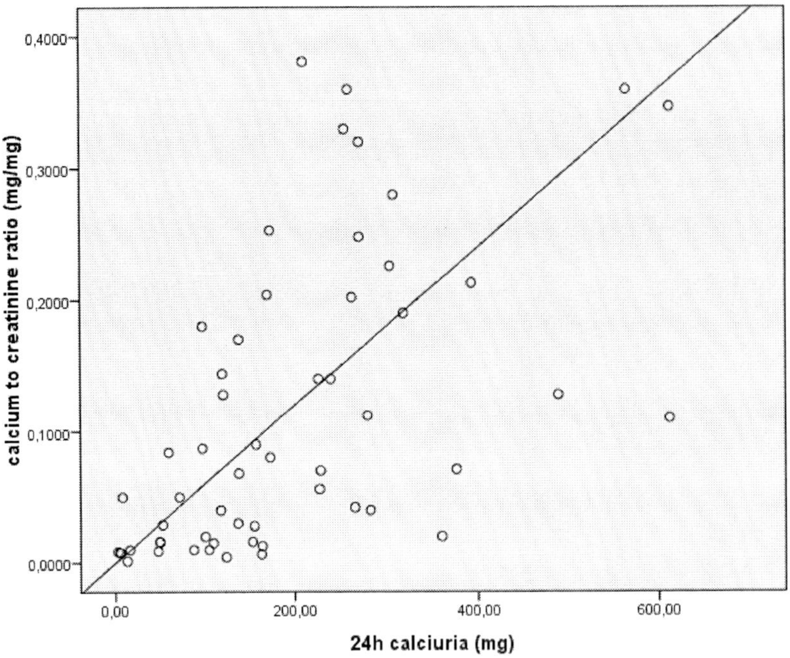

Figure 2. Correlation of 24-hour calciuria and calcium-to-creatinine ratio.

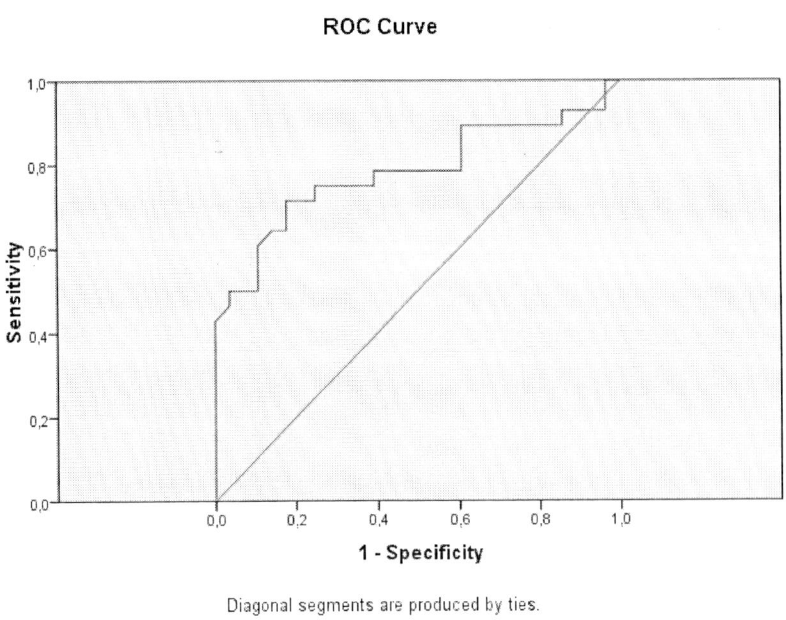

Figure 3. ROC curve of calcium-to-creatinine ratio for preeclampsia diagnosis: area under the curve 0.792, $p < 0.0001$.

Discussion

This study assessed the relationship between hypocalciuria, represented by the CCR measured in urine spot, and preeclampsia. The findings indicated that this ratio can probably differentiate between severe preeclampsia and chronic hypertension, and between severe preeclampsia and normal pregnancy, as well as separating severe and mild cases of preeclampsia. According to our results, 24-hour calciuria could not be used to distinguish severe from mild preeclampsia.

The predictive diagnosis of preeclampsia and a differential diagnosis from other forms of hypertension can be difficult to accomplish at first clinical presentation, especially in the presence of proteinuria. The identification of markers has been the objective of many researchers.

Twenty-four hour calciuria has been used as an indicator of disease, but sometimes a prompt examination or a rapid test is required for monitoring high-risk pregnancies: the CCR seems to be a good candidate for use in both cases. Our observations are in accord with those of the other investigators who have suggested that hypocalciuria can be used as a diagnostic test for differentiating among the various forms of hypertension in pregnancy. Huikeshoven concluded that measuring urinary calcium excretion may be valuable to provide care for and to study pregnant patients with hypertensive disorders, and that 24-hour urinary calcium excretion can be estimated from a single voided urine sample [95]. Our findings indicated no difference between the subjects with chronic hypertension and the controls. Frenkel et al. showed that the CCR was lowest in preeclampsia (0.049 ± 0.03), intermediate in chronic hypertensives (0.15 ± 0.09), and highest in normotensives (0.231 ± 0.17) [87]. The CCR may be a useful potential screening test for preeclampsia. The contradictory results among some studies may be a result of differences in sample size, prevalence of preeclampsia, diagnosis criteria and population ethnicity.

Calcium-to-creatinine ratio in isolated urine is found to be significantly lower in the second trimester and is reported to be an effective marker in predicting preeclampsia. The determination of this rate in the first trimester is found to be limited value for identifying patients with high risk of developing the disease [84]. Sanchez-Ramos, in a prospective study, measured the calciuria in the three gestational trimesters: the patients who later developed preeclampsia excreted less calcium than the others [96].

Kazerooni et al measured the ratio in 102 pregnant patients between 20-24 gestational weeks: 94 persisted normotensive and 8 developed preeclampsia. The values of the CCR were different between the groups: 0.306 ± 0.27 mg/mg for preeclampsia and 0.52 ± 0.3 mg/mg for normotensive patients. A ROC Curve, with a cutoff point of 0.229, showed sensitivity, specificity, positive and negative predictive values of 75%, 77.7%, 20.7% and 97%, respectively [97]. Mandira et al showed a progressive hypocalciuria in patients that became preeclamptics between 32 and 40 weeks of gestational age, analyzing 24-hour calciuria and CCR [98].

Rizk found that the area under a ROC Curve, with the gold standard for diagnosis being 24-hour proteinuria, was 0.82 for the protein-to-creatinine ratio and 0.55 for the calcium-to-creatinine ratio; the latter was non-significant [44]. This information shows that the CCR is not a good diagnostic test, but can serve as a good auxiliary test to differentiate the forms of hypertension, although it is no substitute for the protein-to-creatinine ratio. Nevertheless, the correlation of the CCR and 24-hour calciuria seems to be, although rather high as in our paper, not as strong as the PCR ratio and 24-hour proteinuria.

Ozcan found a cutoff value of 0.066 for a sensitivity of 75%, specificity of 86%, positive and negative predictive values of 55% and 95% to diagnose preeclampsia with this ratio. Preeclamptic patients showed a ratio of 0.0475 ± 0.0260, compared with the control group which showed a ratio of 0.1466 ± 0.1353 [88].

Despite these papers, Sauden et al. did not recommend the use of this ratio as a screening test for preeclampsia: the value of 0.10 showed a sensitivity of only 68% and specificity of 70%. The emergence of preeclampsia was preceded by 12 days with a low CCR [89]. Smith-Adijé, in turn, concluded that the ratio did not provide any additional advantage compared to the 24-hour calciuria [90]. Raniollo et al, making a follow-up of 456 pregnant women between 20-30 gestational weeks, don't find a significant difference in the CCR between the subject that became preeclampsia, gestational hypertension or that persisted normotensives (0.49 ± 0.32 mg/mg, 0.57 ± 0.41 mg/mg, 0.52 ± 0.32 mg/mg), with variations in calcium levels interpopulation and intrapopulation [99]. Backer and Hackett didn't find significant predictive values. Suarez et al showed a significant difference in the CCR between the groups: 0.29 (0.26-0.32) and 0.23 (0.14-0.32) mg/mg for normotensive and preeclamptic patients, respectively. The values found in the study showed relative risks for preeclampsia development, when dosed between 17-20 weeks, of 3.6 with 24-hour calciuria, 4.9 for urinary excretion of calcium (value value divided for weight) and 3.1 for the analyzed ratio [100]. Himgire found that urinary calcium alone could be taken as high risk factor for prediction of preeclampsia ($p<0.001$), demonstrating accuracy of 71% [101]. Studies that included women with gestational hypertension reported a urine calcium excretion in this population similar to that of the normal pregnant women [102-104].

Analyzing the correlation between 24-h calciuria and the ratio in a urine spot indicated that the calciuria levels vary during the day, which does not occur in pregnant women with protein-to-creatinine urine [46]. Some studies that did not show favorable results collected urine in the morning. On other hand, the correlation between 24-hour calciuria and the CCR is real only within certain limited values, as in proteinuria, which is not correlated with the protein-to-creatinine ratio in cases where the proteinuria is higher than 1 or 2 g [60,61].

Our observation that preeclamptic patients have hypocalciuria is in accord with records from other investigators. These authors suggested that urinary calcium excretion levels may serve as a diagnostic tool for differentiating among the various forms of hypertension in pregnancy. This might be explained by an increase in tubular calcium reabsorption rather than a decrease in glomerular filtration, since similar creatinine clearance values were found among the groups. An overlap of values in laboratory tests is expected in preeclampsia, as a clinical syndrome with such an extensive diversity of clinical signs. Even in classical measurements such as uric acid, or in more recently developed measurements such as placental growth factor (PIGF), values will overlap in borderline clinical cases. Although the case-control study is not the most appropriate method, this kind of research will generate lines of inquiry to justify a study with more subjects, with the objective of calculating the sensitivity and specificity of the test. The number of subjects in this study was calculated based on a previous study, to attain the desired level of statistical difference.

Calcium intake was not controlled, but in a previous study in the same population it was concluded that patients with severe preeclampsia have a reduced calcium intake when compared with mild preeclampsia or normal pregnancies [105]. The calcium intake did not differ among the patients who were hospitalized. There was no control of calcium intake in patients who collected their urine at home.

Suarez et al found lower calcium urinary excretion like risk factor for preeclampsia development when done between 17-20 weeks, with 80% of the patients with hypocalciuria becoming preeclamptic patients [106], as Sirohiwal who had showed a decrease in 24-hour urinary calcium and increase in protein between 20-28 weeks gestation like risk factors of preeclampsia [72]. Identifying women with gestation hypertension who are likely to progress to preeclampsia would allow better counseling and closer monitoring.

Conclusion

In conclusion, calciuria, as demonstrated in most reports, is lower in preeclampsia. A single urine spot can possibly estimate this value, and is helpful to diagnose hypertension diseases. Calciuria levels can also estimate the chance that the disease will develop, as a preeclampsia predictor, which was shown in some reports [96,97,99,107,108,109]., but was not the objective of our research. The cutoff point, however, still has to be defined, and varied among studies, as seen in Table 4.

Table 4. Calcium-to-creatinine ratio in the papers

Authors (year)	PE	CH	NP
Huikeshoven et al (1990)	0.03 ± 0.03	0.20 ± 0.18	0.44 ± 0.32
Frenkel et al (1991)	0.049 ± 0.03	0.15 ± 0.09	0.23 ± 0.17
Raniollo et al (1993)	0.049 ± 0.32		0.52 ± 0.32
Ozcan et al (1995)	0.047 ± 0.026		0.1466 ± 0.1353
Suarez et al (1996)	0.23 (0.14-0.32)		0.29 (0.26-0.32)
Izumi et al (1997)	0.121 ± 0.63		0.158 ± 0.239
Sauden et al (1998)	0.07 (0.04-0.09)		
Kazerooni et al (2003)	0.306 ± 0.27		0.52 ± 0.3
Smith-Adijé et al (2006)	0.2 ± 0.2		0.6 ± 0.4
Mandira et al (2008)	0.12 ± 0.11		0.21 ± 0.10
McGrowder et al (2009)	0.17 ± 0.03		0.45 ± 0.08
Gasnier et al	Severe PE 0.0108 (0-0.14) Mild PE 0.05 (0.01-0.36)	0.14 (0.02-0.38)	0.0995 (0.04-0.23)

PE – preeclampsia, CH – chronic hypertension, NP – normal pregnancy.

References

[1] NHBPEWG, Report of the National High Blood Pressure Education Program Working Group on High Blood Pressure in Pregnancy, *Am. J. Obstet. Gynecol.* 183(1) (2000) S1–S22.

[2] Brown MA, Hague WM, Higgins J, et al. The detection, investigation and management of hypertension in pregnancy. *Aust. N. Z. J. Obstet. Gynaecol.* 2000; 40: 133-155.

[3] Brown MA, Lindheimer M, de Swiet M, et al. The classification and diagnosis of the hypertensive disorders of pregnancy: statement from the International Society for the Study of Hypertension in Pregnancy. *Hypertens Pregnancy* 2001; 20: IX-XIV.

[4] Ray J, Vasishta K, Kaur S, Majumdar S, Sawhney H. Calcium metabolism in preeclampsia. *Int. J. Gynecol. Obstet.* 1999;66:245–50.

[5] Lindheimer MD, Umans JG. Explaining and predicting preeclampsia. *N. Engl. J. Med.* 2006; 355(10): 1056-8.

[6] Sibai B, Dekker G, Kupferminc M. Pre-eclampsia. *Lancet* 2005; 365(9461): 785-99.

[7] Wagner LK. Diagnosis and management of preeclampsia. *Am. Farm Physician* 2004; 70(12): 2317-24.

[8] North RA, Taylor RS, Schellenberg JC. Evaluation of a definition of preeclampsia. *Br. J. Obstet. Gyneacol.* 1999; 106: 767-773.

[9] Sibai BM, Abdela TM, Anderson GD. Pregnancy outcome in 211 patients with mild chronic hypertension. *Obstet. Gynecol.* 1983; 61: 571-6.

[10] Ferrazani S, Caruso A, Carrolis S, Martino IV and Mancuso S. Proteinuria and outcome of 444 pregnancies complicated by hypertension. *Am. J. Obstet. Gynecol.* 1990; 162: 366-371.

[11] Hayashi M, Ueda Y, Hoshimoto K, Ota Y, Fukasawa I, Sumori K, Kaneko I, Abe S, Uno M, Ohkura T and Inaba N. Changes in urinary excretion of six biochemical parameters in normotensive pregnancy and preeclampsia. *Am. J. Kidney Dis.* 2002; 39(2): 392-40.

[12] Fisher KA et al. Hypertension in pregnancy. Clinical pathological correlations and late prognosis. Medicine 1981; v.60: 267.

[13] Alvarez RR. Hypertensive disorders in pregnancy: toxemias of pregnancy, preeclampsia, eclampsia. In: Alvarez, RR. The Kidney in Pregnancy. New York, Wiley, first edition, 1976: 113-1.

[14] Dunlop D, Davidson JM. Renal haemodynamics and tubular function in human pregnancy. *Baillière's Clin. Obstet. Gynaecol.* 1987; 1:769-788.

[15] Toback FG, Hall PW and Lindheimer MD. Effect of posture on urinary protein patterns in nonpregnant, pregnant and toxemic women. *Obstet. Gynecol.* 1970; 35(5): 765-68.

[16] Chappel L, Poulton L, Halligan A, Shennan AH. Lack of consistency in research papers over the definition of pre-eclampsia. *Br. J. Obstet. Gynaecol.* 1999; 106: 983-5.

[17] Lindheimer MD and Kanter D. Interpreting abnormal proteinuria in pregnancy. *Obstet. Gynecol.* 2010; 115: 365-75.

[18] Maybury H, Waugh J. Proteinuria in pregnancy – just what is significant? *Fetal and Maternal Medicine Review* 2004; 16: 71-95.

[19] Higby K, Suiter C, Phelps J, et al. Normal values of urinary albumin and total protein excretion during pregnancy. *Am. J. Obstet. Gynecol.* 1994; 71: 984-9.

[20] Kuo VSKoumanantakis G, Gallery EDM. Proteinuria and its assessment in normal and hypertensive pregnancy. *Am. J. Obstet. Gynecol.* 1992; 167: 723-8.

[21] Page EW, Christianson R. Influence of blood pressure changes with and without proteinuria upon outcome of pregnancy. *Am. J. Obstet. and Gynecol.* 1976; 126: 821-9.

[22] Schiff E, Friedman AS, Kao L, Sibai BM. The importance of urinary protein excretion during conservative management of severe preeclampsia. *Am. J. Obstet. Gynecol.* 1996; 175: 1313-6.

[23] Seshadri L, Venkataraman I. Hypertension in pregnancy outcomes, proteinuric versus nonproteinuric. *The Journal of Reproductive Medicine* 1997; 42: 88-90.

[24] Sibai BM, Lidheimer MD, Hauth J, Caritis S, Van Dorstein P, et al. Risks factors for preeclampsia, abruption placentae and adverse neonatal outcomes among women with chronic hypertension. *N. Engl. J. Med.* 1998; 339: 667-71.

[25] Hall DR, Odentaal HJ, Steyn DW, Grové D. Urinary protein excretion and expectant management of early onset, severe preeclampsia. Internat *J. Gynecol. Obstet.* 2002; 77: 1-6.

[26] Buchbinder A, Sibai BM, Caritis S, MacPherson C, Hauth J, Lindheimer MD, et al. Adverse perinatal outcomes are significantly higher in severe gestational hypertension than in mild preeclampsia. *Am. J. Obstet. Gynecol.* 2002; 186: 66-71.

[27] Martins-Costa SH, Vettorazzi J, Valerio EG, Ramos JGL, Barros EG, et al. Protein creatinine ratio in random urine sample of hypertensive pregnant womenÇ maternal and perinatal outcomes. *Hypertens Pregnancy* 2011, 30(3): 331-7.

[28] Thangaratinam S, Coomarasamy A, O'Mahony F, Sharp S, Zamora J, Klan KS, et al. Estimation of proteinuria as a predictor of complications of preeclampsia: a systematic review. *BMC Med.* 2009, March 24: 7-10.

[29] Sasaki M, Pugia MJ, Parker DR, Kuromoto K, Furukawa I, Konishi I. Measurement of the albumin content of urinary protein using dipsticks. *J. Clin. Lab. Anal.* 1999; 13(5): 246-50.

[30] Agarwal R, Panesar A, Lewis RR. Dipstick proteinuria: can it guide hypertension management? *Am. J. Kidney Dis.* 2002; 39(6): 1190-5.

[31] Meyer NL, Mercer BM, Friedman AS, SIBAI BM. Urinary dipstick protein: a poor prediction of absent or severe proteinuria. *Am. J. Obstet. Gynecol.* 1994; 170: 137-41.

[32] Phelan LK, Brown MA, Davis GK, Mangos G. A prospective study of the impact of automated dipstick urinalysis on the diagnosis of preeclampsia. *Hypertension in Pregnancy* 2004; 23(2): 135-42.

[33] Bell SC, Halligan AW, Martin A, Ashmore J, Shennan AH, Lambert PC, et al. The role of observer error in antenatal dipstick proteinuria analysis. *Br. J. Obstet. Gynaecol.* 1999; 106(11): 1177-80.

[34] Halligan AW, Bell SC, Taylor DJ. Dipstick proteinuria: caveat emptor. *Br. J. Obstet. Gyneacol.* 1999; 106(11): 1113-5.

[35] Waugh JS, Justin CT, Divakaran TG, Khan KS, Kilby MD. Accuracy of urinalysis dipstick techniques in predicting significant proteinuria in pregnancy. *Obst. Gynecol.* 2004ç 103(4)Ç 769-77.

[36] Kieler H.; Zettergren T.; Svensson H.; Dickman P.W.; Larsson A.. Assessing urinary albumin excretion in pre-eclamtic women: Wich sample to use? *BJOG*, 2003; 110 (1):12-17.

[37] Shaw AB, Risdon P, Lewis-Jackson JD. Protein creatinine index and Albustix in assessment of proteinuria. *Br. Med. J. (Clin. Res. Ed)* 1983; 287(6397): 929-32.

[38] Roy C, Boyce T, Dodd C, Bosio P, Waugh J. Protein creatinine ratio dipsticks are effective in reducing false positive and false negative rates when screening for proteinuria in normotensive women. *Hypertension in Pregnancy* 2004; 23(Suppl 1): 36.

[39] Côté AM, Lam E, von Dadelszen P, Magee LA. Accuracy of the 24-hour urine collection in hypertensive women. *Hypertension in Pregnancy* 2006; 25(Suppl): 230.

[40] Ramos JGL, Martins-Costa SH, Mathias MM, Guerin YL, Barros EG. Urinary protein/creatinine ratio in hypertensive women. *Hypertension in Pregnancy* 1999; 18(3): 209-18.

[41] Rodriguez-Thompson D, Lieberman ES. Use of a random urinary protein-to-creatinine ratio for the diagnosis of significant proteinuria during pregnancy. *Am. J. Obstet. Gynecol.* 2001; 185(4): 808-11.

[42] Neithardt AB, Dooley SL, Borensztajn J. Prediction of 24-hour protein excretion in pregnancy with a single voided urine protein-creatinine ratio. *Am. J. Obstet. Gynecol.* 2002; 186: 883-6.

[43] Yamasmit W, Chaitongwongwathana S, Charoenvidhya D, Uerpairojki B, Tolosa J. Random urinary protein-to-creatinine ratio for prediction of significant proteinuria in women with preeclampsia. *J. Mater. Fetal Neonatal Med.* 2004; 16(5): 227-9.

[44] Blackburn C, Powrie RO, Phipps M, Sung J, Weitzen S, Rosene-Montella K. Urinary protein-to-creatinine ratio is a clinically useful test in pregnancy. *Hypertension in Pregnancy* 2004; 23:37.

[45] Rizk DE, Agarwal MM, Pathan JY, Obineche EN. Predicting proteinuria in hypertensive pregnancies with urinary protein-creatinine or calcium-creatinine ratio. *J Perinatol.* 2007; 27(5): 272-7.

[46] Leãnos-Miranda A, Marquez-Acosta J, Romero-Arauz F, Cárdenas-Mondrágon GM, Rivera-Leãnos R, Isordia-Salas I, Ulloa-Aguirre A. Protein:creatinine ratio in random urine samples is a reliable marker of increased 24-hour protein excretion in hospitalized women with hypertensive disorders of pregnancy. *Clinical Chemistry* 2007; 53(9): 1623-7.

[47] Valerio EG, Ramos JGL, Martins-Costa SM, Müller ALL. Variation in the urinary protein/creatinine ratio at four different periods of the day in hypertensive pregnant women. *Hypertension in Pregnancy* 2005; 24: 213-21.

[48] Yamasmit W, Wongkitisophon K, Charoenvidhya D, Uerpairojki B, Chaitongwongwatthana S. Correlation between random urinary protein-to-creatinine ratio and quantitation of proteinuria in preeclampsia. *J. Med. Assoc. Thai.* 2003; 86 (1): 69-73.

[49] Côté AM, Brown M, Halsted AC, Daldelszen PV, Linston RM, Magee LA. Should the urinary spot protein/creatinine ratio (PCR) be used as a diagnostic test in hypertensive pregnant women: a systematic review. *Hypertension in Pregnancy* 2004; 23(Suppl 1): 36.

[50] Misiani R, Marchesi D, Tiraboschi G, Gualandris L, Pagni R, Goglio A, et al. Urinary albumin excretion in normal pregnancy and pregnancy-induced hypertension. *Nephron* 1991; 59: 416-22.

[51] Côté AM, Brown MA, Lam E, von Dadelszen P, Firoz T, Liston RM, Magee LA. Diagnostic accuracy of urinary spot protein:creatinine ratio for proteinuria in hypertensive pregnant women: systematic review. *BMJ* 2008; online publication.
[52] Ginsberg JM, Chang BS, Matarese RA, Garella S. Use of single voided urine samples to estimate quantitative proteinuria. *N. Engl. J. Med.* 1983; 309: 1543-6.
[53] Lindheimer MD, Taler SJ, Cunningham FG. Hypertension in Pregnancy. *J. Am. Soc. Hypertens* 2008; 2(6): 484-94.
[54] National Kidney Foundation. K/DOQI clinical practice guidelines for chronic kidney disease: evaluation, classification and stratification. *Am. J. Kidney Dis.* 2002; 39(2 Suppl 1): S1-266.
[55] Vassalotti JA, Stevens LA, Levey AS. Testing for chronic kidney disease: a position statement from the National Kidney Foundation. *Am. J. Kidney Dis* 2007; 50: 169-80.
[56] Morales JV, Weber R, Wagner MB, Barros EJ. Is morning urinary protein/creatinine ratio a reliable estimator of 24-hour proteinuria in patients with glomerulonephritis and different levels of renal function? *J. Nephrol.* 2004; 17(5): 666-72.
[57] Price CP, Newall RG, Boyd JC. Use of protein:creatinine ratio measurements on random urine samples for prediction of significant proteinuria: a systematic review. *Clinical Chemistry* 2005; 51(9): 1577-86.
[58] Lane C, Brown M, Dunsmuir W, Kelly J, Mangos G. Can spot urin protein/creatinine ratio replace 24 h urine protein in usual clinical nephrology? *Nephrology (Carlton)* 2006; 11: 245-9.
[59] Wikström A-K, Wikström J, Larsson A, Olovsson M. Random albumin/creatinine ratio for quantification of proteinuria in manifest pre-eclampsia. *BJOG* 2006; 113: 930-4.
[60] Boler L, Edward AZ, Gleicher N. Quantitation of proteinuria in pregnancy by the use of single voided urine samples. *Obstet. Gynecol.* 1987:70–99.
[61] Jaschevatzky OE, Rosenberg RP, Shalit A, Zonder HB, Grunstein S.Protein / creatinine ratio in random urine specimens for quantization of proteinuria in preeclampsia. *Obstet. Gynecol.* 1990;75:604.
[62] Antunes VVH, Veronese FJV, Morales JV. Diagnostic accuracy of the protein/creatinine ratio in urine samples to estimate 24-h proteinuria in patients with primary glomerulopathies: a longitudinal study. *Nephrol. Dial. Transpl.* 2008; 23(7): 2242-6.
[63] Cunningham FG, Gant NF, Leveno KJ, Gilstrap III, Hauth JC, Wenstron KD. Hypertensive disorders in pregnancy. In: Cunningham et al, Williams Obstetrics 21ª ed, McGraw-Hill Companies, 2001; 567-618.
[64] Adelberg AM, Miller J, Doerzbacher M, Lambers DS. Correlation of quantitative protein measurements in 8-, 12-, and 24-hour urine samples for the diagnosis of preeclampsia. *Am. J. Obstet. Gynecol.* 2001; 185: 804-7.
[65] Evans W, Lensmeyer JP, Kirby RS, Malnory ME, Broekhuizen FF. Two-hour urine collection for evaluating renal function correlates with 24-hour urine collection in pregnant patients. *J. Matern Fetal Med.* 2000; 9: 233-7.
[66] Rinehart BK, Terrone DA, Larmon JE, Perry KG Jr, Martin RW, Martin JN Jr. A 12-hour urine collection accurately assesses proteinuria in the hospitalized hypertensive gravid. *J. Perinatol.* 1999; 19: 556-8.

[67] Somanathan N, Farrell T, Galimberti A. A comparison between 24-hour and 2-hour urine collection for the determination of proteinuria. *J. Obstet. Gynaecol.* 2003; 23: 378-80.

[68] Wongkitisophon K, Phupong V, Yamasmit W, Pansin P, Tannirandom Y, Charoenvidhya D. Correlation ofr 4- and 24-hour urine protein in women with initially diagnosed hypertensive disorders in pregnancy. *J. Med. Assoc. Thai.* 2003; 86: 529-34.

[69] Ingec M, Nazik H, Kadanali S. Urinary calcium excretion in severe preeclampsia and eclampsia. *Clin Chem Lab Med* 2006;44(1):51–3.

[70] Al-Mait AM, Petrulius AS, Amini SB, Mann LI. Hypocalciuria can differentiate preeclampsia from chronic hypertension in the third trimester. *J. Mate–Fetal Neonat. Med.* 1993;2(1):300–4.

[71] Segovia BL, Vega IT, Villarreal EC, Licona NA. Hypocalciuria during pregnancy as a risk factor of preeclampsia. *Ginecol. Obstet. Mex.* 2004;72:570–4.

[72] Sirohiwal D, Dahyla K, Khaneja N. Use of 24-hour urinary protein and calcium for prediction of preeclampsia. *Taiwanese Journal of Obstetrics and Gynecology* 2009;48(2):113–5.

[73] Halhali A, Diaz L, Avila E, Ariza AC, Garabedian M, Larrea F. Decreased fractional urinary calcium excretion and serum 1,25- dihydroxyvitamin D and IGF-I levels in preeclampsia. *J. Steroid Biochem. Mol. Biol.* 2007;103(3-5):803–6.

[74] Ramos JG, Martins-Costa SH, Vettorazzi J, Vettori DV, Louzado M, Dornelles MS, Bastos M. Calciuria levels in pregnant women with high blood pressure. *Revista HCPA* 2000;20(2):103–7.

[75] Cross NA, Hilman LS, Allen SH, Krause GF, Vieira NE. Calcium homeostasis and bone metabolism during pregnancy, lactation and postweaning: A longitudinal study. *Am. J. Clin. Nutr.* 1995; 61: 514-23.

[76] Gertner JM, Counstan DR, Kliger AS, Mallette LE, Ravin N, Broadus AE. Pregnancy as state of physiologic absorptive hypercalciuria. *Am. J. Med.* 1986; 81: 451-6.

[77] Hutchesson ACJ, Macintosh MC, Duncan SLB, Forrest ARW. Hypocalciuria and hypertension in pregnancy: A prospective study. *Clin. Exp. Hypertens* 1990; B9: 115-34.

[78] Covi G, Corsato M, Paluani F, Marcolongo A, Minuz P, Lechi A. Reduced urinary excretion of calcium in pregnancy-induced hypertension: Relationship to renal prostaglandin excretion. *Hypertens Pregnancy* 1990; 9: 151-67.

[79] Tolaymat A, Sanchez-Ramos L, Yergey AL, Vieira NE, Abrams AS, Edelstein P. Pathophysiology of hypocalciuria in preeclampsia: Measurement of intestinal calcium absorption. *Obstet. Gynecol.* 1994; 83: 239-43.

[80] Bilgin T, Kutlu O, Kimya Y, Kuçukkomurcu S, Uncu G. Urine calcium excretion in preeclampsia. *T. Klin. Jinekol. Obstet.* 2000; 10: 29-32.

[81] Van Overloop B, Treisser A, Coumaros G, Schleiffer R, Gairard A. Decreased ionized calcium and increased parathyroid hormone in the serum of mild gestational hypertensive patients at the third trimester: A link between calcium metabolism and hypertension in pregnancy. *Hypertens Pregnancy* 1992; 11: 233-47.

[82] Ray J, Vasishta K, Kaur S, Majumdar S, Sawhney H. Calcium metabolism in pre-eclampsia. Int. J. Gynecol. Obstet. 1999; 66: 245-50.

[83] Seely EW, Wood RJ, Brown EM, Graves SW. Lower serum ionized calcium and abnormal calciotropic hormone levels in preeclampsia. *J. Clin. Endocrinol. Metab.* 1992; 74: 1436-40.

[84] Izumi A, Minakami H, Kuwata T, Sato I. Calcium-to-creatinine ratio in spot urine samples in early pregnancy and its relation to the development of preeclampsia. *Metabolism* 1997; 46: 1107-8.

[85] Adamova Z, Ozkan S, Khalil RA. Vascular and cellular calcium in normal and hypertensive pregnancy. *Curr. Clin. Pharmacol. 2009; 4(3): 172-90.*

[86] McGrowder D, Williams A, Gordon L, Crawford T, Alexander-Lindo R, Irving R, Hamilton M, Fraser YTP. Hypocalciuria in preeclampsia and gestational hypertension due to decreased fractional excretion of calcium. *Arch. Med. Sci.* 2009; 5(1):80–5.

[87] Frenkel Y, Barkai G, Mashiach S, Dolev E, Zimlichman R, Weiss M. Hypocalciuria of preeclampsia is independent of parathyroid hormone level. *Obstet.* 1991;77:689–91.

[88] Ozcan T, Kaleli B, Ozeren M, Turan C, Zorlu G. Urinary calcium to creatinine ratio for predicting preeclampsia. *Am. J. Perinatol.* 1995; 12(5):349–51.

[89] Saudan PJ, Shaw L, Brown MA. Urinary calcium / creatinine ratio as a predictor of preeclampsia. *Am. J. Hypertension* 1998; 11:839–43.

[90] Szmidt-Adijé V, Vendittelli F, David S, Bredent-Bangou J, Janky E. Calciuria and preeclampsia: a case-control study. *Eur. J. Obstet. Gynecol. Reprod. Biol.* 2006;125(2):193–8.

[91] Nielsen TF, Rylander R. Urinary calcium and magnesium excretion relates to increase in blood pressure during pregnancy. *Arch. Gynecol. Obstet.* 2010;283(3):443–7.

[92] B.E. Metzger, D.R. Coustan, Summary and recommendations of the Fourth International Workshop-Conference on Gestational DiabetesMellitus, The Organizing Committee, *Diabetes Care* 21(2) (1998) B161–B167.

[93] Kasiske BL, Keane WF. Laboratory assessment of renal disease: clearance urinalysis and renal biopsy. In: Brenner BM, editor. The Kidney. Philadelphia: WB Saunders; 1996. p. 1137–74.

[94] Ramos JGL, Martins-Costa SH, Kessler JB, Costa CA, Barros EG. Calciuria and preeclampsia. Braz. *J. Med. Biol. Res.* 1998;31:519–22.

[95] Huikeshoven FJM, Zuijderhoudt FMJ. Hypocalciuria in hypertensive disorder in pregnancy and how to measure it. *Eur. J. Obstet. Gynecol. Reprod. Biol.* 1990;36(1-2):81–5.

[96] Sanchez-Ramos L, Jones D, Cullen MT., Kaunitz AM. Urinary calcium as early marker for preeclampsia. *Obstet. Gynecol.* 1991; 77: 685-8.

[97] Kazerooni T, Hamze-Nejadi S. Calcium to creatinine ratio in a spot sample of urine for early prediction of preeclampsia. *International J. Gynecol. Obstet.* 2003; 80(3): 279-83.

[98] Mandira D, Sudhir A, Mamtaz S. Urinary calcium levels in preeclampsia. *J. Obstet. Gynecol. India* 2008;58(4):308–11.

[99] Raniolo E, Phillipou G. Prediction of pregnancy-induced hypertension by means of urinary calcium: creatinine ratio. *Medical J. Australia* 1991; 158(2): 98-100.

[100] Baker PN, Hackett GA. The use of urinary albumin/creatinine ratio and calcium/creatinine ratio as screening tests for pregnancy-induced hypertension. *Obstet. Gynecol.* 1994; 83: 745-49.

[101] Himgire JR. Estimation of urinary calcium as a predictor of pre-eclampsia. Online publication 2011: http://hdl.handle.net/123456789/ 4730.

[102] Taufield PA, Alles KL, Resnick LM, Druzin ML, Gertner JM, Laragh JH. Hypocalciuria in preeclampsia. *N. Eng. J. Med.* 1987;316:715–8.

[103] Sanchez-Ramos L, Sandroni FJA, Kaunitz AM. Calcium excretion in preeclampsia. *Obstet. Gynecol.* 1991;77:510–3.

[104] Graves SW, Wood RJ, Brown EM, et al. Calcium and calciotropic hormones in transient hypertension of pregnancy versus preeclampsia. *Hypertension in Pregnancy* 1994;12:87–95.

[105] Ramos JGL, Brietzke E, Martins-Costa S, Vettorazzi JS, Barros E, Carvalho C. Reduced calcium intake is reduced in women with preeclampsia. *Hypertens Pregnancy* 2006;25:229–39.

[106] VR, Trelles JG, Miyahira JM. Urinary calcium in asymptomatic primigravidas who later developed preeclampsia. *Obstet. Gynecol.* 1996;87(1):79–82.

[107] Rodriguez JG, Avendano R, Inzunza B. Hypocalciuria in preeclampsia. *Chil. Obstet. Gynecol.* 1993;58(6):470–4.

[108] Suarez VR, Trelles JG, Miyahira JM. Urinary calcium in asymptomatic primigravidas who later developed preeclampsia. *Obstet. Gynecol.* 1996;87(1):79–82.

[109] Kazemi AFN, Sehhatie F, Sattarzade N, Mameghani ME. The predictive value of urinary calcium to creatinine ratio, roll-over test and BMI in early diagnosis of preeclampsia. *Res. J. Biol. Sci.* 2010; 5(2): 183-6.

In: Creatinine
Editors: I. H. Perkins and C. M. Chapman

ISBN: 978-1-62257-475-9

Chapter II

Creatinine: Production, Physiology and Diagnostic Use in Kidney Diseases

Pierre Delanaye[1,*], Emmanuelle Vidal-Petiot[2] and Martin Flamant[2,3]

[1]Department of Nephrology-Dialysis-Transplantation, University of Liège, CHU Sart Tilman, Liège, Belgium
[2]Department of Renal Physiology, Hôpital Bichat, AP-HP, Paris, France
[3]Inserm U699, University Paris Diderot, Paris, France

Abstract

Plasma creatinine is one of the most frequently prescribed blood tests in clinical practice. Indeed, although it has used for many decades, it remains the reference marker to assess renal function. In this chapter, we propose to detail the physiological aspects that explain that creatinine is a relatively good marker of endogenous glomerular filtration. We will review the determinants of plasma creatinine independent of GFR, in terms of muscle production, non-renal clearance and tubular secretion. The value and limitations of the urinary clearance of creatinine will be discussed. We will present the formulas derived from serum creatinine to estimate GFR.

1. Introduction

The word "creatinine" was probably used for the first time by Justus von Liebig in 1847. This German Chemist was thus describing the product obtained from heating creatine with mineral salts [1]. Nowadays, serum creatinine is one of the most frequently prescribed analyses in Clinical Chemistry. However, historically, serum blood urea nitrogen (BUN) was first used to evaluate renal function. The term "clearance" was used for the first time by the American scientist Eggert Möller about urea clearance [2]. Serum creatinine and creatinine

* Address correspondence to: Pierre Delanaye, Service de Dialyse, CHU Sart Tilman, 4000 Liège, Belgium; Tel: ++32-43667317; Fax: ++32-43667405; E-mail: pierre_delanaye@yahoo.fr.

clearance were firstly used to evaluate renal function by the Danish Physiologists Rehberg and Holten in the mid-twenties. In this article, the authors had already suggested that creatinine is secreted by renal tubules [3]. The interest in this renal marker was then admitted and the superiority over BUN was accepted [4]. To estimate glomerular filtration rate (GFR), the first physiologists used perfusion of creatinine to increase its plasma concentration and make its measurement easier [3; 5]. Indeed, until that time, the real presence of creatinine in serum was even questioned [6; 7]. Endogenous creatinine clearance was first studied at the end of the thirties notably after improvement in creatinine measurement [8].

Serum creatinine is the only renal plasma biomarker used in daily clinical practice to estimate GFR. However, good interpretation of the creatinine result remains sometimes problematic. There are physiological reasons to explain these difficulties (serum creatinine is not an "ideal" renal marker). In this chapter, we will successively review:

- creatinine physiology compared to the physiology of an ideal GFR marker
- variations of serum creatinine not due to GFR variations (physiological and analytical interferences)
- strengths and limitations of creatinine clearance to estimate GFR
- strengths and limitations of creatinine-based equations to estimate GFR

2. Creatinine Physiology

2.1. Creatine and Creatinine

The molecular weight of creatinine is 113 Daltons. Creatinine is the anhydric catabolite of creatine and phosphocreatine. Creatinine is a catabolite final product and has no physiological role. To better approach the physiology of creatinine, it is thus important to better understand creatine. Creatine is synthesized by two successive steps. The first step is a reaction between glycine and arginine, which are converted into guanidinoacetic acid *via* a transamidase enzyme. This reaction takes place in kidneys, small intestine, pancreas, spleen, brain, breast and liver. In the liver, guanidinoacetic acid is then methylated from S-adenosylmethionin to give creatine [9]. Creatine is then transferred to other organs (brain, liver and kidney). However, the vast majority of creatine (98%) is found in muscles where it is phosphorylated by creatine kinase into phosphocreatine. Phosphocreatine is a highly energetic product which appears essential for muscle contraction [10]. Creatinine is thus synthesized from creatine by a non-enzymatic and irreversible reaction [11]. Under particular circumstances, it seems that creatinine can also be synthesized from phosphocreatine. Each day, 1 to 2% of the muscular creatine is converted into creatinine [9]. From these physiologic data, it is obvious that serum creatinine concentration is highly dependent on muscular mass [9; 12; 13]. Differences in muscular mass largely explain differences observed in creatinine concentrations according to gender, age and ethnicity [12; 14]. We will now discuss the physiology of creatinine in the light of the characteristics of an ideal biomarker of GFR, i.e. freely filtrated (with no binding to proteins) through the glomerulus, produced at a constant rate, neither secreted nor reabsorbed by the tubules, with no extra-renal excretion, and easy to measure in blood and urine [4]. First of all, it is well demonstrated that creatinine is freely filtered because of its low molecular weight and the absence of binding to proteins [12].

2.2. Is the Creatinine Production Really Constant and Similar between Individuals?

In the steady-state, the serum creatinine concentration remains stable in each subject because the daily production of creatinine from muscular creatine is constant [15]. In the absence of extra-renal excretion, renal excretion thus reflects the global creatinine production [12]. If the global creatine concentration is constant in healthy subjects, the "level of steady state" may be highly variable according to some muscular pathologies (infectious, genetic, immune and degenerative myopathies, hyperthyroidism, para- or quadriplegia, chronic steroid therapy [16-19]) or, from a larger point of view, in all diseases with anorexia and muscular mass decrease (cirrhosis, intensive care etc) [10; 15; 20]. In these situations, serum creatinine will decrease (or will not increase) although GFR is actually decreasing [12]. In the same way, creatinine production tends to decrease with age [12]. However, this decrease in serum creatinine is compensated by a physiologic decrease of GFR [12; 14; 21]. In children, variations in "normal" serum creatinine concentrations are observed according to growth and progressive gain of muscular mass. This observation can be a source of confusion because normal reference values vary according to age in Pediatrics [22]. Some authors have also suggested that the creatinine production may be decreased in cirrhotic patients, not only because muscular mass is decreased, but also because creatine is synthesized at a lower rate by the cirrhotic liver [10; 23]. There are also pathological situations where the conversion rate of creatine to creatinine (normally at 1 to 2%) is modified [12; 24]. Such variations in the rate of conversion are however very difficult to study. For example, in case of rhabdomyolysis, the increase in serum creatinine is higher and faster than in other causes of acute renal failure. Some authors hypothesize that the production of creatinine from muscular creatine and phosphocreatine could explain this observation. An opposite example is the potential decreased conversion rate of creatine to creatinine which has been suggested in cirrhotic subjects [25].

2.3. Is Muscle the Only Source of Creatinine?

Creatine and creatinine can also come from food. Serum creatinine concentration increases after meals. An intake of non cooked beef will bring 3.5 to 5 mg of creatinine by gram of lean beef [12]. Ingestion of 1 gram of pure creatine increases the creatine pool, and the creatinine urinary excretion might increase up to 25% [12; 24]. The quantity of creatinine in non-cooked meals is negligible but cooking will convert 15 to 65% of creatine into creatinine, which will be then absorbed by gastrointestinal tract and excreted by the kidneys [9; 24; 26]. The net effect of a meal on serum creatinine concentrations remains a matter of debate. According to different studies, variations observed range, from 10 to 100% [27; 28]. This effect is probably different from one subject to another. Explanations for such discrepancies between studies are multiple: (i) intestinal absorption is variable (75 à 80%) [29], (ii) GFR also increases after ingestion of a meal rich in proteins (and this variation is not taken into account in most of the studies) [12]. The effect of pure creatine intake (by some athletes) on serum creatinine is not well known but an increase of 27 μmol/L has been observed after ingestion of 20 grams of creatine [30]. Daily ingestion of 5 grams of creatine during a 12-week period has no significant effect on GFR measured by a reference method, or on plasma serum creatinine [31].

According to these potential variations, it could be better to measure fasting serum creatinine (or at least, not after a meal rich in meat). This suggestion is however poorly taken into account in daily practice.

2.4. Is Creatinine Secreted by Renal Tubules?

The tubular secretion of creatinine has been known for more than one century and is one of the major limitations of its use as a GFR biomarker [4; 5; 8; 12; 32-37]. The tubular secretion of creatinine occurs via an organic cation transporter localized to the proximal tubule (Organic Cation Transporteur type 2 or OCT2) [38]. Since creatinine was used as a GFR marker in the 1920's, the tubular secretion of creatinine has been suspected because creatinine clearance overestimates inulin clearance, the historical reference method to measure GFR. The overestimation of GFR with the clearance of creatinine, when assessed as a ratio, is higher in lower GFR values [3; 5; 8]. The creatinine clearance on inulin clearance ratio varies from 1 to 1.4. From these data, it has been concluded that 10 to 40% of creatinine is secreted by the tubules [4; 5;8; 32; 33; 36; 37]. This ratio can increase over 2 in severe chronic kidney disease (CKD) [5; 33-36]. For some authors, nephrotic proteinuria could increase the creatinine secretion, independently of GFR level [39]. This last assertion is however still a matter of debate [40]. In African-American subjects, the creatinine secretion could be less important compared to Caucasians. It has been suggested that the faster increase of serum creatinine in African-Americans could thus be linked to a lesser creatinine secretion (and not a faster decrease of GFR) [41-45]. This last observation in African-American is however still debated. Recently, it has also been suggested that creatinine secretion could be higher in male and in healthy subject with higher body mass index, suggesting that creatinine supply might set the creatinine tubular secretion [37].

It is important to underline some characteristics of this tubular secretion. First, tubular secretion is highly variable between individuals (high inter-individual variability). Second, this secretion is impossible to predict. Third, the day-to-day intra-individual variability is far from negligible and tubular secretion could even vary during diurnal cycle [12; 14; 32; 46]. Tubular creatinine secretion can also be blocked by some therapies, which induce an increase in serum creatinine without any change in GFR (see below).

2.5. Is Creatinine Reabsorbed by Renal Tubules?

It has been shown that creatinine clearance can sometimes be less than the inulin clearance, for low values of GFR [4; 47]. This suggested the possibility of a renal tubular reabsorption of creatinine in advanced renal failure [47; 48]. Despite this, to date, no carrier for creatinine reabsorption has been described. Thus, the hypothesis of passive transport has been discussed [49]. More likely, these observations are related to the imprecision of the assay of creatinine with the methods that were used, and not to reabsorption of creatinine.

2.6. Is Creatinine Excretion Only Renal?

Using creatinine clearance as a marker of GFR obviously implies that constant creatinine production is equivalent to its urinary excretion [12]. Indeed, in the healthy or moderate CKD subjects, there is no, or very negligible, extra-renal excretion of creatinine [50]). However, in advanced CKD, creatinine excretion is not only renal [51]. Mitch described a decreased excretion of 66% [51] which seems independent of any decrease in muscular mass or in creatinine production [52]. In these patients with very severe CKD, serum creatinine concentration is lower than expected, according to their GFR and muscular mass [51]. The authors have hypothesized that bacteria from the intestinal flora could activate a creatininase in the presence of very high concentrations of creatinine. This hypothesis remains however somewhat speculative, not easy to prove and, once again, will impact creatinine results only in the lowest GFR values, which is probably less relevant from a clinical point of view [53].

2.7. Is the Measurement of Creatinine in Serum Reliable?

Creatinine can be measured in serum and urine by several methods. High liquid performance chromatography and, still more, methods based on mass spectrometric are considered as reference methods [54]. However, they are not adapted for the daily practice. Nowadays, two main methods are proposed by laboratories to measure creatinine: the method derived from the Jaffe reaction and the enzymatic method. In 1886, Jaffe described the reaction between picrate and creatinine. In an alkaline milieu, reaction between picrate and creatinine in urine gives a red-orange product [55]. In 1905, Folin was the first author to effectively quantify creatinine in urine by colorimetry [56]. Detection and quantification of creatinine in plasma has been debated for a long time until it was proven in the thirties [7; 26]. As early as 1924, Abderhalden has shown that plasma proteins interfere with the colorimetric dosage of creatinine yielding falsly increased concentrations [57]. These historical difficulties in measuring serum creatinine are a good illustration of the problematic of these plasma components interfering with creatinine measurement, namely the "pseudochromogens". These pseudochromogens (acetoacetate, pyruvate, ketonic acids, proteins, glucose and ascorbic acid) are numerous and take part in 15-20% of the Jaffe reaction if serum creatinine is in the normal range [6; 12; 32; 58]. However, the exact concentration is unpredictable in a given subject [59]. Different improvements have been proposed to limit this pseudochromogen effect [13; 60-63]. One of the most improvements is the concept of kinetic measurement. Several authors have actually demonstrated the interest of measuring the reaction not at the end but during the Jaffe reaction. These methods are called "kinetic" methods [13;60-63]. Globally, the colorimetric measurement is done between 20 and 120 seconds even if differences exist according to the manufacturer. Two types of interferences are thus improved: acetoacetate and proteins. Actually, acetoacetate (especially high in the plasma if ketoacidosis [61; 64]) react with picrate strongly and very quickly. If the optic measurement is made after 20 seconds and using the measurement as a blank, the interference with acetoacetate is largely decreased because the acetoacetate-picrate reaction is already finished at this time [60; 61; 63]. On the other hand, proteins and glucose react very slowly with picrate. A relatively rapid lecture of the reaction will thus decrease the interferences with these components [60; 63].

More recently, several manufacturers have introduced the concept of "compensated" creatinine. This concept was first proposed by Roche Diagnostics [65]. The concept is to recalibrate the assay by systematically subtracting 27 µmol/L to all creatinine results. The 27 µmol/L concentration is meant to reflect the mean concentration of pseudochromogens in the plasma. This is a purely mathematical compensation which does not reflect the "true" concentration of pseudochromogens. This true concentration remains unpredictable for a given subject and may actually vary between 0 and 44 µmol/L [66]. Moreover, this mathematical compensation is probably not accurate for very low creatinine concentrations, especially in Pediatrics or Neonatology [67]. Nowadays, other manufacturers use such a mathematical compensation. The way the compensation is applied may differ depending on manufacturers which may be a source of confusion.

The first enzymatic dosage has been described in 1937 but these methods were only available in clinical practice fifty years later. Nowadays, enzymatic measurement of creatinine is based on successive enzymatic steps. Two main types of reactions have been described: creatinine amidohydrolase or iminohydrolase [68]. Enzymatic methods are now considered to be more accurate and precise than Jaffe methods. The enzymatic methods are thus recommended even if they are more costly [13; 69-71].

As expected, results given by enzymatic and Jaffe methods are different [72; 73]. In the same way, reference normal values are lower with the enzymatic than with the Jaffe methods [74]. There is also a great heterogeneity in the results observed with the same method according to the manufacturers. Nowadays, there are several automates and the number of different assays is now very high [72; 73]. The same comment can be made for the enzymatic methods [54]. Consequences of this lack of homogenous calibration are far from negligible, especially for the estimation of GFR by the creatinine-based equations [75-78]. Very recently, improvements have been made by manufacturers to standardize creatinine measurements. In this context, development of a reference method which is strong, reproducible and traceable is an essential step. The method now considered as the reference is the isotope dilution mass spectrometry (IDMS) method [54; 79]. It is now recommended that all creatinine measurements are IDMS-traceable. Once again, this traceability is of the highest importance in the context of creatinine-based equations [80;81]. Recently, the IDMS traceability and the high analytical performances of enzymatic methods available in Europe and China have been confirmed [70; 71; 82].

3. Diagnostic Tool in Kidney Disease

3.1. Sensitivity of Serum Creatinine and GFR-Creatinine Relationship

As already discussed, a correct interpretation of a creatinine measurement remains delicate because creatinine concentration is dependent not only on GFR but also on muscular mass and, therefore, on gender, age and ethnicity. Defining normal reference values is thus not so easy and should take into account all these variables. To simplify, only gender (and sometimes ethnicity [83]) differences are often taken into consideration in adult populations in daily practice [67].

Serum creatinine lacks sensitivity to detect early CKD stages. In other words, if serum creatinine increases above the normal reference range, it implies that GFR has already decreased by, at least, 50% [3; 12; 14; 33; 84; 85]. Bröchner-Mortensen has shown that 60% of patients with moderate CKD (defined in this study by a GFR of 50 to 70% of the normal range) have however a serum creatinine concentration in the normal range of the laboratory [85].

Shemesh has shown in 26 CKD patients (mean GFR at 49±6 mL/min) that despite an improving GFR (inulin clearance increasing of 33% in 3 to 12 months), serum creatinine will decrease only in 13% of the patients (creatinine remains stable in 14 patients) [33]. This lack of sensitivity is even more striking in patients with loss of muscular mass. Papadakis has thus shown that 57% of cirrhotic patients with ascite have normal creatinine values although the mean measured GFR is 32 mL/min [25]. We also demonstrated the very poor sensitivity of serum creatinine to detect GFR below 60 mL/min in patients with anorexia nervosa [20].

We also want to insist on the following point. The relationship between serum creatinine and GFR is not linear but exponential (Figure 1) [32; 86]. Keeping this in mind is fundamental for a good interpretation of the creatinine result. Indeed, this exponential relation implies that a little change in creatinine level will have great consequences in terms of GFR at low creatinine levels, although the same creatinine variation in higher ranges will be negligible in terms of GFR. In other words, if serum creatinine increases from 50 to 100 μmol/L, GFR decreases by 50%. Such a 50% decrease will be equivalent to an increase from 400 to 800 μmol/L in a CKD patient. This exponential relationship will have practical implications for the precision and the interpretation of creatinine-based equations used to estimate GFR [81].

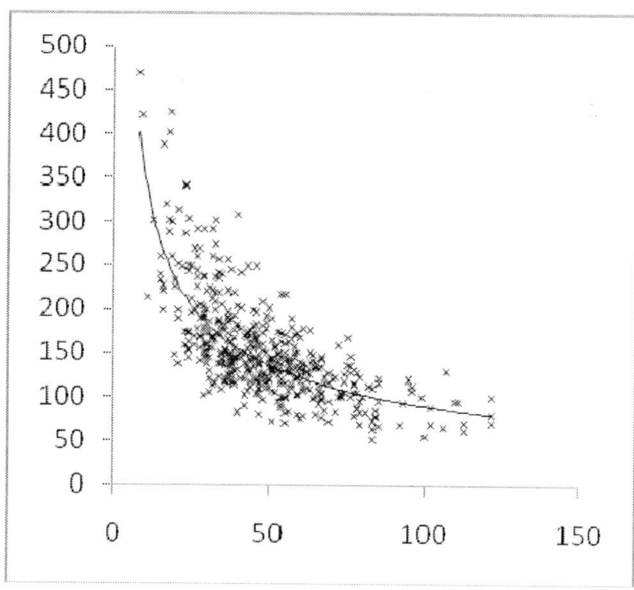

Figure 1. Relationship between serum creatinine and GFR.

3.2. Serum Creatinine in Acute Kidney Injury

If a rapid decline in GFR occurs (as in acute kidney injury), serum creatinine interpretation is even more complicated. Indeed, creatinine production is constant and its volume of distribution is large. After acute renal injury, a new steady-state must be reached. The increase in serum creatinine will thus be progressive over 2 or 3 days. Waikar and Bonventre have recently studied the creatinine kinetic during acute kidney injury. They have demonstrated that the net increase in serum creatinine depends on the initial creatinine concentration.

Therefore, 24 hours after the creatinine clearance has decreased by 90%, serum creatinine concentration increased by 246% in healthy subject, 174% in patients with GFR between 60 and 90 m//min, 92% in CKD patients with GFR between 30 and 60 mL/min, and only 47% for CKD patients with GFR below 30 mL/min [87]. In acute renal failure, serum creatinine must be interpreted with circumspection and this is reinforced by the fact that patients with acute renal failure, notably in intensive care units, have also frequently a decreased muscular mass.

4. Changes in Serum Creatinine Independent on GFR Variations: Analytical and Therapy-Related Interferences

4.1. Analytical Interference with Bilirubin

Icterus associated with high bilirubin concentrations is a frequent cause of analytical interferences in creatinine measurement. Such interferences have been described with automated methods either with Jaffe or enzymatic methods. These interferences are multiple and complex [13; 23]. In 1976, Watkins has first described the negative interference (i.e. results lower than expected) observed with an automatic measurement of serum creatinine [88]. Nevertheless, this type of interference seems very dependent on the creatinine assay used.

The interference is not linked to reagents, to pH reaction or to the picrate concentration but rather to the alkaline milieu used, the reaction time and the reaction temperature [89]. However, differences observed between automates and methods are not clearly understood. If an interference occurs, it will be dependent on bilirubin concentration but not on serum creatinine concentration [89]. Bilirubin can also induce negative interferences with enzymatic methods and especially in enzymatic methods based on creatinine amidohydrolase [69; 90]. We also note the absence of interferences observed in enzymatic methods based on creatinine iminohydrolase.

The best study on bilirubin interferences is actually very recent [70]. The authors have studied the adjunction of bilirubin to pediatric samples in 15 different assays (4 enzymatic and 11 Jaffe). No significant interference was observed in the four enzymatic methods although a relevant interference was evidenced only in 3 Jaffe methods. These "optimistic" results probably illustrate the improvements in creatinine measurements regarding the interference with bilirubin [70].

4.2. Analytical Interferences Between Jaffe Methods and Cephalosporins

Cephalosporins are classically presented as a source of interferences for the measurement of creatinine by the Jaffe methods. Some cephalosporins (cephalotin and cefoxitin) can be considered as strong pseudochromogens. However, the "new" cephalosporins, still used in clinical practice in 2012, seem free from such interferences. The interferences with cephalosporins can be thus considered historical [91].

4.3. Interferences «at High Concentrations»

Interferences are sometimes observed for enzymatic methods with some therapies but only at very high concentrations (higher than usual therapeutic concentrations). In other words, these negative interferences are only relevant when samples are taken by error on the therapy perfusion line. Such interferences have been described with lidocaïn, metamizol, ascorbate, dopamin, dobutamin and acetylcysteine [92-95].

4.4. Interferences with 5-Flucytosine

The molecular structure of the antifungal therapy 5-flucytosine is similar to creatinine. 5-flucytosine induced a very strong interference with the creatinine enzymatic measurement based on the creatinine iminohydrolase. Interference was so strong that creatinine measurement has been recommended to monitor 5-flucytosine plasma concentrations [96].

4.5. Cimetidine, Trimethoprim, Fibrates and Vitamin D

Since 1976, cimetidine has been known to significantly increase the plasma creatinine concentrations. This increase in plasma creatinine is due to a selective blockade of the creatinine tubular secretion by cimetidine [97]. This tubular blockade is strong but time-limited regarding the half-life of cimetidine (1.8 hours). The cimetidine effect is linked to its charge and molecular structure. This is not a "class effect" and ranitidine does not modify serum creatinine [98].

Trimethoprim can increase the serum creatinine concentration. Once again, this increase in creatinine concentration is independent of any GFR change but is explained by the blockade of tubular secretion of creatinine [99-101]. At usual doses, the increase of creatinine ranges from 10 to 20% in healthy subjects but can reach 30% in CKD patients. Trimethoprim effect is rapid (within 2 to 6 hours after intake) and can last from 8.8 to 17.3 hours according to the half-life of the molecule (this duration is doubled or tripled in case of CKD). Trimethoprim in monotherapy is not nephrotoxic [99-102]. However, trimethoprim combined with sulfamethoxazole (also known as co-trimoxazole) can be nephrotoxic when used at inappropriate dosage in CKD patients [100; 101; 103].

Fibrates are agents currently used in patients with dyslipidemia. In 1993, Devuyst first described an increase in serum creatinine by 10% in renal grafted patient treated by fibrates [104]. The same kinds of observations have been then published by others [105]. However, some researchers have well demonstrated that GFR is not modified under fibrates therapy although serum creatinine increases. The physiological explanation for this increase in serum creatinine is however still discussed. Fibrates could act on the conversion rate of creatine into creatinine [106; 107]. We have to note that nephrotoxicity or glomerular heamodynamic changes induced by fibrates is not totally excluded as some authors have demonstrated that serum creatinine does not always decrease after stopping the therapy [108] and others have also demonstrated that cystatin C (another renal biomarker for GFR estimation) also increases during fibrate therapy [109].

Some authors have recently suggested that vitamin D receptor activation (notably by selective activator like paricalcitol) could increase serum creatinine (and consequently decrease GFR estimated by creatinine clearance) [110-112]. One study suggested an inhibition of tubular secretion of creatinine [112], although the other favored an increase in creatinine production rate [110]. Recently, Agarwal studied the effect of paricalcitol (2 µg for 7 days) in 16 CKD patients (mean GFR measured by iothalamate at 48 mL/min). The authors demonstrated that measured GFR was not modified by therapy although serum creatinine concentrations significantly increased ($p=0.03$) during therapy exposition (this effect is reversible one week after therapy cessation). Creatinine clearance remained stable as well and creatinine excretion significantly increased. The authors thus suggested that vitamin D activation by paricalcitol was due to an increased creatinine production (probably *via* the action of paricalcitol on muscular metabolism), with no effect on "true" GFR [113]. These results must be confirmed because the exact mechanism on serum creatinine metabolism is still unknown. Moreover, the authors also demonstrated an increased BUN concentration during therapy, which is intriguing. The net effect on serum creatinine is actually relatively limited (even if statistically significant) with a slope of creatinine only at 0.01 mg/dL.

5. Creatinine Clearance

5.1. Creatinine Clearance: Strength and Limitations

Creatinine clearance is a relatively easy method to estimate GFR. For this reason, it is still commonly used nowadays. However, we have already underlined the main physiological limitation of this measurement which is the creatinine tubular secretion. Creatinine clearance thus systematically overestimates measured GFR. This overestimation is relatively higher for low GFR levels. The tubular secretion is variable from one subject to another and is absolutely unpredictable [12; 32]. This limitation has been described in numerous studies comparing creatinine clearance with measured GFR [33; 114].

Analytical limitations also exist to limit creatinine clearance use in daily practice. The most important analytical limitation is the high inter- and intra-individual variation of creatinine clearance [12; 14]. Biological variation (intra-individual variation) of creatinine clearance ranges from 5 to 15% [115].

Analytical limitations of creatinine clearance are thus linked to biological variations in creatinine excretion, to physiological variations in tubular secretion and to analytical variations in the measurement of serum and urinary creatinine [116]. Nevertheless, the most important limitation could be linked to the imprecision and errors in urine collections [86;

117]. Errors in urine collection can lead to intra-individual variations reaching 70% [14]. In the context of a clinical trial (where subjects are trained), Toto estimated that 16% of urine collections are erroneous [118]. Regarding pitfalls with 24h urine collections, some authors have found a higher precision with creatinine clearance measured on a shorter timing (two hours) [37]. Additional studies seem however necessary.

Because of these limitations, creatinine clearance is no longer recommended to estimate GFR. The lack of accuracy is especially relevant for follow-up of patients or in longitudinal trials studying GFR slopes. Up to now, creatinine clearance may be useful for patients with abnormal muscular mass (anorexia, paraplegia, amputation) because creatinine-based equations are then particularly inaccurate [119]. However, even in these specific clinical situations, a "true" GFR measurement by a reference method is more accurate.

5.2. Creatinine Clearance with Cimetidine

As mentioned above, cimetidine is able to block creatinine tubular secretion. Blocking this secretion with cimetidine has thus logically been proposed to improve precision and accuracy of creatinine clearance. Of course, it has been first tested that cimetidine has no effect on GFR [33; 34]. In 1986, Shemesh is the first author to propose cimetidine with urine collection to better estimated GFR. In 12 CKD patients, GFR and 4 hours creatinine clearance were simultaneously measured before and after intravenous injection of cimetidine (300 mg). He showed that GFR was not modified by cimetidine but the creatinine clearance on inulin clearance ratio significantly decreased (from 1.67±0.1 to 1.16±0.06). These interesting preliminary results have since been confirmed by other authors [34; 120]. However, strong differences are observed between cimetidine protocols (dosage and timing). The complete blockade of secretion is not proven.

The protocol proposed by van Acker is certainly one of the most interesting: one *per os* dose of 1200 mg and clearance measurement between the 3rd and 6th hour following the intake [14; 34]. However, this protocol remains relatively cumbersome (even if it is one of the simplest protocols published up to now). Errors in urine collection are not ruled out. Therefore, even if the creatinine clearance with cimetidine is well known by the nephrologic community, this GFR estimation method remains poorly used both in clinical practice and in clinical trials.

5.3. Combined Urea and Creatinine Clearance

Urea clearance is known to underestimate GFR. Combined urea and creatinine clearance has thus been proposed to estimate GFR. The GFR overestimation by the creatinine clearance would be compensated by the GFR underestimation of the urea clearance [35; 121]. In 1967, Lubowitz was the first to study and advocate for this combined clearances [121]. Thereafter, other authors have however shown some discrepant results [35; 121-123]. In conclusion, it seems that such a combined clearance has an interest only for estimation of low GFR levels (below 20 mL/min/1.73 m^2) [35]. Moreover, we think that the physiological basis for such a combined clearance is very poor (only a compensation of two successive errors) [14].

Nowadays, it seems that, for the estimation of GFR, combined urea and creatinine clearance has no adding value compared to serum creatinine and to creatinine-based equations [14; 86; 118; 119].

6. Creatinine-Based Equations

Because serum creatinine concentration is influenced by age, gender and ethnicity, some authors have proposed a different approach using only serum creatinine and «correcting» its concentration value according to «normal» reference values proposed in different populations (of age, gender and ethnicity) [124-126]. Other authors proposed equations to directly estimate GFR or creatinine clearance, integrating these parameters. In all these equations, it remains important to underline that serum creatinine is the most powerful variable. Moreover, among the proposed equations, three are most often used in clinical practice (Table 1): the Cockcroft equation, published in 1976 [127], the Modification of Diet in Renal Disease study (MDRD) equation, published in 1999 [128] and the Chronic Kidney Disease Epidemiology Collaboration (CKD-EPI) equation, published by the same leader authors in 2009 [129]. The Cockcroft equation has been built from a relatively limited sample (n=249), compared to the MDRD (n=1628) and the CKD-EPI (n=5504) equations. Also in favor of the MDRD and CKD-EPI equations, is the fact that they have been built and validated in comparison to GFR measured by a reference method (iothalamate), whereas Cockcroft is, *sensu stricto*, an estimation of creatinine clearance, not an estimation of GFR. Most of the external validation studies showed a better performance of the two new equations compared to the Cockcroft one [128; 130; 131]. The Cockcroft equation lacks overall precision and is especially inaccurate in obese and elderly populations [128; 130; 132; 133]. All the variables, both in the MDRD and CKD-EPI equations, are directly available in the laboratories which are thus able to give an automated GFR estimation when serum creatinine is measured [134]. Moreover, the two recent equations have been designed to be used with IDMS traceable creatinine [71; 78; 135-137].

Even if performances of the MDRD study equation were better than those of the Cockcroft one, this equation also has limitations. Indeed, this equation has been developed from patients in the MDRD study cohort who all suffered from CKD. Their mean GFR measured by iothalamate clearance was 40 mL/min/1.73 m^2 [123]. However, there is evidence that the relationship between serum creatinine and GFR is not identical in CKD patients and healthy subjects [81; 138-140]. Therefore, it was not surprising that most of the studies demonstrated a bias in healthy subjects for whom the MDRD study equation tends to systematically underestimate measured GFR [130; 131; 140-144]. The main reason why the new CKD-EPI equation has been developed is thus to improve the performance of the GFR estimation in the higher levels of GFR, i.e. for GFR above 60 mL/min/1.73 m^2 [129].

The CKD-EPI equation has been built from the development data set including 5504 subjects and thus validated in an internal validation data set including 2750 subjects. Moreover, the equation was also validated in an "external" validation data set (n=3896). The samples, both of development and validation data sets, were thus much more important than for the MDRD study equation. Importantly according to the limitations of the MDRD study equation, a substantial proportion of subjects included in these data sets had measured GFR above 60 mL/min/1.73 m². Most of these patients were potential kidney donors. Logically, the mean GFR in this study was at 68±40 mL/min/1.73 m², thus higher than in the MDRD study.

As expected, the performance of the new equation was globally better than for the MDRD study equation. For example, in the external validation data set, the median bias and the 30% accuracy (defined as the percentage of subjects with eGFR between ±30% of measured GFR) for the MDRD and the CKD-EPI equations were -5.5 *versus* -2.5 mL/min/1.73 m², and 81 *versus* 84%, respectively.

As expected also, the performance of the new equation was especially better for GFR above 60 mL/min/1.73 m² [129; 145]. It must however be underlined that the improved performance of the CKD-EPI equation was essentially due to a better bias although precision remained comparable and, maybe, suboptimal, especially in the high GFR values [146]. Performances in some specific subgroups also remained suboptimal, notably in subjects with low body mass index. The problematic of the ethnic coefficients is also important and is not fully resolved by the data from the CKD-EPI group [147]. Briefly, we think the AA ethnic factor remains too high, especially in the low creatinine values [43]. In the same way, we are not fully convinced by the data about the Asian coefficient proposed by the CKD-EPI group [147], even if, according to other authors, we could maybe agree with the assertion that the Asian ethnic coefficient could be close to 1 [147-149]. Some authors have clearly confirmed the first data published by the CKD-EPI group [150-155] although others found no clear adding value [156] [157] [158] [159] [153; 160-162] [163-167].

The most interesting study on the relative performances of the MDRD and CKD-EPIequations is certainly the one published in 2011 by Murata *et al* from the Mayo clinic [167]. It was a powerful study as 5238 patients were included. The authors have analyzed the results both globally and according to health status: Therefore, results were analyzed globally but also according to 5 subgroups: potential kidney donors, donors after the nephrectomy, native CKD, renal transplanted and nonkidney transplanted. The vast majority were Caucasian (only 98 AA).

Analyzing bias and accuracy, the authors confirmed that the CKD-EPI equation underestimated to a lesser degree measured GFR in kidney donors before and after donation. However, the performance of the CKD-EPI equation was not better and even slightly worse compared to the MDRD in the three other types of patients ("the CKD patients") at least for eGFR under 90 mL/min/1.73 m² [167].

In summary, the CKD-EPI equation is an evolution, not a revolution. Indeed, the precision of this equation remains suboptimal mainly in higher GFR and, for example, it is still not recommended to use this GFR estimation to decide if a subject is a good candidate for living kidney donation [168]. Moreover, we must admit that one important publication demonstrated a lower performance (with a significant overestimation) in CKD patients [167]. This overestimation in CKD stages could be the "price to pay" for a better performance in higher GFR level.

In the same way, it must be underlined that the creatinine-based equations are estimations and these estimations may be particularly flawed and source of errors in very specific patients: hyperfiltrating diabetic patients [160; 162; 169], cirrhotic [170;171], renal transplanted [164; 165; 167], elderly [167; 171], anorectic [171]. In these situations, there is no miracle and using the CKD-EPI equation will not give accurate results (and sometimes the estimation will even be worse than with the MDRD study equation). In these specific populations, measuring GFR is still recommended [168].

Table 1. The MDRD and the CKD-EPI equations. SCr=serum creatinine

Cockcroft equation
$$\text{GFR (mL/min)} = \frac{(140 - \text{Age}) \times \text{Weight (kg)}}{7{,}2 \times \text{SCr (mg/dL)}} \times 0{,}85 \text{ if woman}$$
IDMS traceable MDRD study equation
$\text{GFR (mL/min/1.73m}^2) = 175 \times \text{SCr (mg/dL)}^{-1.154} \times \text{Age}^{-0.203} \times 0.742$ (if woman)
X 1.21 if African American
CKD-EPI equation
Women:
if creatinine<0.7 mg/dL:
$\text{GFR (mL/min/1.73m}^2)=144 \times \text{SCr}/0.7^{-0.329} \times 0.993^{\text{age}}$
if creatinine>0.7 mg/dL:
$\text{GFR (mL/min/1.73m}^2)=144 \times \text{SCr}/0.7^{-1.209} \times 0.993^{\text{age}}$
Men:
if creatinine<0.9 mg/dL:
$\text{GFR (mL/min/1.73m}^2)=141 \times \text{SCr}/0.9^{-0.411} \times 0.993^{\text{age}}$
if creatinine>0.9 mg/dL:
$\text{GFR (mL/min/1.73m}^2)=141 \times \text{SCr}/0.9^{-1.209} \times 0.993^{\text{age}}$
166 replaced 144 and 163 replaced 141 if African American

Conclusion

Serum creatinine is still the key biomarker to estimate GFR in clinical practice. In this chapter, we have stressed on the limitations of serum creatinine. Nevertheless, we have also to underline the strengths of this renal biomarker. Serum creatinine measurement is cheap, analytical performances are high (especially for enzymatic methods) and its specificity to detect CKD is relatively good (few false-positive).

Nowadays, the creatinine-based equations, especially MDRD and CKD-EPI are used worldwide to estimate GFR [123; 129; 172; 173]. These equations have replaced creatinine clearance to estimate GFR in daily practice. However, one must keep in mind that serum creatinine is the factor in the MDRD study equation with the greatest mathematical importance. Therefore, precision of the MDRD study equation is very dependent on serum creatinine precision [43; 81; 174]. The precision of Jaffe methods does not permit to give, with an absolute precision, a MDRD study equation results over 60 mL/min. This 60 mL/min limit could certainly be increased to 80 or 90 mL/min/1.73 m² if enzymatic IDMS traceable methods were systematically used [78; 80; 81; 174; 175]. Moreover, at the patient-level, we have to keep in mind the limitations of serum creatinine, especially limitations due to the impact of muscular mass. In other words, it is useless to expect satisfying performances for the creatinine-based equation in specific populations where serum creatinine is known to be misleading. Classical examples are patients with anorexia nervosa, renal transplantation, liver transplantation, cirrhosis etc [176-180]. In these specific patients, measuring creatinine clearance may have adding value but, from our point of view, it is clear that measuring GFR by a reference method should also be considered.

References

[1] Liebig J. Kreatin und Kreatinin, Bestandtheile des Harns der Menschen. *J. Prakt. Chem.* 1847;40:288-92.

[2] Möller E, McIntosh JF, Van Slycke DD. Studies of urea excretion. II. Relationship between urine volume and the rate of urea excretion by normal adults. *J. Clin. Invest.* 1929;6:427-65.

[3] Rehberg PB. Studies on Kidney Function: The Rate of Filtration and Reabsorption in the Human Kidney. *Biochem. J.* 1926;20:447-60.

[4] Smith HW: The kidney: Structure and function in health and disease. New York, Oxford University Press Inc, 1951.

[5] Shannon JA. The renal excretion of creatinine in man. *J. Clin. Invest.* 1935; 14 : 403-10.

[6] Danielson IS. On the presence of creatinine in blood. *J. Biol. Chem.* 1936;113: 181-95.

[7] Gaebler OH. Further studies of blood creatinine. *J. Biol. Chem.* 1930;89:451-66.

[8] Miller BF, Winkler AW. The renal excretion of endogenous creatinine in man. Comparison with exogenous creatinine and inulin. *J. Clin. Invest.* 1938; 17:31-40.

[9] Heymsfield SB, Arteaga C, McManus C, Smith J, Moffitt S. Measurement of muscle mass in humans: validity of the 24-hour urinary creatinine method. *Am. J. Clin. Nutr.* 1983;37:478-94.

[10] Cocchetto DM, Tschanz C, Bjornsson TD. Decreased rate of creatinine production in patients with hepatic disease: implications for estimation of creatinine clearance. *Ther. Drug Monit.* 1983;5:161-8.

[11] Borsook H, Dubnoff JW. The hydrolysis of phosphocreatine and the origin of urinary creatinine. *J. Biol. Chem.* 1947;168:493-510.

[12] Perrone RD, Madias NE, Levey AS. Serum creatinine as an index of renal function: new insights into old concepts. *Clin. Chem.* 1992; 38: 1933-53.

[13] Spencer K. Analytical reviews in clinical biochemistry: the estimation of creatinine. *Ann. Clin. Biochem.* 1986;23 (Pt 1):1-25.

[14] Walser M. Assessing renal function from creatinine measurements in adults with chronic renal failure. *Am. J. Kidney Dis.* 1998; 32: 23-31.

[15] Shaffer P. The excretion of kreatinine and kreatin in health and disease. *Am. J. Physiol.* 1908; 23:1-22.

[16] Horber FF, Scheidegger J, Frey FJ. Overestimation of renal function in glucocorticosteroid treated patients. *Eur. J. Clin. Pharmacol.* 1985;28: 537-41.

[17] Kasiske BL. Creatinine excretion after renal transplantation. *Transplantation* 1989;48: 424-8.

[18] Friedman RB, Anderson RE, Entine SM, Hirshberg SB. Effects of diseases on clinical laboratory tests. *Clin. Chem.* 1980;26:1D-476D.

[19] Mohler JL, Barton SD, Blouin RA, Cowen DL, Flanigan RC. The evaluation of creatinine clearance in spinal cord injury patients. *J. Urol.* 1986;136:366-9.

[20] Delanaye P, Cavalier E, Radermecker RP, Paquot N, Depas G, Chapelle JP, Scheen AJ, Krzesinski JM. Cystatin C or Creatinine for Detection of Stage 3 Chronic Kidney Disease in Anorexia Nervosa. *Nephron. Clin. Pract.* 2008;110:c158-c163.

[21] Davies DF, Shock NW. Age changes in glomerular filtration rate, effective renal plasma flow, and tubular excretory capacity in adult males. *J. Clin. Invest.* 1950;29:496-507.

[22] Schwartz GJ, Haycock GB, Spitzer A. Plasma creatinine and urea concentration in children: normal values for age and sex. *J. Pediatr.* 1976;88:828-30.

[23] Delanghe JR, Louagie HK, De Buyzere ML, Leroux-Roels GG. Glomerular filtration rate and creatinine production in adult icteric patients. *Clin. Chim. Acta* 1994; 224: 33-44.

[24] Crim MC, Calloway DH, Margen S. Creatine metabolism in men: creatine pool size and turnover in relation to creatine intake. *J. Nutr.* 1976; 106:371-81.

[25] Papadakis MA, Arieff AI. Unpredictability of clinical evaluation of renal function in cirrhosis. Prospective study. *Am. J. Med.* 1987;82:945-52.

[26] Hayman JM, Johnston SM, Bender JA. On the presence of creatinine in blood. *J. Biol. Chem.* 1935;108:675-91.

[27] Preiss DJ, Godber IM, Lamb EJ, Dalton RN, Gunn IR. The influence of a cooked-meat meal on estimated glomerular filtration rate. *Ann. Clin. Biochem.* 2007;44:35-42.

[28] Mayersohn M, Conrad KA, Achari R. The influence of a cooked meat meal on creatinine plasma concentration and creatinine clearance. *Br. J. Clin. Pharmacol.* 1983;15:227-30.

[29] Dominguez R, Pomerene E. Recovery of creatinine after ingestion and after intravenous injection in man. *Proc. Soc. Exp. Biol. Med.* 1945; 58:26-9.

[30] Pline KA, Smith CL. The effect of creatine intake on renal function. *Ann. Pharmacother.* 2005;39:1093-6.

[31] Gualano B, Ugrinowitsch C, Novaes RB, Artioli GG, Shimizu MH, Seguro AC, Harris RC, Lancha AH, Jr. Effects of creatine supplementation on renal function: a randomized, double-blind, placebo-controlled clinical trial. *Eur. J. Appl. Physiol.* 2008;103:33-40.

[32] Bauer JH, Brooks CS, Burch RN. Clinical appraisal of creatinine clearance as a measurement of glomerular filtration rate. *Am. J. Kidney Dis.* 1982;2:337-46.

[33] Shemesh O, Golbetz H, Kriss JP, Myers BD. Limitations of creatinine as a filtration marker in glomerulopathic patients. *Kidney Int.* 1985;28: 830-8.

[34] van Acker BA, Koomen GC, Koopman MG, de Waart DR, Arisz L. Creatinine clearance during cimetidine administration for measurement of glomerular filtration rate. *Lancet* 1992;340:1326-9.

[35] Bauer JH, Brooks CS, Burch RN. Renal function studies in man with advanced renal insufficiency. *Am. J. Kidney Dis.* 1982;2:30-5.

[36] DeSanto NG, Coppola S, Anastasio P, Coscarella G, Capasso G, Bellini L, Santangelo R, Massimo L, Siciliano A. Predicted creatinine clearance to assess glomerular filtration rate in chronic renal disease in humans. *Am. J. Nephrol.* 1991;11:181-5.

[37] Sinkeler SJ, Visser FW, Krikken JA, Stegeman CA, Homan van der Heide JJ, Navis G. Higher body mass index is associated with higher fractional creatinine excretion in healthy subjects. *Nephrol. Dial. Transplant.* 2011;26:3181-8.

[38] Urakami Y, Kimura N, Okuda M, Inui K. Creatinine transport by basolateral organic cation transporter hOCT2 in the human kidney. *Pharm. Res.* 2004;21:976-81.

[39] Berlyne GM, Varley H, Nilwarangkur S, Hoerni M. Endogenous-creatinine clearance and glomerular-filtration rate. *Lancet* 1964; 22: 874-6.

[40] Hilton PJ, Roth Z, Lavender S, Jones NF. Creatinine clearance in patients with proteinuria. *Lancet* 1969;2:1215-6.

[41] Hsu CY, Chertow GM, Curhan GC. Methodological issues in studying the epidemiology of mild to moderate chronic renal insufficiency. *Kidney Int.* 2002;61:1567-76.

[42] Coresh J, Toto RD, Kirk KA, Whelton PK, Massry S, Jones C, Agodoa L, Van Lente F. Creatinine clearance as a measure of GFR in screenees for the African-American Study of Kidney Disease and Hypertension pilot study. *Am. J. Kidney Dis.* 1998;32:32-42.

[43] Delanaye P, Mariat C, Maillard N, Krzesinski JM, Cavalier E. Are the creatinine-based equations accurate to estimate glomerular filtration rate in african american populations? *Clin. J. Am. Soc. Nephrol.* 2011; 6: 906-12.

[44] Goldwasser P, Aboul-Magd A, Maru M. Race and creatinine excretion in chronic renal insufficiency. *Am. J. Kidney Dis.* 1997;30:16-22.

[45] Jacobs DR, Jr., Murtaugh MA, Steffes M, Yu X, Roseman J, Goetz FC. Gender- and race-specific determination of albumin excretion rate using albumin-to-creatinine ratio in single, untimed urine specimens: the Coronary Artery Risk Development in Young Adults Study. *Am. J. Epidemiol.* 2002;155:1114-9.

[46] van Acker BA, Koomen GC, Koopman MG, Krediet RT, Arisz L. Discrepancy between circadian rhythms of inulin and creatinine clearance. *J. Lab. Clin. Med.* 1992; 120: 400-10.

[47] MCCance RA, Widdowson EM. Functional disorganization of the kidney in disease. *J. Physiol.* 1939;95:36-44.

[48] Miller BF, Leaf A, Mamby AR, Miller Z. Validity of the endogenous creatinine clearance as a measure of glomerular filtration rate in the diseased human kidney. *J. Clin. Invest.* 1952;31:309-13.

[49] Levinsky NG, Berliner RW. Changes in composition of the urine in ureter and bladder at low urine flow. *Am. J. Physiol.* 1959;196:549-53.

[50] Crim MC, Calloway DH, Margen S. Creatine metabolism in men: urinary creatine and creatinine excretions with creatine feeding. *J. Nutr.* 1975;105:428-38.

[51] Mitch WE, Walser M. A proposed mechanism for reduced creatinine excretion in severe chronic renal failure. *Nephron.* 1978;21:248-54.

[52] Mitch WE, Collier VU, Walser M. Creatinine metabolism in chronic renal failure. *Clin. Sci. (Lond)* 1980;58:327-35.

[53] Jones JD, Burnett PC. Implication of creatinine and gut flora in the uremic syndrome: induction of "creatininase" in colon contents of the rat by dietary creatinine. Clin. Chem. 1972;18:280-4.

[54] Thienpont LM, Van Landuyt KG, Stockl D, De Leenheer AP. Candidate reference method for determining serum creatinine by isocratic HPLC: validation with isotope dilution gas chromatography-mass spectrometry and application for accuracy assessment of routine test kits. *Clin. Chem.* 1995; 41:995-1003.

[55] Jaffe M. Ueber den Neiderschlag, welchen Pikrinsäre in normalen Harn erzeugt und über eine neue Reaktion des Kreatinins. *Z. Physiol. Chem.* 1886; 10:391-400.

[56] Folin O. Approximately complete analyses of thirty "normal" urines. *Am. J. Physiol.* 1905;13:45-65.

[57] Abderhalden E, Komm E. Uber die Anhydridstrukter der Proteine. *Z. Physiol. Chem.* 1924;139:181.

[58] Hunter A, Campbell WR. The probable accuracy, in whole blood and plasma, of colorimetric determinations of creatinine and creatine. *J. Biol. Chem.* 1917;32:195-231.

[59] Miller BF, Dubos R. Studies on the presence of creatinine in human blood. *J. Biol. Chem.* 1937;121:447-56.

[60] Cook JG. Factors influencing the assay of creatinine. *Ann. Clin. Biochem.* 1975; 12: 219-32.

[61] Fabiny DL, Ertingshausen G. Automated reaction-rate method for determination of serum creatinine with the CentrifiChem. *Clin. Chem.* 1971; 17:696-700.

[62] Lustgarten JA, Wenk RE. Simple, rapid, kinetic method for serum creatinine measurement. *Clin. Chem.* 1972;18:1419-22.

[63] Bowers LD, Wong ET. Kinetic serum creatinine assays. II. A critical evaluation and review. *Clin. Chem.* 1980;26:555-61.

[64] Gerard SK, Khayam-Bashi H. Characterization of creatinine error in ketotic patients. A prospective comparison of alkaline picrate methods with an enzymatic method. *Am. J. Clin. Pathol.* 1985;84:659-64.

[65] Mazzachi BC, Peake MJ, Ehrhardt V. Reference range and method comparison studies for enzymatic and Jaffe creatinine assays in plasma and serum and early morning urine. *Clin. Lab.* 2000;46:53-5.

[66] Parry DM. Use of single-value protein compensation of the Jaffe creatinine assay contributes to clinically significant inaccuracy in results. *Clin. Chem.* 2008;54:215-6.

[67] Ceriotti F, Boyd JC, Klein G, Henny J, Queralto J, Kairisto V, Panteghini M. Reference intervals for serum creatinine concentrations: assessment of available data for global application. *Clin. Chem.* 2008; 54:559-66.

[68] Suzuki M. Purification and some properties of sarcosine oxidase from Corynebacterium sp. U-96. *J. Biochem.* 1981;89:599-607.

[69] Fossati P, Prencipe L, Berti G. Enzymic creatinine assay: a new colorimetric method based on hydrogen peroxide measurement. *Clin. Chem.* 1983;29:1494-6.

[70] Cobbaert CM, Baadenhuijsen H, Weykamp CW. Prime time for enzymatic creatinine methods in pediatrics. *Clin. Chem.* 2009; 55: 549-58.

[71] Pieroni L, Delanaye P, Boutten A, Bargnoux AS, Rozet E, Delatour V, Carlier MC, Hanser AM, Cavalier E, Froissart M, Cristol JP. A multicentric evaluation of IDMS-traceable creatinine enzymatic assays. *Clin. Chim. Acta* 2011;412:2070-5.

[72] Van Lente F, Suit P. Assessment of renal function by serum creatinine and creatinine clearance: glomerular filtration rate estimated by four procedures. *Clin. Chem.* 1989;35:2326-30.

[73] Fossati P, Ponti M, Passoni G, Tarenghi G, Melzi d'Eril GV, Prencipe L,. A step forward in enzymatic measurement of creatinine. *Clin. Chem.* 1994;40:130-7.

[74] Junge W, Wilke B, Halabi A, Klein G. Determination of reference intervals for serum creatinine, creatinine excretion and creatinine clearance with an enzymatic and a modified Jaffe method. *Clin. Chim. Acta* 2004;344:137-48.

[75] Myers GL, Miller WG, Coresh J, Fleming J, Greenberg N, Greene T, Hostetter T, Levey AS, Panteghini M, Welch M, Eckfeldt JH. Recommendations for improving serum creatinine measurement: a report from the laboratory working group of the national kidney disease education program. *Clin. Chem.* 2006;52:5-18.

[76] Seronie-Vivien S, Galteau MM, Carlier MC, Hadj-Aissa A, Hanser AM, Hym B, Marchal A, Michotey O, Pouteil-Noble C, Sternberg M, Perret-Liaudet A. Impact of

standardized calibration on the inter-assay variation of 14 automated assays for the measurement of creatinine in human serum. *Clin. Chem. Lab. Med.* 2005;43:1227-33.

[77] Delanaye P, Cavalier E, Chapelle JP, Krzesinski JM. Importance of the creatinine calibration in the estimation of GFR by MDRD equation. *Nephrol. Dial. Transplant* 2006;21:1130.

[78] Murthy K, Stevens LA, Stark PC, Levey AS. Variation in the serum creatinine assay calibration: a practical application to glomerular filtration rate estimation. *Kidney Int.* 2005;68:1884-7.

[79] Bjorkhem I, Blomstrand R, Ohman G. Mass fragmentography of creatinine proposed as a reference method. *Clin. Chem.* 1977; 23: 2114-21.

[80] Seronie-Vivien S, Pieroni L, Galteau MM, Carlier MC, Hanser AM, Cristol JP. Evolution des modalités d'évaluation de la fonction rénale basée sur la créatinine entre 2005 et 2008: conséquences pour les biologistes. *Ann. Biol. Clin. (Paris)* 2008; 66: 263-8.

[81] Delanaye P, Cohen EP. Formula-based estimates of the GFR: equations variable and uncertain. *Nephron. Clin. Pract.* 2008;110:c48-c53.

[82] Liu Y, Xu GB. Trueness investigation of routine creatinine assays on nine homogeneous systems in Beijing demonstrates an encouraging outcome that meets clinical requirements. *Chin. Med. J. (Engl.)* 2010; 123: 2364-9.

[83] Wang X, Xu G, Li H, Liu Y, Wang F. Reference intervals for serum creatinine with enzymatic assay and evaluation of four equations to estimate glomerular filtration rate in a healthy Chinese adult population. *Clin. Chim. Acta* 2011;412:1793-7.

[84] Couchoud C, Pozet N, Labeeuw M, Pouteil-Noble C. Screening early renal failure: cut-off values for serum creatinine as an indicator of renal impairment. *Kidney Int.* 1999;55:1878-84.

[85] Brochner-Mortensen J, Jensen S, Rodbro P. Assessment of renal function from plasma creatinine in adult patients. *Scand. J. Urol. Nephrol.* 1977;11:263-70.

[86] Morgan DB, Dillon S, Payne RB. The assessment of glomerular function: creatinine clearance or plasma creatinine? *Postgrad. Med. J.* 1978; 54:302-10.

[87] Waikar SS, Bonventre JV. Creatinine kinetics and the definition of acute kidney injury. *J. Am. Soc. Nephrol.* 2009;20:672-9.

[88] Watkins RE, Feldkamp CS, Thibert RJ, Zak B. Interesting interferences in a direct serum creatinine reaction. *Microchem. J.* 1976;21:370-84.

[89] Knapp ML, Hadid O. Investigations into negative interference by jaundiced plasma in kinetic Jaffe methods for plasma creatinine determination. *Ann. Clin. Biochem.* 1987;24 (Pt 1):85-97.

[90] Lindback B, Bergman A. A new commercial method for the enzymatic determination of creatinine in serum and urine evaluated: comparison with a kinetic Jaffe method and isotope dilution-mass spectrometry. *Clin. Chem.* 1989;35:835-7.

[91] Kroll MH, Elin RJ. Mechanism of cefoxitin and cephalothin interference with the Jaffe method for creatinine. *Clin. Chem.* 1983;29:2044-8.

[92] Daly TM, Kempe KC, Scott MG. "Bouncing" creatinine levels. *N. Engl. J. Med.* 1996;334:1749-50.

[93] Lognard M, Cavalier E, Chapelle JP, Lambermont B, Krzesinski JM, Delanaye P. Acetylcysteine and enzymatic creatinine: beware of laboratory artefact! *Intensive Care Med.* 2008;34:973-4.

[94] Bagnoud MA, Reymond JP. Interference of metamizol (dipyrone) on the determination of creatinine with the Kodak dry chemistry slide comparison with the enzymatic method from Boehringer. *Eur. J. Clin. Chem. Clin. Biochem.* 1993;31:753-7.

[95] Saenger AK, Lockwood C, Snozek CL, Milz TC, Karon BS, Scott MG, Jaffe AS. Catecholamine interference in enzymatic creatinine assays. *Clin. Chem.* 2009; 55: 1732-6.

[96] Toffaletti J, Blosser N, Hall T, Smith S, Tompkins D. An automated dry-slide enzymatic method evaluated for measurement of creatinine in serum. *Clin. Chem.* 1983; 29:684-7.

[97] Larsson R, Bodemar G, Kagedal B. The effect of cimetidine, a new histamine H2-receptor antagonist, on renal function. *Acta Med. Scand.* 1979;205:87-9.

[98] van den Berg JG, Koopman MG, Arisz L. Ranitidine has no influence on tubular creatinine secretion. *Nephron*. 1996;74:705-8.

[99] Berglund F, Killander J, Pompeius R. Effect of trimethoprim-sulfamethoxazole on the renal excretion of creatinine in man. *J. Urol.* 1975; 114:802-8.

[100] Trollfors B, Wahl M, Alestig K. Co-trimoxazole, creatinine and renal function. *J. Infect.* 1980;2:221-6.

[101] Delanaye P, Mariat C, Cavalier E, Maillard N, Krzesinski JM, White CA. Trimethoprim, Creatinine and Creatinine-Based Equations. *Nephron. Clin. Pract.* 2011;119:c187-c194.

[102] Berglund F. Urinary excretion patterns for substances with simultaneous secretion and reabsorption by active transport. *Acta Physiol. Scand.* 1961; 52:276-90.

[103] Rudra T, Webb DB, Evans AG. Acute tubular necrosis following co-trimoxazole therapy. *Nephron* 1989;53:85-6.

[104] Devuyst O, Goffin E, Pirson Y, van Ypersele dS. Creatinine rise after fibrate therapy in renal graft recipients. *Lancet* 1993;341:840.

[105] Broeders N, Knoop C, Antoine M, Tielemans C, Abramowicz D. Fibrate-induced increase in blood urea and creatinine: is gemfibrozil the only innocuous agent? *Nephrol. Dial. Transplant.* 2000;15:1993-9.

[106] Hottelart C, el Esper N, Rose F, Achard JM, Fournier A. Fenofibrate increases creatininemia by increasing metabolic production of creatinine. *Nephron* 2002; 92: 536-41.

[107] Ansquer JC, Dalton RN, Causse E, Crimet D, Le Malicot K, Foucher C. Effect of fenofibrate on kidney function: a 6-week randomized crossover trial in healthy people. *Am. J. Kidney Dis.* 2008;51:904-13.

[108] Polanco N, Hernandez E, Gonzalez E, Gutierrez ME, Bello I, Gutierrez-Millet V, Garcia F, Morales E, Praga M. [Fibrate-induced deterioration of renal function]. *Nefrologia* 2009;29:208-13.

[109] Forsblom C, Hiukka A, Leinonen ES, Sundvall J, Groop PH, Taskinen MR. Effects of long-term fenofibrate treatment on markers of renal function in type 2 diabetes: the FIELD Helsinki substudy. *Diabetes Care* 2010; 33:215-20.

[110] Bertoli M, Luisetto G, Ruffatti A, Urso M, Romagnoli G. Renal function during calcitriol therapy in chronic renal failure. *Clin. Nephrol.* 1990; 33:98-102.

[111] de Zeeuw D., Agarwal R, Amdahl M, Audhya P, Coyne D, Garimella T, Parving HH, Pritchett Y, Remuzzi G, Ritz E, Andress D. Selective vitamin D receptor activation

with paricalcitol for reduction of albuminuria in patients with type 2 diabetes (VITAL study): a randomised controlled trial. *Lancet* 2010;376:1543-51.

[112] Perez A, Raab R, Chen TC, Turner A, Holick MF. Safety and efficacy of oral calcitriol (1,25-dihydroxyvitamin D3) for the treatment of psoriasis. *Br. J. Dermatol.* 1996;134:1070-8.

[113] Agarwal R, Hynson JE, Hecht TJ, Light RP, Sinha AD. Short-term vitamin D receptor activation increases serum creatinine due to increased production with no effect on the glomerular filtration rate. *Kidney Int.* 2011;80:1073-9.

[114] Bauer C, Melamed ML, Hostetter TH. Staging of chronic kidney disease: time for a course correction. *J. Am. Soc. Nephrol.* 2008; 19: 844-6.

[115] Greenblatt DJ, Ransil BJ, Harmatz JS, Smith TW, Duhme DW, Koch-Weser J. Variability of 24-hour urinary creatinine excretion by normal subjects. *J. Clin. Pharmacol.* 1976;16:321-8.

[116] Ransil BJ, Greenblatt DJ, Koch-Weser J. Evidence for systematic temporal variation in 24-hour urinary creatinine excretion. *J. Clin. Pharmacol.* 1977;17:108-19.

[117] Brochner-Mortensen J, Rodbro P. Selection of routine method for determination of glomerular filtration rate in adult patients. *Scand. J. Clin. Lab. Invest.* 1976;36:35-43.

[118] Toto RD, Kirk KA, Coresh J, Jones C, Appel L, Wright J, Campese V, Olutade B, Agodoa L. Evaluation of serum creatinine for estimating glomerular filtration rate in African Americans with hypertensive nephrosclerosis: results from the African-American Study of Kidney Disease and Hypertension (AASK) Pilot Study. *J. Am. Soc. Nephrol.* 1997; 8:279-87.

[119] National Kidney Foundation. K/DOQI clinical practice guidelines for chronic kidney disease: evaluation, classification, and stratification. *Am. J. Kidney Dis.* 2002; 39: S1-266.

[120] Hilbrands LB, Artz MA, Wetzels JF, Koene RA. Cimetidine improves the reliability of creatinine as a marker of glomerular filtration. *Kidney Int.* 1991;40:1171-6.

[121] Lubowitz H, Slatopolsky E, Shankel S, Rieselbach RE, Bricker NS. Glomerular filtration rate. Determination in patients with chronic renal disease. *JAMA* 1967; 199:252-6.

[122] Lavender S, Hilton PJ, Jones NF. The measurement of glomerular filtration-rate in renal disease. *Lancet* 1969;2:1216-8.

[123] Levey AS, Bosch JP, Lewis JB, Greene T, Rogers N, Roth D. A more accurate method to estimate glomerular filtration rate from serum creatinine: a new prediction equation. Modification of Diet in Renal Disease Study Group. *Ann. Intern. Med.* 1999; 130: 461-70.

[124] Pottel H, Vrydags N, Mahieu B, Vandewynckele E, Croes K, Martens F. Establishing age/sex related serum creatinine reference intervals from hospital laboratory data based on different statistical methods. *Clin. Chim. Acta* 2008;396:49-55.

[125] Pottel H, Martens F. Are eGFR equations better than IDMS-traceable serum creatinine in classifying chronic kidney disease? *Scand. J. Clin. Lab. Invest.* 2009;69:550-61.

[126] Pottel H, Hoste L, Delanaye P, Cavalier E, Martens F. Demystifying ethnic/sex differences in kidney function: Is the difference in (estimating) glomerular filtration rate or in serum creatinine concentration? *Clin. Chim. Acta* 2012.

[127] Cockcroft DW, Gault MH. Prediction of creatinine clearance from serum creatinine. *Nephron* 1976;16:31-41.

[128] Levey AS, Coresh J, Greene T, Stevens LA, Zhang YL, Hendriksen S, Kusek JW, Van Lente F. Using standardized serum creatinine values in the modification of diet in renal disease study equation for estimating glomerular filtration rate. *Ann. Intern. Med.* 2006;145:247-54.

[129] Levey AS, Stevens LA, Schmid CH, Zhang YL, Castro AF, III, Feldman HI, Kusek JW, Eggers P, Van Lente F, Greene T, Coresh J. A new equation to estimate glomerular filtration rate. *Ann. Intern. Med.* 2009; 150:604-12.

[130] Froissart M, Rossert J, Jacquot C, Paillard M, Houillier P. Predictive performance of the modification of diet in renal disease and Cockcroft-Gault equations for estimating renal function. *J. Am. Soc. Nephrol.* 2005; 16:763-73.

[131] Poggio ED, Wang X, Greene T, Van Lente F, Hall PM. Performance of the modification of diet in renal disease and Cockcroft-Gault equations in the estimation of GFR in health and in chronic kidney disease. *J. Am. Soc. Nephrol.* 2005;16:459-66.

[132] Rigalleau V, Lasseur C, Perlemoine C, Barthe N, Raffaitin C, Chauveau P, Combe C, Gin H. Cockcroft-Gault formula is biased by body weight in diabetic patients with renal impairment. *Metabolism* 2006;55:108-12.

[133] Stevens LA, Levey AS. Chronic kidney disease in the elderly--how to assess risk. *N. Engl. J. Med.* 2005;352:2122-4.

[134] Levey AS, Stevens LA, Hostetter T. Automatic reporting of estimated glomerular filtration rate--just what the doctor ordered. *Clin. Chem.* 2006; 52:2188-93.

[135] Coresh J, Astor BC, McQuillan G, Kusek J, Greene T, Van Lente F, Levey AS. Calibration and random variation of the serum creatinine assay as critical elements of using equations to estimate glomerular filtration rate. *Am. J. Kidney Dis.* 2002; 39: 920-9.

[136] Myers GL. Standardization of serum creatinine measurement: theory and practice. *Scand. J. Clin. Lab. Invest. Suppl.* 2008;241:57-63.

[137] Stevens LA, Manzi J, Levey AS, Chen J, Deysher AE, Greene T, Poggio ED, Schmid CH, Steffes MW, Zhang YL, Van Lente F, Coresh J. Impact of creatinine calibration on performance of GFR estimating equations in a pooled individual patient database. *Am. J. Kidney Dis.* 2007;50:21-35.

[138] Rule AD, Larson TS, Bergstralh EJ, Slezak JM, Jacobsen SJ, Cosio FG. Using serum creatinine to estimate glomerular filtration rate: accuracy in good health and in chronic kidney disease. *Ann. Intern. Med.* 2004; 141:929-37.

[139] Rule AD, Bergstralh EJ, Slezak JM, Bergert J, Larson TS. Glomerular filtration rate estimated by cystatin C among different clinical presentations. *Kidney Int.* 2006;69:399-405.

[140] Botev R, Mallie JP, Wetzels JF, Couchoud C, Schuck O. The Clinician and Estimation of Glomerular Filtration Rate by Creatinine-based Formulas: Current Limitations and Quo Vadis. *Clin. J. Am. Soc. Nephrol.* 2011;6:937-50.

[141] Ibrahim H, Mondress M, Tello A, Fan Y, Koopmeiners J, Thomas W. An alternative formula to the Cockcroft-Gault and the modification of diet in renal diseases formulas in predicting GFR in individuals with type 1 diabetes. *J. Am. Soc. Nephrol.* 2005;16:1051-60.

[142] Ibrahim HN, Rogers T, Tello A, Matas A. The performance of three serum creatinine-based formulas in estimating GFR in former kidney donors. *Am. J. Transplant.* 2006;6:1479-85.

[143] Issa N, Meyer KH, Arrigain S, Choure G, Fatica RA, Nurko S, Stephany BR, Poggio ED. Evaluation of creatinine-based estimates of glomerular filtration rate in a large cohort of living kidney donors. *Transplantation* 2008;86:223-30.

[144] Rule AD, Gussak HM, Pond GR, Bergstralh EJ, Stegall MD, Cosio FG, Larson TS. Measured and estimated GFR in healthy potential kidney donors. *Am. J. Kidney Dis.* 2004;43:112-9.

[145] Stevens LA, Schmid CH, Greene T, Zhang YL, Beck GJ, Froissart M, Hamm LL, Lewis JB, Mauer M, Navis GJ, Steffes MW, Eggers PW, Coresh J, Levey AS. Comparative performance of the CKD Epidemiology Collaboration (CKD-EPI) and the Modification of Diet in Renal Disease (MDRD) Study equations for estimating GFR levels above 60 mL/min/1.73 m2. *Am. J. Kidney Dis.* 2010;56:486-95.

[146] Delanaye P, Cavalier E, Mariat C, Maillard N, Krzesinski JM. MDRD or CKD-EPI study equations for estimating prevalence of stage 3 CKD in epidemiological studies: which difference? Is this difference relevant? *BMC Nephrol.* 2010;11:8.

[147] Stevens LA, Claybon MA, Schmid CH, Chen J, Horio M, Imai E, Nelson RG, Van DM, Wang HY, Zuo L, Zhang YL, Levey AS. Evaluation of the Chronic Kidney Disease Epidemiology Collaboration equation for estimating the glomerular filtration rate in multiple ethnicities. *Kidney Int.* 2011;79:555-62.

[148] Delanaye P, Cavalier E, Mariat C, Krzesinski JM, Rule AD. Estimating glomerular filtration rate in Asian subjects: where do we stand? *Kidney Int.* 2011;80:439-40.

[149] Teo BW, Xu H, Wang D, Li J, Sinha AK, Shuter B, Sethi S, Lee EJ. GFR estimating equations in a multiethnic Asian population. *Am. J. Kidney Dis.* 2011;58:56-63.

[150] Cirillo M, Lombardi C, Luciano MG, Bilancio G, Anastasio P, De Santo NG. Estimation of GFR: a comparison of new and established equations. *Am. J. Kidney Dis.* 2010;56:802-4.

[151] Soares AA, Eyff TF, Campani RB, Ritter L, Weinert LS, Camargo JL, Silveiro SP. Performance of the CKD Epidemiology Collaboration (CKD-EPI) and the Modification of Diet in Renal Disease (MDRD) Study equations in healthy South Brazilians. *Am. J. Kidney Dis.* 2010; 55: 1162-3.

[152] Orskov B, Borresen ML, Feldt-Rasmussen B, Ostergaard O, Laursen I, Strandgaard S. Estimating glomerular filtration rate using the new CKD-EPI equation and other equations in patients with autosomal dominant polycystic kidney disease. *Am. J. Nephrol.* 2010;31:53-7.

[153] Iliadis F, Didangelos T, Ntemka A, Makedou A, Moralidis E, Gotzamani-Psarakou A, Kouloukourgiotou T, Grekas D. Glomerular filtration rate estimation in patients with type 2 diabetes: creatinine- or cystatin C-based equations? *Diabetologia* 2011; 54: 2987-94.

[154] Lane BR, Demirjian S, Weight CJ, Larson BT, Poggio ED, Campbell SC. Performance of the chronic kidney disease-epidemiology study equations for estimating glomerular filtration rate before and after nephrectomy. *J. Urol.* 2010;183:896-901.

[155] White CA, Akbari A, Doucette S, Fergusson D, Knoll GA. Estimating glomerular filtration rate in kidney transplantation: is the new chronic kidney disease epidemiology collaboration equation any better? *Clin. Chem.* 2010;56:474-7.

[156] Eriksen BO, Mathisen UD, Melsom T, Ingebretsen OC, Jenssen TG, Njolstad I, Solbu MD, Toft I. Cystatin C is not a better estimator of GFR than plasma creatinine in the general population. *Kidney Int.* 2010; 78:1305-11.

[157] Nyman U, Grubb A, Sterner G, Bjork J. The CKD-EPI and MDRD equations to estimate GFR. Validation in the Swedish Lund-Malmo Study cohort. *Scand. J. Clin. Lab. Invest.* 2011;71:129-38.

[158] Michels WM, Grootendorst DC, Verduijn M, Elliott EG, Dekker FW, Krediet RT. Performance of the Cockcroft-Gault, MDRD, and new CKD-EPI formulas in relation to GFR, age, and body size. *Clin. J. Am. Soc. Nephrol.* 2010;5:1003-9.

[159] Tent H, Rook M, Stevens LA, van Son WJ, van Pelt LJ, Hofker HS, Ploeg RJ, van der Heide JJ, Navis G. Renal function equations before and after living kidney donation: a within-individual comparison of performance at different levels of renal function. *Clin. J. Am. Soc. Nephrol.* 2010;5:1960-8.

[160] Nair S, Hardy KJ, Wilding JP. The Chronic Kidney Disease Epidemiology Collaboration (CKD-EPI) formula performs worse than the Modification of Diet in Renal Disease (MDRD) equation in estimating glomerular filtration rate in Type 2 diabetic chronic kidney disease. *Diabet. Med.* 2011;28:1279.

[161] Rognant N, Lemoine S, Laville M, Hadj-Aissa A, Dubourg L. Performance of the chronic kidney disease epidemiology collaboration equation to estimate glomerular filtration rate in diabetic patients. *Diabetes Care* 2011;34:1320-2.

[162] Silveiro SP, Araujo GN, Ferreira MN, Souza FD, Yamaguchi HM, Camargo EG. Chronic Kidney Disease Epidemiology Collaboration (CKD-EPI) equation pronouncedly underestimates glomerular filtration rate in type 2 diabetes. *Diabetes Care* 2011;34:2353-5.

[163] Bargnoux AS, Servel AC, Pieroni L, Dupuy AM, Badiou S, Garrigue V, Mourad G, Cristol JP. Accuracy of GFR predictive equations in renal transplantation: Validation of a new turbidimetric cystatin C assay on Architect c8000(R). *Clin. Biochem.* 2012;45:151-3.

[164] Kukla A, El-Shahawi Y, Leister E, Kasiske B, Mauer M, Matas A, Ibrahim HN. GFR-estimating models in kidney transplant recipients on a steroid-free regimen. *Nephrol. Dial. Transplant.* 2010;25:1653-61.

[165] Poge U, Gerhardt T, Stoffel-Wagner B, Sauerbruch T, Woitas RP. Validation of the CKD-EPI formula in patients after renal transplantation. *Nephrol. Dial. Transplant.* 2011;26:4104-8.

[166] Buron F, Hadj-Aissa A, Dubourg L, Morelon E, Steghens JP, Ducher M, Fauvel JP. Estimating glomerular filtration rate in kidney transplant recipients: performance over time of four creatinine-based formulas. *Transplantation* 2011;92:1005-11.

[167] Murata K, Baumann NA, Saenger AK, Larson TS, Rule AD, Lieske JC. Relative Performance of the MDRD and CKD-EPI Equations for Estimating Glomerular Filtration Rate among Patients with Varied Clinical Presentations. *Clin. J. Am. Soc. Nephrol.* 2011;6:1963-72.

[168] Stevens LA, Levey AS. Measured GFR as a confirmatory test for estimated GFR. *J. Am. Soc. Nephrol.* 2009;20:2305-13.

[169] Camargo EG, Soares AA, Detanico AB, Weinert LS, Veronese FV, Gomes EC, Silveiro SP. The Chronic Kidney Disease Epidemiology Collaboration (CKD-EPI) equation is less accurate in patients with Type 2 diabetes when compared with healthy individuals. *Diabet Med.* 2011; 28:90-5.

[170] Xirouchakis E, Marelli L, Cholongitas E, Manousou P, Calvaruso V, Pleguezuelo M, Guerrini GP, Maimone S, Kerry A, Hajjawi M, Nair D, Thomas M, Patch D, Burroughs

AK. Comparison of cystatin C and creatinine-based glomerular filtration rate formulas with 51Cr-EDTA clearance in patients with cirrhosis. *Clin. J. Am. Soc. Nephrol.* 2011;6: 84-92.
[171] Segarra A, de la Torre J, Ramos N, Quiroz A, Garjau M, Torres I, Azancot MA, Lopez M, Sobrado A. Assessing glomerular filtration rate in hospitalized patients: a comparison between CKD-EPI and four cystatin C-based equations. *Clin. J. Am. Soc. Nephrol.* 2011;6:2411-20.
[172] Levey AS, de Jong PE, Coresh J, El NM, Astor BC, Matsushita K, Gansevoort RT, Kasiske BL, Eckardt KU. The definition, classification, and prognosis of chronic kidney disease: a KDIGO Controversies Conference report. *Kidney Int.* 2011;80:17-28.
[173] Stevens LA, Coresh J, Greene T, Levey AS. Assessing kidney function - Measured and estimated glomerular filtration rate. *N. Engl. J. Med.* 2006; 354:2473-83.
[174] Delanaye P, Cavalier E, Krzesinski JM, Chapelle JP. Why the MDRD equation should not be used in patients with normal renal function (and normal creatinine values)? *Clin. Nephrol.* 2006;66:147-8.
[175] Levey AS, Eckardt KU, Tsukamoto Y, Levin A, Coresh J, Rossert J, de Zeeuw D, Hostetter TH, Lameire N, Eknoyan G. Definition and classification of chronic kidney disease: a position statement from Kidney Disease: Improving Global Outcomes (KDIGO). *Kidney Int.* 2005;67:2089-100.
[176] Delanaye P, Nellessen E, Grosch S, Depas G, Cavalier E, Defraigne JO, Chapelle JP, Krzesinski JM, Lancellotti P. Creatinine-based formulae for the estimation of glomerular filtration rate in heart transplant recipients. *Clin. Transplant.* 2006; 20: 596-603.
[177] Delanaye P, Cavalier E, Radermecker RP, Paquot N, Depas G, Chapelle JP, Scheen AJ, Krzesinski JM. Estimation of GFR by different creatinine- and cystatin-C-based equations in anorexia nervosa. *Clin. Nephrol.* 2009;71:482-91.
[178] Poggio ED, Nef PC, Wang X, Greene T, Van Lente F, Dennis VW, Hall PM. Performance of the Cockcroft-Gault and modification of diet in renal disease equations in estimating GFR in ill hospitalized patients. *Am. J. Kidney Dis.* 2005;46:242-52.
[179] Skluzacek PA, Szewc RG, Nolan CR, III, Riley DJ, Lee S, Pergola PE. Prediction of GFR in liver transplant candidates. *Am. J. Kidney Dis.* 2003;42:1169-76.
[180] White CA, Huang D, Akbari A, Garland J, Knoll GA. Performance of creatinine-based estimates of GFR in kidney transplant recipients: a systematic review. *Am. J. Kidney Dis.* 2008;51:1005-15.

In: Creatinine
Editors: I. H. Perkins and C. M. Chapman

ISBN: 978-1-62257-475-9

Chapter III

Serum Creatinine: It's Source, Interpretation and Effect on the Management of Renal and Hepatic Diseases

Christopher M. Moore*[1]*, Omar Lateef*[2] *and David H. Van Thiel*[1]*
[1]Section of Hepatology
[2]Section of Pulmonary and Critical Care,
Rush University Medical Center, Chicago, Illinois

Abstract

Chronic kidney disease (CKD) comprises a spectrum of pathology with significant medical and financial burden, affecting at least 26 million individuals in the United States. The staging of CKD has implications upon the utilization of medical therapeutics and procedural interventions, including renal replacement therapies such as hemodialysis and transplantation. The ability to measure CKD is based upon many parameters, an important one being the glomerular filtration rate (GFR). The assessment of GFR, despite numerous iterations, still for practical reasons, relies heavily upon the serum creatinine level, a suboptimal marker. Creatinine exists within a complex biology wherein its serum level is affected by intrinsic factors such as age and nutritional status, and extrinsic factors such as medications and other forms of iatrogenic intervention. Furthermore, the nature of the creatinine assays themselves are non-standardized, and their ability to sense true creatinine concentrations are affected at times quite severely by non-creatinine chromogens. Unfortunately many clinical decisions are made with the simple assumption that the reported serum creatinine level truly represents an *in vivo* level and that by extension the severity of CKD. Beyond the immediate consequences of this assumption, the long-term consequences can be quite significant. Medical surveillance, specific pharmacologic and procedural replacement therapies, including transplantation of a kidney and simultaneous liver-kidney transplantation rest in large

* Correspondence to: David H Van Thiel, MD Section of Hepatology, Department of Medicine, Rush University Medical Center, Chicago, Illinois 60612, Phone: 13125633937, Email: david_vanthiel@rush.edu.

measure upon the serum creatinine level and its expression of kidney function. Implementation of therapy can be life-extending, however, unfortunately in other cases, medically-deserving patients are denied treatment given the limitations and/or mis-allocation of these resources based upon the same creatinine measurement. In this review, the complexities of creatinine analysis, it's evolving role in assessing kidney function, and it's ultimate effect upon renal and liver replacement therapies will be discussed.

Origin of Serum Creatinine and Its Characteristics in Healthy and Diseased States

Creatinine is a relatively small molecule of 113 Daltons that forms from the spontaneous breakdown of creatine-phosphate [1]. The creatine molecule was originally identified by Michel Chevreul in 1832, who isolated it from skeletal muscle and aptly named it in reference to the Greek word "*kreas*" meaning "flesh" [2]. Creatine itself is derived from either carnivorous ingestion or through endogenous production in liver and kidney via utilization of arginine, glycine and methionine. Approximately 95% of creatine is localized to skeletal muscle where it serves as a high-energy carrier for replenishing ATP storage, in the form of creatine-phosphate [3].

In the musculature, creatinine is produced at a relatively constant rate, and in healthy or chronic kidney disease (CKD) patients maintains a stable serum level given its fairly uniform excretion rate [1, 4-5]. By extension, alterations in the production or excretion mechanisms will then change the creatinine level to reflect the sum of their independent directions and magnitudes. For example, in sepsis serum creatinine levels can be severely impaired for a number of reasons including decreased production in muscles and malnutrition, giving a false sense of kidney function in the acute setting [6]. In healthy states, creatinine is mainly excreted (cleared) renally with 85% of it being filtered and the remainder being secreted by the proximal tubules. Therefore, the creatinine clearance (CrCl) overestimates the true GFR as a function of the tubular secretion of creatinine [1]. In progressive stages of CKD, the amount of creatinine secreted by the tubules represents a larger percentage contribution towards the total amount excreted and as a result the implied GFR is even less accurate, being over-estimated. Creatinine is excreted in the urine at approximately 20-25 mg/kg/day in males and 10-15 mg/kg/day in females, and traditionally given this stable rate has been used as a guide to assess the accuracy of the measured total 24-hour urinary outputs, e.g. volume as well as the amount of proteinuria [7-8]. However, in various degrees of CKD the serum creatinine rises as the GFR decreases, and non-renal patterns of excretion become important, and are to a degree dependent upon intestinal bacterial degradation [1]. In so far as muscle mass and dietary proclivities are also reflected in age, gender, race and nutritional status, these constitutional factors will ultimately affect baseline serum creatinine levels across the lifetime of an individual and range across a heterogenous population.

Superimposed upon these basic constitutional factors and the intrinsic properties of the chronically diseased kidney, other systemic diseases processes can also significantly alter serum creatinine levels and thus affect the calculated GFR. Beyond the obvious manifestation of dialysis-dependent kidney disease in which there is volume overload and azotemia from insufficient filtration and secretion of substances by the nephrons, notable are cases of congestive heart failure and cirrhosis both of which subject the patient to a functionally postrenal venous congestion and/or pre-renal hypoperfusion state of the kidney [9-10]. It is important to note that in the setting of hemodialysis (HD) or any other type of renal replacement therapy (RRT), serum creatinine is essentially useless as a marker for GFR for obvious reasons.

In the setting of these systemic diseases, two general results are incurred: (1) not only is more creatinine retained in the body due to failure of renal excretion; (2) the actual serum level in the body given the enlarged volume of distribution and altered oncotic properties of low albumin/edematous states can underestimate the GFR; (3) conversely, depending upon the severity of volume overload, the weight factor in these equations may be inordinately high having presupposed to detect muscle mass when indeed there is rather just an abundance of fluid, thus manifesting an over-estimate of GFR. Indeed these volume states within the intra- and extra-vascular compartments, are quite volatile given the day-to-day decompensated nature of these diseases and the level of iatrogenic interference upon them, i.e. aggressive diuresis, paracentesis, vasopressor or inotropic therapeutics as the specific case may warrant [11-13]. These concerns are significant and common and suggest that the GFR and by extension kidney function must be carefully calculated.

The Importance of Creatinine in Kidney Disease

Creatinine is notable not for what it is, but rather what it has been touted to represent, namely a principal actor in defining the GFR as a marker of kidney function in both relatively stable healthy and chronic disease states, i.e. CKD [1, 5, 9]. This assumption rests the idea that creatinine is unerringly produced, mainly filtered and measured in a fairly consistent manner without being interfered upon by other factors. In a sense, creatinine is supposed to be inert. However with the complexities of even a relatively healthy patient, whether it is in relation to age or medication use, thia assumption is altered in non-predictable ways, thus limiting what can be inferred from the measurement of this single parameter as regards to GFR and ultimately kidney function. Beyond creatinine, many other variables have been rightly taken into account to assess GFR, as noted in the iterations of the various modified diet in renal disease (MDRD) equations [14]. These equations, of which creatinine is a heavily weighted variable, are meant to reflect a complex biology, and in the clinical sphere to extrapolate not only disease prognosis but also justify interventions which can be life extending, but are themselves not without attendant morbidity and significant cost. Given these facts, it is quite useful to understand the scope and limits of the serum creatinine measurement and its relationship to the presence of kidney and/or liver disease in order to grasp the assumptions upon which various clinical decisions rests [1, 14-16].

CKD is unfortunately a rather large problem, with approximately 26 million individuals affected in the United States [4]. This number is expected to continue to increase given the increasing prevalence of diabetes mellitus (DM), hypertension and obesity within the population. In 2007 over 35 billion dollars was allocated to the end-stage renal disease (ESRD) program. Given this rather large medical and financial burden of CKD and the threat of further rationing of medical care, an accurate assessment of kidney function, to prognosticate disease severity, prevent worsening disease and allocate precious resources is essential [1, 17].

With the limitations described, the GFR is an excellent, albeit imperfect marker for overall kidney function. CKD quantitates the end result of either sustained local kidney injury, like renal artery stenosis or drug toxicity, or systemic-wide injury like DM and hypertension. CKD comprises 5 stages of disease severity, based heavily, but not exclusively upon the calculated notion of GFR, ranging from stage 1 which is ≥ 90ml/min/1.73 m^2 to stage 5 which is < 15 ml/min/1.73 m^2 [18]. Over the years, the GFR has been assessed by numerous mathematical equations, comprising a number of important individual and epidemiologic markers. The serum creatinine level is fundamental to all of these equations [19]. The National Kidney Foundation suggests a sustained decrease of function (stage 3 ≤ 60 ml/min 1.73 m^2) over time, for at least 3 months, or signs of structural (e.g abnormal renal biopsy or imaging) or functional (albuminuria/proteinuria) abnormalities regardless of the GFR, to establish a diagnosis of CKD [18]. This definition was chosen as a GFR at this level reflects an overall 50% loss of renal function, and that the accuracy of standard GFR equations also becomes difficult beyond this level. CKD stage 5 is also synonymous with the (older) U.S. government designated term ESRD, which after legal extensions to the Medicare bill in 1973, was invoked for individuals under the age of 65 to receive financial coverage for HD or other RRTs [20]. Notably those with CKD stage 5, as their clinical status dictates, may not necessarily be on RRTs, although certainly eligible if need be.

Acute kidney injury (AKI) is an exceedingly common phenomenon which is marked by an acute rise in creatinine, usually defined as ≥ 0.5 mg/dl within 2 weeks, from baseline with associated markers such as a reduced urinary output and/or an abnormal urinary sediment or proteinuria. AKI results from a number of both local and systemic insults, ranging from ischemia, infectious causes and drug or contrast-induced toxicity [21-22]. However standard definitions with regard to absolute changes in creatinine should be taken with caution for the following reasons. It is important to note that AKI can arise either within a healthy or CKD state and because the baseline serum creatinine is dependent on a number of constitutional factors (*vide infra*), it is not the absolute value that is important in making the diagnosis of AKI but rather the absolute change in value (at low creatinine levels) or changes in laboratory and clinical data (at higher values) in general. Take for instance the following examples: If a patient had a baseline creatinine of 5.0 mg/dl and it rises to 5.5 mg/dl, technically there is an injury and indeed GFR will decrease by a few points, whereas a serum creatinine change of 0.5 mg/dl to 1.0 mg/dl would reflect a 50% loss of GFR. In both cases the absolute change in serum creatinine levels are the same and would fit the definition, yet it is not uniformly obvious that the former case has any clinical relevance *a priori*, whereas it is very likely that the latter case would.

In this setting, GFR and hence true kidney function, is impossible to quantitate in any simple way utilizing traditional laboratory methods. Importantly, serum creatinine levels tend to lag behind true GFR in the setting of both worsening and resolving injury [4]. In such cases, it is likely more appropriate to track the rate of creatinine change, urinary volume output or changes in other urinary markers as measures of the AKI trajectory or recovery rather than using of a mathematical equation that inaccurately estimates the GFR.

The Importance of Creatinine in Liver Disease

It has become doctrine that the serum creatinine level, despite it's imperfections as a GFR marker, has been recognized as the clinical gold standard of kidney function [1, 4, 18, 21]. Moreover it has been appreciated that the serum creatinine also reflects global systemic dysfunction and likelihood of mortality.

This concept is manifestly true in liver disease in particular, where all patients, who are deemed eligible for liver transplantation (LT), e.g. for common chronic liver diseases (CLD) such as alcoholic or hepatitis C associated cirrhosis, have their three-month mortality assessed quantitatively using the Model for end-stage liver disease (MELD) score [23-25].

The MELD score was originally utilized in 2000 to predict the survival of patients undergoing a transvenous intrahepatic portosystemic shunt (TIPS) procedure in the setting of refractory variceal bleeding [25-27].

It was subsequently validated in 2002 for use in LT prognostication, given the inadequacies of the older methods of "wait-list time" and "status level" [23]. The components of the MELD score consist of the serum bilirubin, creatinine and INR values. The implications of these parameters will be more fully discussed in the following sections (*vide infra*) [10]. Given the myriad of functions that the liver performs, e.g. volume regulation, immune function, coagulation, xenobiotic excretion and energy metabolism, it is not surprising that its dysfunction leads to systemic consequences that directly affect the kidney and the assessment of kidney function.

Pertinent to this review, cirrhosis is associated with an effective pre-renal state through a number of pathophysiologic mechanisms. Through malnutrition, either by decreased oral intake or cachectic hypermetabolism, and the failed synthetic capability of the liver, the absolute serum albumin amount is depressed [27]. Albumin, as the main oncotic factor in the serum is critical to in the principle of volume distribution, and as such its loss may allow for increased filtration of the plasma volume into so called "third spaces" particularly the interstitium, leading to edema and anasarca, or into the peritoneum, leading to ascites. Siimilarly so, the interstitium is also a dynamic environment and it's own hydrostatic and osmotic forces will contend with the those of the vasculature. This third space volume expansion can be substantial, and as has been alluded above, alters the baseline concentration of serum molecules, including creatinine and albumin itself. The resultant decreased intravascular volume is sensed by the kidney manifested in a compensatory induction of the renin-angiotensin-aldosterone system (RAAS) in an effort to increase vascular tone and volume. Concurrently, the enhanced concentration of substances such as nitric oxide (NO) in the splanchnic circulation, resulting from the hypertensive portal circulation and impaired flow through the liver, leads to further vasodilation and an enhancement of the functional pre-renal state [11-13].

These mechanisms generate an environment in which there is in fact a total body hypervolemic state, albeit maldistributed, with concurrent inadequacy to meet the perfusion needs of the kidney [25]. As a result, the GFR, by definition, is decreased and suffers in-step with the variability of the CLD volume status, which is rather delicate. The resultant low perfusion state of the kidney leads to both AKI and CKD, depending on the duration and severity of the insult. The clinical diagnosis of kidney function in this setting is by-and-large based upon alterations of the serum value of creatinine, and to a lesser but more accurate extent on urinary output and other markers to include proteinuria or renal biopsy. More recently, other serum molecules to include cystatin C have also been studied for their utility in assessing renal function in this setting and will be discussed further (*vide infra*) [28].

It then becomes obvious that in a complex disease state like CLD, the assessment of kidney function is a difficult one [10]. Not only are the absolute quantities of molecules like creatinine diminished, but their concentrations in serum are in a state of flux. As will be detailed, the creatinine level taken as accurate laboratory value for assessing the GFR and implied kidney function has significant prognostic value and even more profound implications relative to the application of aggressive treatments [23].

Creatinine and Iatrogenic Interference

As has been noted, a small percentage of creatinine is secreted by the proximal tubules, however other medications also compete for this same pathway, in particular cimetidine and trimethoprim [1, 29]. In this setting serum creatinine levels will rise (having been outcompeted for the transporter site), and the calculated CrCl falls necessarily while the actual GFR is unchanged. However the serum creatinine level and resultant equations used to calculate GFR suggest that an insult to kidney function has occurred. There is no implemented standard correction factor for the serum creatinine value when these medications are used other than a sense of clinical caution [9-10].

Furthermore, in the setting of CKD, particularly HD or in decompensated cirrhosis, overall total body volume is an important variable of concern given the effects it has on quality-of-life, morbidity and mortality. Total body volume can be manipulated through decreased intake or nature of the type of intake, in particular a low salt diet, or through mechanisms of fluid removal. Fluid removal can follow the natural course of urination with iatrogenic assistance of diuretics, renal replacement therapies like HD or percutaneous drainage of third space volumes such as the peritoneum (ascites) or pleural cavities (hepatohydrothroax). In patients with CKD and/or cirrhosis, fluid removal through urination may be inadequate or altogether absent, either through effective destruction of a significant population of nephrons in primary CKD, or through the inability of the blood in the vascular volume to meet the nephrons as observed in cirrhosis. Indeed, it is just as likely in such patients that the causes of inadequate urination are complex and intertwined as has been discussed (*vide supra*). In so far as these cases are beyond the body's ability to self-regulate, iatrogenic assistance effectively becomes a chronic process until some form of definitive therapy like solitary kidney transplantation (SKT) or LT is prescribed [24, 30-31].

Given the potency of current pharmacologic therapies such as furosemide, spironolactone and other agents, the delicacy of the volume state in these patients and the concentration of measured molecules in the serum can be strikingly manipulated over a period of hours. The creatinine level, depending on the nuance of therapy can either be normalized (as volume overload has been alleviated and more of the intravascular volume is now able to meet the kidneys), or worsened with over diuresis (a reduction in the amount of the intravascular volume that meets the kidneys). In the setting of AKI and CKD, whether or not with associated CLD, these are important daily concerns for patients and clinicians involved in the evaluation and treatment of an elevated serum creatinine level. The interpretation of the biologic state, i.e. assessment of the serum creatinine value is real although it may not accurately reflect the underlying disease processes. Nonetheless, it certainly affects the perceived disease state and by implication the prognosis and either the aggressiveness or lack thereof to a specific patient [9].

Based upon the initial state of disease, implied by the aggregate assessment of clinical, laboratory and imaging data, the physician has the ability to maintain or improve a patient's condition limited by the motivation to do so given specific concerns: In the final analysis the question becomes in cases of advanced kidney and/or liver disease, should all means of medical interference be implemented for hopeful immediate and sustained benefit, or should a modicum of restraint be initiated given that in fact deteriorization, or perceived deteriorization, of the clinical state would allow for expedited routing to the definitive treatment of transplantation, which the individual would inevitably need in the future? Given the morbidity, mortality and substantial costs with medical and to a greater extent surgical procedures, these are critical concerns and generate a number of conflicting ethical values for clinicians. Our code of *primum non nocere* in absolute terms is over-ridden by our utilitarian ethic of possible immediate harm, e.g. hypoxemia from fluid overload or infection from diminished immune function of the liver, through de-escalation of therapy or lack thereof, in an effort to receive potential long-term gain. In the domain of LT in particular just as the limitations and manipulations of the true and perceived creatinine values are understood in regards to the effect on the MELD score, so too but to a more limited extent are the concerns of the INR value as well [32].

Specifically, there is significant variability in the assays for INR among different institutions, and like creatinine these results have implications for higher MELD scores and thus eligibility for more immediate transplantation. Additionally, just as the serum creatinine will be truly effected by medications like cimetidine that inhibit it's secretion, without altering the true GFR and the implied kidney function, INR can be altered through the use of agents like coumadin, which inhibit the activation of the coagulation factors, without altering the intrinsic synthetic capacity of the liver for which the INR is supposed to measure [33-35].

It is well recognized that the diseased liver is in an altered coagulation state, and that despite suggestions that concerns for thrombosis may be obviated by "auto-anticoagulation" which is certainly inaccurate given the understanding that the array of pro- and anti-coagulant factors present in liver disease patients, e.g. for instance protein C levels and activity, antithrombin and a host of other factors, are not equally assessed or measured utilizing the standard assays in routine clinical practice [36]. Furthermore, the decision to anticoagulate a cirrhotic and how aggressively, is ultimately a subjective, although not unreasoned analysis, just like assessment of an individual's volume status.

As a result, the implementation of medical or other therapeutic interventions is affected importantly by personal proclivities.

The Limitations of Creatinine Assays

Creatinine is unfortunately measured in non-standard ways by either colorimetric or enzymatic methods, both of which are nevertheless simple in process and low in cost [5, 10, 15]. These methods utilize the Jaffe reaction, wherein creatinine binds with an alkaline picrate to form a Janovski complex which is then measured at 520 nm [9]. However, many other compounds can mimic or interfere with this reaction.

There is ample evidence that so called non-creatinine chromogens can cause both positive interference (perceived elevated creatinine levels) as seen with glucose, uric acid and ketoacids, and negative interference (perceived depressed creatinine levels) as seen with elevated bilirubin levels whether conjugated or not [9, 37].

In fact there appears to be an inverse correlation of serum creatinine values with increasing bilirubin levels. Worse, the precision of these creatinine measurements (variability) becomes less with increasing bilirubin levels beyond 3.7 mg/dl [10]. This dynamic effect upon creatinine is not addressed in routine clinical practice regarding CKD alone nor more importantly in the setting of chronic liver disease (CLD). Various modifications to the Jaffe method have been implemented to try to correct for these factors but they are costly and laborious and as a result have not been widely implemented. More fundamentally disturbing is the fact that there is no reference standard for creatinine that is in universal use.

As Cholangitas *et al* have noted, various GFR equations, like the MDRD were validated utilizing the standard of only one company [9-10]. However, upon implementation of this MDRD equation in hospitals across the country, a number of companies each with their own creatinine standard are in use. Thus, these technologies of GFR assessment are in a sense being misused and their results construed to be accurate. Unfortunately, there is no simple solution to this problem.

The Measurement of GFR

The accurate measurement of GFR and by extension kidney function has undoubtedly been quite difficult to capture [1, 4, 16]. Over the years, it has become increasingly clear relative to the GFR, there is an intricate relationship between constitutional factors such as age and ethnicity, in combination with more labile factors that include volume status and medications that affect the the serum creatinine level [14]. Furthermore, the accuracy and reproducibility of obtaining a serum creatinine value is impaired by the nature of the various assays themselves [1]. Indeed, the more we look into the true nature of creatinine and by extension GFR, the more unstable they seem to be, and that rather than developing a reasonable generalization, have in fact identified increasing limitations in the assessment of a given serum level.

Ideally when assessing GFR one would seek a perfect marker, one that it is indeed inert: 1) generated at a constant rate; 2) filtered through the glomerulus into the tubules, and neither secreted nor re-absorbed; 3) not affected by endogenous or exogenous chemicals in the serum or in the laboratory assay; and 4) that can be measured accurately and precisely, at low cost and minimal laboratory effort. There are indeed markers that fulfill many but not all of these criteria [9-10, 37]. Each of these markers has been utilized as the 'gold standard' when they are described in the literature. These markers are invariably exogenous compounds such as inulin, non-radioactive contrast media like iohexol, and radioisotopes such as ^{125}I-iothalamate. However, each is costly and their measurement is labor intensive, and therefore none of them are routinely used in clinical practice. Furthermore, each is known to be unreliable in patients with third space issues such as edema and ascites; the very patients in whom an assessment of GFR is critical for both prognostic and therapeutic purposes [37-39]. Thus, in interpreting a given calculated GFR value, clinicians are left with trying to accurately define the principles and parameters of the markers used to assess the GFR and their relevance to a given patient with an abnormal physiology.

As noted, the measured CrCl is larger than the actual GFR, and was initially assessed with a 24-hour urine collection. It was found however that this method underestimates the GFR in children, and that it was impractical in uniform implementation given errors in measurement of urine volume and/or it's incomplete collection. Moreover, this method does not account for the inherent limitations in the actual serum creatinine assessment, nor does it take into account the constitutional epidemiolgoic factors such as age, weight and ethnicity that affect the serum creatinine level. Advances were made by Cockcroft and Gault in 1976 with their eponymous equation, the Cockcroft-Gault (CG) equation which improved the clinical assessment of the GFR beyond that achieved with a 24-hour creatinine collection [40]. They assessed 249 relatively healthy males ranging in age from 18-92 years old. Their equation incorporates corrective factors such as age, weight and gender for a more comprehensive assessment of the calculated CrCl and by extension GFR. Subsequently, it has was validated more broadly such that it had been until lately the principal method for the clinical assessment of GFR and CKD, for pharmacologic studies, and eligibility of patients to be accepted into ESRD programs such as HD [4, 41]. The CG equation however does not take into account body surface area, ethnicity nor obviate the implicit concerns of chemical interference upon the serum creatinine measurement (nor do any of the other more recent GFR equations).

In 1999 Levey *et al* published the Modified diet in renal disease (MDRD) study in which 7 different GFR equations, including the CG equation, were analyzed in 1628 patients, with 1 equation being found to be highly accurate at calculating the GFR utilizing 6 variables: serum creatinine, age, gender, ethnicity, blood urea nitrogen (BUN), and serum albumin [14]. It is notable that the initial MDRD study was limited in its analysis of sub-populations, excluding those of extreme age (< 18 or > 70 years of age), individuals without CKD, or DM and distinguishing between individuals with type 1 and those with type 2 on insulin, renal transplant recipients, and individuals of black ethnicity. Subsequent studies however have to an extent validated its use in these additional groups, however its true utility in patients without CKD remains to be determined, and indeed likely underestimates GFR in healthy individuals. Further modifications to the MDRD equation, such as the removal of the BUN and albumin variables and the standardization of the serum creatinine assays in 2006, made the accurate estimation of GFR even better (lowered GFR estimates ~ 6%), and easier to calculate, such that the National Kidney Foundation Kidney Disease Outcomes Quality Initiative (NKF-KDOQI) advocated for its primary use in assessing CKD staging [4, 42]. The current MDRD iteration utilizes the four variable equation, herein referred to as the MDRD-4V.

Most recently, Levey *et al* in 2009 published the Chronic Kidney Disease Epidemiology collaboration (CKD-EPI) research group's results utilizing the CKD-EPI creatinine equation designed in response to concerns about the MDRD equation, that despite having gained large usage and acceptance within the preceding ten years, nevertheless underestimated GFR at higher values, those > 60 ml/min/1.73 m^2 [43]. The result being that for patients with more mild or no CKD they were identified as having a more functional impairment than in fact was present. The CKD-EPI equation assessed similar factors to the MDRD-4V including serum creatinine, age, gender and ethnicity in 8254 patients in 10 studies, and 3896 patients in 16 studies that was used for subsequent validation. Importantly, they used a "spline factor" for creatinine, wherein mathematically, the creatinine value carried a lesser weight relative to the GFR at lower levels of creatinine than at higher levels. The CKD-EPI equation was utilized within the framework of National Health and Nutrition Examination Survey (NHANES), and predicted a median estimated GFR elevation of 9.5 ml/min/1.73m^2, thus decreasing the prevalence of CKD within the United States population by 1.6%. Furthermore, the number of CKD patients consisting of woman and Caucasian patients was decreased, while the number of elderly patients with CKD remained similar to that obtained with the MDRD-4V equation.

Given the proliferation of GFR equations, and the importance of their calculated results, it is worthwhile to examine them in parallel [4, 19, 44]. A recent study in 2010 analyzed CG, MDRD-4V and CKD-EPI creatinine equations [20]. They defined bias as the mean difference from the estimated GFR to the measured GFR, and accuracy represented the percentage of estimated GFR within 30% of measured GFR. GFR was determined through the use of the iothalamate marker standard. Both the MDRD-4V and the CKD-EPI equations were found to be more accurate than the CG equation in assessing true GFR in all of the subgroups studied, with the CKD-EPI equations performing slightly better overall compared to the MDRD-4V equation, although not significantly. In particular the CKD-EPI had a tighter fit for GFRs $\geq$ 90 ml/min/1.73m^2 compared to the MDRD-4V which was better at GFR levels ranging from 15-29 ml/min/1.73m^2.

It was noted that in the elderly and/or those with low body weights, no significant bias was evident among any of the three equations, thus it was concluded that the CG was a reasonable and simpler alternative in these cases.

There clearly has been a substantial improvement in the accuracy and precision of GFR estimates through a better understanding of the biologic complexity of creatinine and it's measurement and interpretation [44]. It is clear that better estimates of GFR and thus by implication kidney function have a number of consequences for individuals as well as populations. CKD is known to be associated with an increased morbidity and mortality rate that is scaled relative to the degree of renal impairment.

As a result our medical societies have developed guidelines related to blood pressure management, restrictions and/or reductions in the use of certain medications, the application of certain medications, the use of routine laboratory and/or imaging surveillance, and also the utilization of renal and/or liver replacement therapies to include transplantation (*vida infra*). On a national and even global scale, the assessment of GFR, has major and life-long implications for the intensity of medical therapy, quality-of-life and cost utilization [18, 45-46].

As the most recent data utilizing the CKD-EPI equations would suggest, it is quite possible that many patients have been given erroneous diagnoses of CKD severity and as a result have been inappropriately managed to a degree, with risks attendant upon such therapeutic and diagnostic interventions relative to their perceived stage of renal function, with a resultant mis-allocation of limited resources at an increased cost [23, 44]. This concern must of course be tempered by the understanding that clinical assessment and action take these numeric results into consideration and are not driven exclusively by them.

The Effects of Serum Creatinine on Renal and Liver Replacement Therapies

The maturation of transplant surgery and hepatology combined with powerful immunosuppressive therapies, like cyclosporine and tacrolimus, has made LT a universally accepted procedure for end-stage liver disease as well as fulminant hepatic failure. The widespread utilization of LT has created a natural strain upon the pool of liver donors, and somewhat unexpectedly more recently a strain upon the kidney transplantation and specifically the kidney donor pool in part as a result of the weight given the serum creatinine value within the calculated MELD score [23, 25, 47]. Despite the complexities in assessing the true serum creatinine level in individuals with advanced liver disease, it nevertheless remains the main factor upon which kidney function is qualitatively and quantitatively assessed in such patients. As alluded to above, the MELD score is validated to rank eligible CLD and acute liver failure patients for LT. The MELD score is calculated utilizing an equation consisting of the serum bilirubin, creatinine and INR levels. The total score ranges from 6 to 40, using only whole numbers, and successfully prognosticates 3 month non-transplant mortality [25-26]. The MELD score has a utilitarian aim of allocating livers to those patients who would most benefit from a LT. It's utilization has achieved this goal to some degree by lowering mortality on the wait-list, lowering wait-list time to LT while not increasing post-transplant mortality. In the setting of HD, the MELD score is minimally scored at 20, beyond whatever contribution the INR and bilirubin provide. In those with AKI or CKD not on HD, the maximum value for creatinine that can be used to calculate the MELD score is 4 mg/dl. As a result, the value of a serum creatinine level, whether the patient is on HD or not, can have life-altering results as a function of determining the availability of a liver allograft to a particular patient [48]. To take a relevant example given data already presented, there are CLD patients with significant elevations in bilirubin, but given the negative interference of it upon the creatinine measurement, the calculated MELD scores are falsely depressed [9-10]. Thus, these patients are given a false representation of how ill they really are and awarded lower priority score.

Expanding further upon the relationship of liver and renal disease in the context of transplantation, it is noted that a substantial number of post-LT patients will incur a degree of renal injury, identified by an increase in the serum creatinine [27, 30-31, 38]. Current data suggest that 10% of liver transplant recipients will develop ESRD during the first 10 years post-transplant and that approximately 25% will experience AKI immediately post-liver transplant [38]. With time, it is estimated that liver transplant recipient's lose 40-50% of their renal function post-transplant as a consequence of their requirement for a calcineurin inhibitor, various hemodynamic problems, the presence of hypertension and/or diabetes or the natural progression of their underlying pre-transplant renal disease [38]. Importantly, those that do develop CKD post-LT have a 4.5 fold greater risk of death compared to those that do not.

Given the important nature of kidney function in the MELD era, reflected in monitoring the serum creatinine value, both before and after liver LT, important clinical results have occurred, these include: (1) an increased rate (and overuse) of simultaneous of liver and kidney transplant (SLKT) procedures [23-24, 30-31]; and resultantly, (2) a reduction in the available donor kidney pool for use in SKT [23, 31]. Importantly, the increase in SLKT procedures has occurred without a change in patient survival while, not unexpectedly, markedly increasing the length of post-transplant hospitalization, the overall cost of LT, and the utilization of RRTs [30-31, 47]. When reviewing the data available on greater than 19,000 LTs, nearly 34,000 SKT and 1,000 SLKTs between 1987 and 2006, no benefit of SLKT compared to LT alone was identified [49]. In fact, the SLKT survival rate actually declined from a high of 87% in 2002 to a low of 76% in 2005 while no difference in the survival rate for LT alone was seen during the same time period [49]. In particular, these SKLT patients as described in other studies as well, characteristically have more advanced liver disease and as a result receive better quality liver allografts, having a donor risk index of 1.55 versus 1.66 compared to those receiving a LT alone [39, 49]. Most unfortunate was the finding that the kidney graft survival was worse at one year in SLKT recipients than in those receiving a SKT (77% vs. 89%) [49]. Importantly, the only sub-group of SLKT patients, who benefited in terms of survival were those who had been on HD for a period of > 3 months [39].

It is important to recognize that patients receiving a SKT or SLKT may differ markedly in terms of their degree and kind of renal impairment. Furthermore, there are no specific and uniform criteria in place for SLKT allocation. Specifically a study by Thompson *et al.* noted that while 100% of SKT patients in this population are on HD, i.e. with GFRs $\leq$ 15 ml/min/1.73 m^2 at the time of transplantation, only 60% of those receiving a SLKT had been on HD at the time of transplant. The reason for this marked difference is that in order to receive a SKT, one had to have a documented GFR < 20 mL/min/1.73 m^2 while no GFR threshold existed for those receiving a SLKT [23].

As a result in the absence of specific criteria for SLKT, the number of individuals receiving these surgeries has increased in the MELD era [39-40, 50]. It should be noted that in the SKT population generally, it is not necessarily the case that that those with CKD stage 5, i.e. < 15 ml/min/1.73 m^2 were on HD or similar modality prior to transplantation. Again, that determination is clinical, and in fact SKTs are done prior to these modalities as well.

It is effectively the situation that without standardized indications and despite and evidence of sub-optimal outcomes, kidneys are being inadequately prioritized towards one population, i.e. those receiving a SLKT, who may or may not benefit from the procedure, from another population, i.e. the SKT patients, who certainly would.

Given all of this data, various groups have tried to suggest methods for a more appropriate prioritization and equitable distribution of a donor kidney amongst these various groups competing for a kidney allograft. For instance, Pichler *et al.* reported their experience with renal biopsies in LT candidates and suggested that a SLKT was only indicated in those with a renal biopsy that had one or more of the following pathologic findings; greater than 40% global glomerulosclerosis, greater than 30% interstitial fibrosis or severe glomerular injury [50]. It has been noted that the degree of interstitial fibrosis in particular may be one of the best prognostic markers for renal function available. More broadly, when the liver allocations committee presented their report on the use of SLKT in 2007, the consensus was that the procedure was only appropriate if the measured CrCl was < 30 mL/min and the patient had required at least 6 weeks of HD therapy [47]. It is hoped that these measures will not only appropriately stratify the best patients for this intense dual surgery, but also decrease the number and types of post-operative complications while simultaneously reducing the substantial cost, and conserving the pool of donor kidneys for the SKT population.

A Replacement Marker for Creatinine

Despite the strength of serum creatinine on it's own and it's utilization within more comprehensive structures like the MDRD equations to assess GFR and ultimately kidney function, it has nevertheless left the medical community wanting [1, 4, 9-10, 19, 28]. Researchers have continued to seek out other endogenous compounds with both minimal chemical interference and continuous tight correlations with measured GFR despite the variations and vicissitudes of including healthy and diseased patients in the population studied [28]. One such marker is cystatin C, originally described in 1961 as gamma-trace protein by Grubb *et al.* who noted that it was elevated in patients with various degrees of renal impairment [51]. Subsequent investigation has shown it to be 13 kDa protein that function as a major extracellular protease inhibitor. It is produced in all nucleated cells and maintains a fairly constant concentration in the blood, and unlike creatinine, has not been found to be affected by gender, muscle mass, or diet. Cystatin C is freely filtered through the glomerulus, without any component of tubular secretion although some re-absorption and metabolism occurs within the proximal tubules [28, 51-53]. Overall studies have shown a correlation of 94% between standard measures of GFR and cystatin C levels. Cystatin C although commercially available is considerably more costly in that it's assay reagent cost per unit is \$3.75 compared to \$0.20 for creatinine [54]. Measured cystatin C is also known to be altered by medications that include angiotension converting enzyme inhibitors and calcinuerin inhibitors. These agents are quite commonly utilized in both pre- and post-SKT, LT and SLKT patients [55].

A number of groups have assessed the efficacy of cystatin C compared to creatinine in measuring GFR and kidney function. In a meta-analysis reported by Dharnidharka *et al* in 2002 a total of 54 data sets reported in the literature up to and including 2001, comprised 4,492 patients wherein these two compounds were assessed for GFR fitness [53]. The measured correlation coefficient of the reciprocal of serum cystatin C ($r = 0.816$) was compared to the serum creatinine with a r-value $= 0.742$, $p < 0.001$. They importantly noted that while the correlation coefficients demonstrated a linear association, this is not always clinically useful as it may still systematically over- or underestimate the true value. Thus, they also measured receiver operating characteristic area under the curve ROC-AUC, which is considered to be a better assessment of diagnostic accuracy, and yielded mean values for cystatin C of 0.926 vs 0.837 for creatinine ($p < 0.001$). These results suggest that the cystatin C level is better than the creatinine in measuring the GFR and by extension kidney function. As has been noted above, a particularly difficult group to assess for renal function has been those with CLD, in particular those with cirrhosis with or without concomitant renal disease, given the effects upon creatinine production, volume of distribution and assay measurement in this population. Woitas *et al* looked specifically at 44 cirrhotic patients and found an increased accuracy in GFR assessment with cystatin C compared to creatinine, particularly in those with Childs class B and C disease [54]. Given these data, cystatin C presents an emerging alternative to creatinine in assessing GFR, that particularly in those with confounding liver disease, requires further validation.

Conclusion

Creatinine is a simple molecule that is being asked to reveal the complex nature, both accurately and precisely, of GFR and by extension kidney function in quantitative terms. Much research and clinical experience has shown how difficult this task is, and that indeed if creatinine is to be used it must be assessed within a network of endogenous host factors, and framed clinically within the dynamics of complex systemic diseases states, for instance cirrhosis.

This is manifest in the evolution of GFR equations, combining both patient-specific and epidemiologic data into quantitative terms. There has been much progress in estimating the true GFR however the identification and utilization of more inert compounds to replace creatinine in assessing kidney function continues to be a goal. The appropriate assessment of creatinine and its relation to the biochemical environment is one of intrinsic interest, but also strongly motivated by the clinical exigencies of patients and the physicians and surgeons who care for them. Creatinine imbues not only diagnostic and prognostic significance, but as described, e.g. within the MELD score, can propel patients towards extreme therapies with effects upon quality of life, morbidity and mortality, all of which occurs with an intrinsic risk and cost. Thus, a careful analysis of the serum creatinine value in it's principles and parameters of measurement allows for a more complete assessment of the kidney, the liver and the patient. With continuous research and clinical practice, both balancing and compelling each other forward, the hope for further advances in the measurement, interpretation and utilization of serum creatinine levels with be achieved.

References

[1] Stevens LA, Coresh J, Greene T, Levey AS. Assessing kidney function--measured and estimated glomerular filtration rate. *N. Engl. J. Med.* 2006 Jun 8; 354 (23):2473-83.

[2] Needham, D. M. Machina Carnis. *The Biochemistry of Muscular Contraction in Its Historical Development.* Cambridge, UK: Cambridge Univ. Press, 1971. P.79.

[3] da Silva RP, Nissim I, Brosnan ME, Brosnan JT. Creatine synthesis: hepatic metabolism of guanidinoacetate and creatine in the rat in vitro and in vivo. *Am. J. Physiol. Endocrinol. Metab.* 2009 Feb; 296 (2):E256-61. Epub 2008 Nov 18.

[4] Steffl JL, Bennett W, Olyaei AJ. The old and new methods of assessing kidney function. J. Clin. Pharmacol. 2012 Jan; 52 (1 Suppl):63S-71S.

[5] Beddhu S, Samore MH, Roberts MS, Stoddard GJ, Pappas LM, Cheung AK. Creatinine production, nutrition, and glomerular filtration rate estimation. J. Am. Soc. Nephrol. 2003 Apr; 14 (4):1000-5.

[6] Doi K, Yuen PS, Eisner C, Hu X, Leelahavanichkul A, Schnermann. Reduced production of creatinine limits its use as marker of kidney injury in sepsis. *J. Am. Soc. Nephrol.* 2009 Jun; 20 (6):1217-21. Epub 2009 Apr 23.

[7] Landry DW, Bazari H. Approach to the patient with renal disease. In: Goldman L, Schafer AI, eds. *Cecil Medicine.* 24th ed. Philadelphia, Pa: Saunders Elsevier; 2011: chap 116.

[8] Gaspari F, Perico N, Remuzzi G. Timed urine collections are not needed to measure urine protein excretion in clinical practice. *Am. J. Kidney Dis.* 2006 Jan;47(1):1-7.

[9] Cholongitas E, Shusang V, Marelli L, Nair D, Thomas M, Patch D, Burns A, Sweny P, Burroughs AK. Review article: renal function assessment in cirrhosis - difficulties and alternative measurements. *Aliment Pharmacol Ther.* 2007 Oct 1; 26 (7):969-78.

[10] Cholongitas E, Marelli L, Kerry A, Senzolo M, Goodier DW, Nair D, Thomas M, Patch D, Burroughs AK. Different methods of creatinine measurement significantly affect MELD scores. *Liver Transpl.* 2007 Apr;13(4):523-9.

[11] Fernandez-Seara J, Prieto J, Quiroga J, Zozaya JM, Cobos MA, Rodriguez-Eire JL, Garcia-Plaza A, Leal J. Systemic and regional hemodynamics in patients with liver cirrhosis and ascites with and without functional renal failure. *Gastroenterology* 1989 Nov;97(5):1304-12.

[12] Aliaga L, Zozoya JM, Omar M, Mediavilla JD, Prieto J. Interrelationships between systemic hemodynamics, urinary sodium excretion, and renin-angiotensin system in cirrhosis. *Acta Gastroenterol. Belg.* 1995 Mar-Apr; 58 (2):213-21.

[13] Arroyo V, Jiménez W. Complications of cirrhosis. II. Renal and circulatory dysfunction. Lights and shadows in an important clinical problem. *J. Hepatol.* 2000; 32 (1 Suppl):157-70.

[14] Levey AS, Bosch JP, Lewis JB, Greene T, Rogers N, Roth D. A more accurate method to estimate glomerular filtration rate from serum creatinine: a new prediction equation. Modification of Diet in Renal Disease Study Group. *Ann. Intern. Med.* 1999 Mar 16;130(6):461-70.

[15] Myers GL, Miller WG, Coresh J, Fleming J, Greenberg N, Greene T, Hostetter T, Levey AS, Panteghini M, Welch M, Eckfeldt JH; National Kidney Disease Education Program Laboratory Working Group. Recommendations for improving serum creatinine measurement: A report from the Laboratory Working Group of the National Kidney Disease Education Program. *Clin. Chem.* 2006 Jan; 52 (1):5-18. Epub 2005 Dec 6.

[16] Chen YW, Chen HH, Wang TE, Chang CW, Chang CW, Wu CJ. Difference between CKD-EPI and MDRD equations in calculating glomerular filtration rate in patients with cirrhosis. *World J. Gastroenterol.* 2011 Oct 28; 17 (40):4532-8.

[17] Collins AJ, Foley RN, Chavers B, Gilbertson D, Herzog C, Johansen K, Kasiske B, Kutner N, Liu J, St Peter W, Guo H, Gustafson S, Heubner B, Lamb K, Li S, Li S, Peng Y, Qiu Y, Roberts T, Skeans M, Snyder J, Solid C, Thompson B, Wang C, Weinhandl E, Zaun D, Arko C, Chen SC, Daniels F, Ebben J, Frazier E, Hanzlik C, Johnson R, Sheets D, Wang X, Forrest B, Constantini E, Everson S, Eggers P, Agodoa L. 'United States Renal Data System 2011 Annual Data Report: Atlas of chronic kidney disease and end-stage renal disease in the United States. *Am. J. Kidney Dis.* 2012 Jan; 59 (1 Suppl 1):A7, e1-420.

[18] Guidelines. http://www.kidney.org/professionals/kdoqi/guidelines_ckd/toc.htm.

[19] Michels WM, Grootendorst DC, Verduijn M, Elliott EG, Dekker FW, Krediet RT. Performance of the Cockcroft-Gault, MDRD, and new CKD-EPI formulas in relation to GFR, age, and body size. *Clin. J. Am. Soc. Nephrol.* 2010 Jun; 5 (6):1003-9. Epub 2010 Mar 18.

[20] http://www.aami.org/publications/HH/Reimbursement.DeOreo.pdf.

[21] Mehta RL, Kellum JA, Shah SV, Molitoris BA, Ronco C, Warnock DG, et al; Acute Kidney Injury Network. Acute Kidney Injury Network: *report of an initiative to improve outcomes in acute kidney injury. Crit Care.* 2007; 11:R31. Available at: http://ccforum.com/content/11/2/R31. Accessed January 12, 2009.

[22] Bellomo R, Ronco C, Kellum JA, Mehta RL, Palevsky P, and the Acute Dialysis Quality Initiative Workgroup. Acute renal failure – definition, outcome measures, animal models, fluid therapy and information technology needs: *the Second International Consensus Conference of the Acute Dialysis Quality Initiative* (ADQI) Group [review] [published online ahead of print May 24, 2004]. *Crit Care.* 2004; 8: R204-R212.

[23] Thompson JA, Lake JR. The impact of MELD allocation on simultaneous liver-kidney transplantation. Curr. Gastroenterol. Rep. 2009 Feb; 11 (1):76-82.

[24] Davis CL, Gonwa TA, Wilkinson AH. Identification of patients best suited for combined liver-kidney transplantation: part II. *Liver Transpl.* 2002 Mar; 8 (3):193-211.

[25] Malinchoc M, Kamath PS, Gordon FD, Peine CJ, Rank J, ter Borg PC. A model to predict poor survival in patients undergoing transjugular intrahepatic portosystemic shunts. *Hepatology.* 2000 Apr;31(4):864-71.

[26] Kamath PS, Wiesner RH, Malinchoc M, Kremers W, Therneau TM, Kosberg CL, D'Amico G, Dickson ER, Kim WR. A model to predict survival in patients with end-stage liver disease. *Hepatology.* 2001 Feb; 33 (2):464-70.

[27] Bosch J, Pizcueta MP, Fernández M, Feu F, Cirera I, Luca A, García-Pagán JC. Hepatic, splanchnic and systemic haemodynamic abnormalities in portal hypertension. *Baillieres Clin. Gastroenterol.* 1992 Sep;6(3):425-36.

[28] Westhuyzen J. Cystatin C: a promising marker and predictor of impaired renal function. Ann. Clin. Lab. Sci. 2006 Autumn; 36 (4):387-94. Review.

[29] Sansoè G, Ferrari A, Castellana CN, Bonardi L, Villa E, Manenti F. Cimetidine administration and tubular creatinine secretion in patients with compensated cirrhosis. *Clin. Sci. (Lond).* 2002 Jan; 102 (1):91-8.

[30] Davis CL, Gonwa TA, Wilkinson AH. Pathophysiology of renal disease associated with liver disorders: implications for liver transplantation. Part I. *Liver Transpl.* 2002 Feb; 8 (2):91-109.

[31] Davis CL, Feng S, Sung R, Wong F, Goodrich NP, Melton LB, Reddy KR, Guidinger MK, Wilkinson A, Lake J. Simultaneous liver-kidney transplantation: evaluation to decision making. *Am. J. Transplant.* 2007 Jul; 7 (7):1702-9. Epub 2007 May 26.

[32] Trotter JF, Brimhall B, Arjal R, Phillips C. Specific laboratory methodologies achieve higher model for endstage liver disease (MELD) scores for patients listed for liver transplantation. *Liver Transpl.* 2004 Aug; 10 (8):995-1000.

[33] Robert A, Chazouillères O. Prothrombin time in liver failure: time, ratio, activity percentage, or international normalized ratio? *Hepatology.* 1996 Dec; 24 (6):1392-4.

[34] Kovacs MJ, Wong A, MacKinnon K, Weir K, Keeney M, Boyle E, Cruickshank M. Assessment of the validity of the INR system for patients with liver impairment. Thromb. Haemost. 1994 Jun; 71 (6): 727-30.

[35] Denson KW, Reed SV, Haddon ME, Woodhams B, Brucato C, Ruiz J. Comparative studies of rabbit and human recombinant tissue factor reagents. *Thromb Res.* 1999 May 15; 94 (4):255-61.

[36] Violi F, Ferro D, Basili S. Coagulopathy of chronic liver disease. *N. Engl. J. Med.* 2011 Oct 13; 365 (15):1453; author reply 1453-4.

[37] Kemperman FA, Weber JA, Gorgels J, van Zanten AP, Krediet RT, Arisz L. The influence of ketoacids on plasma creatinine assays in diabetic ketoacidosis. *J. Intern. Med.* 2000 Dec; 248 (6):511-7.

[38] Ojo AO, Held PJ, Port FK, Wolfe RA, Leichtman AB, Young EW, Arndorfer J, Christensen L, Merion RM. Chronic renal failure after transplantation of a nonrenal organ. N. Engl. J. Med. 2003 Sep 4;349 (10):931-40.

[39] Mindikoglu AL, Raufman JP, Seliger SL, Howell CD, Magder LS. Simultaneous liver-kidney versus liver transplantation alone in patients with end-stage liver disease and kidney dysfunction not on dialysis. *Transplant Proc.* 2011 Sep; 43 (7):2669-77.

[40] Cockcroft DW, Gault MH. Prediction of creatinine clearance from serum creatinine. *Nephron.* 1976; 16 (1):31-41.

[41] U.S. Department of Health and Human Services. HCFA-2728-U4 (4-95). Form Approved: OMB No. 0938-0046, *Health Care Financing Administration.*

[42] Levey AS, Coresh J, Greene T, Stevens LA, Zhang YL, Hendriksen S, Kusek JW, Van Lente F; Chronic Kidney Disease Epidemiology Collaboration. Using standardized serum creatinine values in the modification of diet in renal disease study equation for estimating glomerular filtration rate. *Ann. Intern. Med.* 2006 Aug 15; 145 (4): 247-54.

[43] Levey AS, Stevens LA, Schmid CH, Zhang YL, Castro AF 3rd, Feldman HI, Kusek JW, Eggers P, Van Lente F, Greene T, Coresh J; CKD-EPI (Chronic Kidney Disease Epidemiology Collaboration). A new equation to estimate glomerular filtration rate. *Ann. Intern. Med.* 2009 May 5; 150 (9):604-12.

[44] Murata K, Baumann NA, Saenger AK, Larson TS, Rule AD, Lieske JC. Relative performance of the MDRD and CKD-EPI equations for estimating glomerular filtration rate among patients with varied clinical presentations. Clin. J. Am. Soc. Nephrol. 2011 Aug; 6(8):1963-72. Epub 2011 Jul 7.

[45] Kidney Disease Outcomes Quality Initiative (K/DOQI). K/DOQI clinical practice guidelines on hypertension and antihypertensive agents in chronic kidney disease. *Am. J. Kidney Dis.* 2004 May; 43 (5 Suppl 1):S1-290.

[46] Cameron JS. European best practice guidelines for the management of anaemia in patients with chronic renal failure. *Nephrol. Dial. Transplant.* 1999;14 Suppl 2:61-5.

[47] Eason JD, Gonwa TA, Davis CL, Sung RS, Gerber D, Bloom RD. Proceedings of Consensus Conference on Simultaneous Liver Kidney Transplantation (SLK). *Am. J. Transplant.* 2008 Nov; 8 (11):2243-51. Epub 2008 Sep 19.

[48] Axelrod DA, Koffron AJ, Baker T, Al-Saden P, Dixler I, McNatt G, Sumner S, Vaci M, Abecassis M. The economic impact of MELD on liver transplant centers. *Am. J. Transplant.* 2005 Sep; 5 (9):2297-301.

[49] Locke JE, Warren DS, Singer AL, Segev DL, Simpkins CE, Maley WR, Montgomery RA, Danovitch G, Cameron AM. Declining outcomes in simultaneous liver-kidney transplantation in the MELD era: ineffective usage of renal allografts. *Transplantation* 2008 Apr 15; 85 (7):935-42.

[50] Pichler R, Dittrich MO, Anderson AE *et al.* Prediction of benefit from simultaneous liver–kidney transplantation versus liver-alone transplantation: Potential role for native kidney biopsy. *J. Am. Soc. Nephrol.* 2006; **17**: 795A.

[51] Grubb A, Löfberg H. Human gamma-trace, a basic microprotein: amino acid sequence and presence in the adenohypophysis. *Proc. Natl. Acad. Sci. USA* 1982 May; 79 (9):3024-7.

[52] Fliser D, Ritz E. Serum cystatin C concentration as a marker of renal dysfunction in the elderly. *Am. J. Kidney Dis.* 2001 Jan; 37 (1):79-83.

[53] Dharnidharka VR, Kwon C, Stevens G. Serum cystatin C is superior to serum creatinine as a marker of kidney function: a meta-analysis. *Am. J. Kidney Dis.* 2002 Aug; 40 (2):221-6.

[54] Lamb EJ, O'Riordan SE, Delaney MP. (Cystatin clearance) Kidney function in older people: pathology, assessment and management. Clin. Chim. Acta. 2003 Aug; 334 (1-2):25-40. Review.

[55] Foster J, Reisman W, Lepage N, Filler G. Influence of commonly used drugs on the accuracy of cystatin C-derived glomerular filtration rate. *Pediatr. Nephrol.* 2006 Feb; 21 (2):235-8. Epub 2005 Oct 21.

In: Creatinine
Editors: I. H. Perkins and C. M. Chapman

ISBN: 978-1-62257-475-9

Chapter IV

Evaluation of Renal Function in Patients with Cirrhosis

Evangelos Cholongitas[1], *Elias Xirouchakis*[1], *Evangelos Thalassinos*[1], *Andrew Davenport*[2] *and Andrew K. Burroughs*[1*]

[1]The Royal Free Sheila Sherlock Liver Centre and University Department of Surgery, Royal Free Hospital, London, UK

[2]Department of Renal Medicine, Royal Free Hospital, London, UK

Abstract

Renal function in patients with cirrhosis is an important prognostic factor, both before and following liver transplantation (LT). The importance of renal function is reflected by serum creatinine (Cr) being in the model for end stage liver disease (MELD) score, which predicts the likelihood of death within 3 months for patients on liver transplant waiting lists and is used for prioritization of recipients ("sickest first"). Creatinine is also part of the UKELD score which predicts waiting list mortality over 1 year. Cr is a routine laboratory test and is part of the definitions of acute kidney injury, and hepatorenal syndrome in patients with progressive liver disease. However, it is only an indirect marker of renal function, i.e. of glomerular filtration rate (GFR). Unfortunately, all methods currently in use for assessment of renal function have several limitations and also do not have a good correlation with true GFR. Creatinine estimations are readily available but affected by changes in creatinine generation rate, volume of distribution and assay interference that can affect their interpretation. For example, serum creatinine is dependent upon other factors, including dietary meat, the conversion rate of creatine to creatinine, renal tubular secretion of creatinine, urinary flow rate, hydration status, as well as the total pool of body creatine (total muscle mass). The latter can lead to different Cr concentration between individuals with the same renal function but of different age, race and sex.

* Corresponding Author: Andrew K. Burroughs, FRCP, FMedSci, Professor of Hepatology. Correspondence Address: The Royal Free Sheila Sherlock Liver Centre and Department of Surgery, Royal Free Hospital, Pond Street, Hampstead, London NW3 2QG, UK. Fax Number: 0044 20 74726226, Telephone Number: 0044 20 74726229. E-mail: andrew.burroughs@nhs.net.

Creatinine assays are also subject to interference by chromogens: bilirubin (both conjugated and unconjugated) which typically reduces the creatinine numerical value. In patients with cirrhosis the interference of bilirubin with Cr measurement is a major problem leading to differences in MELD scores up to 7 points, particularly in patients with the highest priority for LT. Modifications to reduce bilirubin interference are used, including enzymatic methods, but these are mostly more expensive and still underestimate creatinine at high bilirubin concentrations..It is important to recognise that there is no universal reference standard for creatinine, and hence, laboratory standardisation of techniques and 'normal' values would be necessary for all liver transplant units to avoid systematic biases in UKELD and MELD-based allocation systems, or others which incorporate Cr values.

Unfortunately, other renal biomarkers, such as cystatin C also have limitations, as cystatin C production is not constant and varies with inflammation. Inulin clearances are impractical in clinical practice. Single bolus isotopic and iodinated radiocontrast methods tend to over estimate "true" GFR in volume expanded patients with ascites, and further inaccuracy is added when attempts are made to correct for body surface area. A recently published modified Tikhonov method may improve isotopic estimation. Further studies are needed in large series of cirrhotic patients to correlate "true" GFR with potential serum or urinary markers, which could result in the creation and validation of more specific mathematical formulae for GFR in patients with cirrhosis.

Abbreviations

MELD:	model for end stage liver disease;
CTP:	Child-Pugh;
Cr:	serum creatinine;
GFR:	glomerular filtration rate;
INR:	international normalised ratio of prothrombin time;
HRS:	Hepatorenal syndrome;
LT:	liver transplantation;
NASH:	non-alcoholic steatohepatitis;
ATN:	acute tubular necrosis;
CKD:	chronic kidney disease;
C-G:	Cockcroft-Gault;
MDRD:	Modification of Diet in Renal Disease;
IDMS:	isotope dilution mass spectroscopy;
CKD-EPI:	Chronic Kidney Disease Epidemiology Collaboration
NGAL:	Neutrophil gelatinase associated lipocalin.

The Prognostic Impact of Renal Dysfunction in Patients with Cirrhosis

Understanding predictive factors for survival in patients with cirrhosis is very useful for therapeutic decision making, including allocation for liver transplantation (LT). Renal dysfunction is strongly associated with increased mortality [1, 2]. Renal function (assessed by serum creatinine estimation) is a well-established independent risk factor predicting mortality in patients with acute or chronic liver disease [3-5], and also following LT and it has a major impact on treatment options for patients with chronic liver disease [6] [7]. This is particularly important, particularly with non-alcoholic steatohepatitis (NASH), which is expected to become the most common indication for LT in the United States, as patients more frequently have raised creatinine and an increased prevalence of chronic kidney disease, compared to other causes aetiologies of chronic liver disease, due to concomitant diabetic nephropathy, hypertensive nephropathy, or renovascular disease [8]. These patients then have more renal dysfunction after LT, which is associated with increased mortality following LT. Renal-sparing immunosuppression regimens after LT may reduce kidney injury, especially in NASH patients [9]. Thus, risk modification is needed to optimize renal function in the pre, peri and postoperative management of LT candidates: this may prevent or delay post-LT end stage renal disease [10]. Lower targets for tacrolimus trough doses have recently been shown to improve graft survival and reduce acute and chronic renal impairment [11].

Hepatorenal syndrome (HRS) is a severe complication of cirrhosis [12]. The definition of HRS uses creatinine both as a major inclusion criteria (> 1.5 mg/dl or 133 umol/l), and also to define HRS type 1 (doubling of creatinine to >2.5 mg/dl within two weeks), and type 2 HRS, which has a slower deterioration in renal function [13]. Survival of patients with cirrhosis and HRS type 1 remains high despite the newer therapies combining terlipressin with daily albumin infusion [13], only approximately 40% respond and survive to 1 month after treatment [14-16]. Patients with HRS who become dependent on haemofiltration (or dialysis) usually remain so until LT or death. Patients with cirrhosis receive therapies and develop complications which increase the risk of renal failure, such as sepsis and hypotensive episodes, which can lead to volume unresponsive acute kidney injury formerly termed acute tubular necrosis (ATN) [16-19].

Table 1. Different methods for estimation of glomerular filtration rate (GFR)

Method	
Clearance of exogenous marker	Inulin Inulin-like polyfructosans Non-radioactive contrast media (iohexol or iothalamate) Radioisotopic methods (^{51}Cr- EDTA, ^{99}Tc-DPTA and ^{125}I-iothalamate)
Serum marker	Creatinine, urea, cystatin C, β_2-microglobin
Creatinine clearance	24h urine collection
Mathematical formulae*	Equations based on serum Cr or Cystatin-C

*For example Cockcroft-Gault (C-G) and Modification of Diet in Renal Disease (MDRD).

C-G: [(140-age (years)) x weight (Kgr)/(0.814 x serum ceatinine (μmol/L)] x (0.85 if female).

MDRD (4-variable) (mL/min/1.73m^2): 186 x [serum creatinine(μmol/L) x 0.0113]$^{-1.154}$ x [age] $^{-0.203}$ x [1.212 if black] x [0.742 if female].

Cr: creatinine.

The Model for End-stage Liver Disease (MELD) is a newer scoring system for severity of liver disease [20], which is used in parallel with the older Child-Pugh (CTP) classification or score [21], or has supplanted it in some centres. The MELD score is considered superior to the Child-Pugh score because it is based on objective and widely available laboratory tests [serum bilirubin, serum creatinine and the international normalised ratio of prothrombin time (INR)] and the incorporation of a marker of renal dysfunction [22]. However, significant variations of MELD score and thus incorrect prioritization for LT occur, due to different laboratory methodologies for INR [23, 24] and serum creatinine (Cr) measurements [25]. In addition, Cr is affect by extra-renal factors, and it is often discrepant in relation to the "true" renal function. Thus, female gender might negatively influence the chances of receiving a liver transplant, compared to men, and Asian candidates have a greater discrepancy between glomerular filtration rate (GFR) and Cr, compared to non-Asian candidates due to differences in body composition, with greater adipose tissue and lower muscle mass [26]. In addition, Cr may weigh too heavily within the MELD score. It is assumed that mortality is constant for Cr less than 1mg/dL or more than 4mg/dL which is likely to be incorrect. A modified MELD score including $\log_e$ [1 + creatinine (mg/dL)] without boundaries and a lower weight for Cr have been proposed [27], but await prospective evaluation. Nevertheless, even after these adjustments, creatinine remains the major prognostic factor in patients with cirrhosis.

Measurement of Glomerular Filtration Rate (Table 1)

Glomerular filtration rate (GFR) is a direct measure of renal function, which becomes abnormal before the onset of symptoms. It correlates with the severity of renal impairment, and is considered the best index of renal function [28]; GFR<60ml/min defines chronic kidney disease (CKD) and represents a 50% or more reduction of normal adult renal function.

Exogenous markers which are only cleared by the kidney are typically considered to be more accurate methods for determining renal function. Inulin clearance is considered as the gold standard for measurement of renal function but cost and technical difficulties limit its use for routine practice [29]. Other direct methods using injected exogenous radiolabelled substances (^{51}Cr-ethylene diamine tetraacetic acid (EDTA), ^{99m}Tc-diethylenetriamine pentaacetate (DPTA) and ^{51}I-iothlamate) or non-radioactive agents (iohexol or iothalamate) are considered as accurate as the inulin clearance method [30]. However all these methods used as the gold standard for measuring GFR, have not been extensively validated in patients with cirrhosis. Indeed in the 2004 British Nuclear Medicine Society Guidelines it is stated that liver failure, ascites, oedema and low clearance status may produce inaccurate clearance values [31] For example ascites has been associated with increased clearance using compartmental models by an average of 16–20 ml/min [32]. Some efforts have been made to overcome these drawbacks, by using delayed sampling but others are needed. For example one of the most important methods to calculate clearance using exogenous markers is ^{51}Cr-EDTA clearance. Typically a single bolus administration is used for ease of use, resulting in an initial peak with redistribution associated with a mono-exponential fall in plasma concentration, as some of the exogenous marker passes from the vascular compartmenting to the interstitial space, which is then followed by a linear decline. However this linear decline is affected by the slower return of the isoptope/marker from the ascitic compartment back into the plasma. GFR is then calculated using the slope-intercept technique, correcting for body surface area, and the fast exponential curve [31]. In patients with cirrhosis, it is necessary to use the three sample method. The ^{51}Cr-EDTA three sample method is performed by sampling blood after single bolus intravenous injection of the tracer at 2, 4, and 6 hours. Another important option to calculate ^{51}Cr-EDTA clearance was developed recently by our group, by the addition of later samples [33]. The clearance method validated used the Tikhonov adaptively regularized gamma variate (Tk-GV) fitting. The Tk-GV results were contrasted with those from mono-exponential fitting. Our results showed that use of Tk-GV has the advantage of increased accuracy for extrapolated clearance while having better precision than that of mono-exponential fitting. It was also significant that the Tk-GV method was valid in patients with liver failure, low GFR and ascites.

Creatinine clearance, using 24 hour urine collections was the standard method for renal function assessment for nephrology patients. However, creatinine clearance underestimates GFR in children and when the serum creatinine levels are high, where re-absorption from the tubules is greater [34]. In adults, creatinine clearance usually overestimates "true" GFR based on inulin clearance. Its limitations are associated not only with the use of serum creatinine in the mathematical equation [$(\text{Urine}_{Cr} \times V_{urine})/\text{Serum}_{Cr}$], but also with the influence of several factors which increase tubular creatinine secretion, including proteinuria, diet (a meat stew, or high meat protein meal can increase 24-hour creatinine clearance by 37%) and extra-renal elimination of creatinine by micro-organisms [35]. Interestingly, a new steady state of creatinine excretion is only achieved after four months following any change in the body creatinine pool. In addition, there may be up to 25% variation in GFR estimation based on creatinine clearance [34], due to incomplete urine collection, errors in urine volume measurements, variations in tubular excretion or re-absorption of creatinine, serum creatinine dilution due to increased fluid retention and other unpredictable factors [28, 36, 37]. Particularly in cirrhosis, creatinine clearance overestimates the "true" GFR [38], due to a combination of the increased proportion of creatinine secreted by the tubule, compared to creatinine filtered by the glomerulus during cirrhosis, and serum creatinine dilution. Thus, there is no evidence that creatinine clearance is superior to serum creatinine in determining renal function in cirrhosis.

To overcome some of the limitations of 24h urine collection, a number of different mathematical formulae have been developed, which incorporate serum creatinine to provide an estimation of GFR (eGFR) trying to overcome some of these limitations of creatinine clearance-based GFR estimation. However, these formulae were developed for a chronic kidney disease population, and not for patients with chronic liver disease, and such have not been validated. These formulae are increasingly used and include the Cockcroft-Gault (C-G) [39] and Modification of Diet in Renal Disease (MDRD) [40] formulae. Others, such as Nankivell, Gates, Jelliffe, Walser, Levey and Wright are recommended for use in particular patients groups. The C-G formula requires serum creatinine, weight, gender and age. The C-G eGFR is within 20% of the reference procedure, which was a duplicate creatinine clearance measured in the original study for GFR estimation. However, only 4% of the reference cohort were women and creatinine was measured on Technicon autoanalyser using Jaffe reagent. This formula does not take into account the ethnic variation in muscle mass. MDRD formula [40] incorporates serum creatinine, ethnicity, gender and age (MDRD-4), or creatinine, ethnicity, gender, age, albumin and urea (MDRD-6). Thus, in contrast to C-G formula, a body weight variable (which is difficult to assess as lean body mass in ascitic and malnourished patients) is not needed, and it uses ethnicity, gender and age and is calculated for 1.73m^2 body surface area; estimated GFR is within 30% of the reference procedure which was ^{125}Iothalamate in 90% of patients (the creatinine measurement used was kinetic Jaffe on Beckman Astra CX3). The accuracy of MDRD has been only estimated on a large scale in patients with CKD. In cirrhosis, although there is discrepancy when compared to ^{125}I-iothalamate [41], MDRD-6 is considered a more accurate formula, compared to C-G, possibly because it incorporates urea and albumin, which are abnormal in cirrhotics and it excludes body weight, a variable which may be difficult to assess in malnourished patients with ascites [42]. However the MDRD-4 formula is typically used to calculate eGFR, as it was as accurate as the original six-variable formula in population screening [43]. However, its usefulness has not been proven in healthy individuals [42, 44], and its accuracy may be lower in specific clinical settings. For example, MDRD is not applicable in children. For the latter, Coulahan-Barratt and Schwartz formulae are considered more accurate [42] and may be superior to ^{99}Tc-DPTA [45]. In kidney transplant patients, the Walser and Jelliffe formulae have been shown to be superior to MDRD [46, 47].

In cirrhosis, C-G and both MDRD formulae typically overestimate true GFR, particularly in those patients below 50 years or with ascites [48]. The MDRD formulae have been reported to overestimate GFR, compared to "true" GFR values of <40 mL/min prior to LT(42). Due to inaccuracies of the MDRD-4 equation in determining renal function in patients with an eGFR>60 ml/min, a new creatinine-based equation known as the Chronic Kidney Disease Epidemiology Collaboration (CKD-EPI) equation, using the same variables with MDRD-4 formula, has been proposed, but its superiority in patients with cirrhosis has not as yet been proven [49]. Nevertheless, the use of such formulae does not overcome the limitations in serum Cr measurement. It has been recommended that creatinine results used for calculating eGFR should be traceable to an isotope dilution mass spectroscopy (IDMS) reference method, and new methods have been developed for the faster and simpler quantification of creatinine, but require further validation [50]. In addition, these formulae have several intrinsic drawbacks due to limitations inherent in the original cohorts from which they were derived (for example the C-G formula was developed in cohorts of healthy men, and might not be suitable in women or other groups of patients) [37, 51]. Importantly, neither C-G nor MDRD were developed in patients with cirrhosis [44, 47]. Recently, we have developed new mathematical formulae specific for patients with cirrhosis, in which we incorporated CTP score [52] and ascites. These formulae showed better agreement with "true" GFR, compared to MDRD formulae, but further validation is needed for final conclusions. Finally, estimates for eGFR are also unreliable in non-steady states, such as acute kidney injury and also muscle wasting disorders due to changing kinetics for creatinine generation and accumulation [53].

Serum Creatinine for Evaluation of Renal Function in Cirrhosis

Creatinine measurement is an inaccurate marker of GFR, partly because creatinine assays are subject to interference by chromogens, bilirubin (both conjugated and unconjugated) typically reducing the numerical value, and making Cr an even less precise surrogate of GFR in jaundiced patients. A modified colourimetric Jaffe reaction is used in most laboratories, which is simple and relatively inexpensive: Cr reacts with alkaline picrate to form an orange red complex (Janovski complex) and is measured spectrophotometrically at 520nm. It is simple, automatized and relatively low cost, and thus used widely. Several modifications have been developed to reduce chromogens, such as bilirubin, glucose, uric acid, ketoacids, pyruvate, and certain antibiotics, which interfere with the Jaffe reaction (including the kinetic alkaline picrate method), and also the introduction of enzymatic methods (using creatininases and creatininase hydrolases), to separate these chromogens, such as acid blanking and absorption techniques with Fuller's earth or Lloyd's reagent, or delayed rate reactions. However, these are laborious and unsuitable for routine use. The kinetic alkaline picrate method is sometimes used giving a differential rate of colour development between Cr and non-creatinine chromogens. Sarcosine is the end product, oxidised to glycine, formaldehyde and hydrogen peroxide. The latter forms a chromogen, the colour intensity being proportional to the starting creatinine.

Dry chemistry systems (e.g. Ortho Diagnostics) are less prone to chromogen interference, but are not suitable for large scale use, are costly, and the equipment is less available. The negative interference of bilirubin, both conjugated and unconjugated, in serum or plasma creatinine measurements by both Jaffe and enzymatic methods is an additional unresolved problem in patients with liver disease. Deproteinisation of samples prior to analysis, has been tried as well as increasing the picrate concentration, use of bilirubin oxidase or addition of potassium ferricyanide, to overcome this in the Jaffe reaction. We recently showed [25] that interference occurs with bilirubin concentrations >62 μmol/L (3.68 mg/dL), resulting in significant differences in Cr values between different methods (modified Jaffe, compensated kinetic Jaffe, enzymatic and standard Jaffe). The standard Jaffe method had the greatest interference with bilirubin, and the modified Jaffe method (addition of potassium ferricyanide) the least interference. Nevertheless, all laboratory assays for Cr gave rise to significantly different MELD scores. If differences in MELD score are only 1-2 points, then this has little clinical impact, but differences of 3 or 4 points which are seen with bilirubin concentrations between 100 μmol/L (5.85 mg/dL) and 200 μmol/L (11.6 mg/dL) are clinically relevant: this interference can result in differences in up to 7 MELD points when bilirubin is >23.4 mg/dL, i.e. those with the highest priority for LT. These results showed that the particular creatinine assay, used in MELD scoring should be taken into account as some patients inadvertently will be discriminated against with respect to others, in terms of priority on a LT waiting list. Similarly starting appropriate therapy with terlipressin could be delayed in a patient with hepatorenal syndrome, whilst awaiting the serum creatinine to reach 1.5 mg/dL [30].

A further problem associated with accuracy and precision of Cr measurements is a lack of universal standard for creatinine. In the UK, National Health Service (NHS) laboratories were sent IDMS standards to develop their correction factors for their own assay. However IDMS standards do not allow for interfering chromogens, and as such there were marked differences in creatinine determination between UK laboratories for patients with chronic liver disease placed on liver transplant waiting lists [54]. In addition, these inaccuracies affect the calculation of MDRD, for which the creatinine measurement method was the Beckman CX3 Jaffe assay [55]. Recently, reporting of estimated GFR, based on MDRD, has been recommended internationally [55]. The IDMS traceable MDRD equation, improves the estimate of GFR when using assays that account for chromogen interference [55].

Creatinine has high specificity but low sensitivity for detection of chronic kidney disease (CKD) [34, 37, 51]. An additional limitation of GFR assessment based on serum creatinine is the fact that, although normally there is a decline in GFR with ageing, there are no differences in creatinine values in the reported normal range between healthy elderly and younger people [53, 56], again suggesting a poor correlation of creatinine with renal function. In addition, creatinine is an insensitive marker for the assessment of severity of acute kidney injury , since anuric patients may have only a modest increase of serum creatinine , even if GFR is almost zero [51]. In fact, most studies have evaluated the correlation between creatinine and GFR in patients with CKD, and not acute kidney injury.

In patients with cirrhosis there are additional reasons why Cr is inadequate for assessment of renal function. These are: a) decreased hepatic production of creatine (reduction in creatine pool), b) the oedematous state with ascites as complication of end stage liver disease, leading to a larger distribution of creatinine in the body and lower serum creatinine concentration [51] and c) use of drugs such as cephalosporins (used as they are non-nephrotoxic) and calcitriol, which affect the tubular secretion of Cr [51]. As a result, in a recent meta-analysis, GFR estimation by inulin clearance was proposed as the only way for accurate assessment of renal function [38], but this remains impractical for routine clinical use.

Factors Affecting Accurate Assessment of Glomerular Filtration Rate (GFR) in Cirrhosis (Tables 2 and 3)

a) Limitations of Exogenous Markers

Clearance of exogenous markers for estimating GFR remains the best method, but these are expensive and impractical for routine clinical use. There are also technical difficulties and potential errors when a single bolus administration is used due to extra-renal clearance, or redistribution of tracer from the plasma volume, leading to an overestimation of plasma clearance compared to renal plasma clearance of about 3.7 ml/min [32].

This overestimation of GFR is higher in patients with oedema, ascites and pleural effusions because of abnormal volumes of distribution, and also can be affected by circulation time. In addition, in patients with cirrhosis and ascites there is redistribution of contrast dye or radionucleotide tracer into the ascitic fluid, and then return of the marker from the ascitic fluid back into the plasma, so changing the slope of the steady part of the decay curve. Thus, bolus administration of exogenous markers tends to over estimate GFR in cirrhosis, by up to 20 ml/min [32], although this could potentially be overcome in part by taking delayed samples.

To exclude these errors, studies have shown that inulin clearance using a constant infusion technique is more reliable than bolus administration [57]. Although, as inulin is a relatively small molecule, it readily redistributes into ascites but then take several hours to fully re-equilibrate and achieve a constant plasma concentration.

These potential errors in estimation of GFR are then compounded when the GFR is corrected for body surface area, as this assumes a normal underlying body composition, whereas patients with cirrhosis and ascites typically have protein energy wasting in keeping with other chronic diseases [58].

Thus, it is not surprising that most studies have shown that these radiocontrast dye and isotopic nucleotides methods also tend to overestimate renal function when compared to inulin infusion clearance measured by constant infusion [57], rather than bolus technique [59]. However the constant inulin infusion technique is based on a stable plasma inulin concentration so that inulin recovered in timed urine collections can be used to estimate GFR. This "gold standard" technique is however time consuming, costly and potentially invasive if bladder catheterisation is required.

Table 2. Characteristics of the established methods for renal function assessment

	Advantages	Disadvantages
Serum marker		
Cr	Widely available	high specificity but low sensitivity for detection of CKD is influenced by several factors unrelated to renal function not early detection of acute renal failure Unreliable in particular group, such as cirrhotics Absence of standardization of the laboratory method Particularly in cirrhotics: is influenced by bilirubin
Clearance of exogenous marker	"gold standard"	technical difficulties expensive impractical for routine use not available in all countries unreliable in patients with oedema, ascites and pleural effusions
Clearance of endogenous marker		
Creatinine (24h urine collection)	More accurate compared to Cr	underestimates GFR in children inconvenient, unpleasant overestimates GFR in proteinuria and renal dysfunction influenced by muscle metabolism and diet, inflammatory disease and malnutrition 25% unexplained variation due to incomplete urine collection and errors in urine volume measurement In cirrhosis: overestimation of GFR
Mathematical formulae based on Cr	easier method compared to 24hr urine collection	The accuracy may be lower in specific clinical settings (none of these have been developed in cirrhotics) unreliable in acute renal failure, muscle wasting disorders Does not overcome the limitations in serum Cr
C-G formula	requires only gender, age, body weight	Not take into account the ethnicity
MDRD formula	body weight is not needed ethnicity, gender and age are taken into account	Has not been extensively validated in patients without CKD 6-variables formula: needs albumin, urea

GFR: glomerular filtration rate, Cr: serum creatinine, C-G: Cockcroft-Gault, MDRD: Modification of Diet in Renal Disease, CKD: chronic kidney disease.

Table 3. Studies comparing different methods for assessment of renal function with a "gold standard" method in cirrhotic patients

Author	Number of patients	"Gold standard" GFR mean±SD (ml/min)	Findings
Proulx NL et al [38], 2005 (meta-analysis)	193	Inulin	Creatinine clearance (24h urine collection) overestimates GFR (particularly in low GFR)
Gonwa T et al [41], 2004	1447	^{125}I-iothalamate (90.7±40.5)	MDRD, C-G: over- and underestimate renal function in GFR<40min/ml and GFR>40ml/min, respectively. MDRD better than C-G
Woitas RP et al [72], 2000	44	Inulin	Cys-C more sensitive than Cr to detect reduced GFR
Orlando R et al 2002 [73]*	36 cirrhotics 56 controls	Inulin	Cys-C more sensitive than Cr and Cr clearance (in both groups)
Demitras S et al [79], 2001	(hepatorenal syndrome) 27	Tc^{99}-DTPA	Cys-C had better correlation with GFR, compared to Cr and Cr clearance
Samyn M et al [86], 2005	62 children	^{51}Cr-EDTA	Cys-C better correlation with GFR, compared to Cr
Poge U et al [83], 2006	44	Inulin (28.3 ml/min/1.73m^2)	Cr and Cys-C overestimate GFR
Skluzacek PA et al [87], 2003		^{125}I-iothalamate (58.2 ±5.1)	MDRD and C-G overestimate GFR MDRD superior to C-G
MacAulay T et al [88], 2006	57	Tc^{99}-DTPA (83 ml/min/1.73m^2	MDRD better correlation and agreement with GFR, compared to G-C and 100/Cr. All methods overestimate GFR

GFR: glomerular filtration rate, Cr: serum creatinine, Cys-C: Cystatin C, C-G: Cockcroft-Gault, MDRD: Modification of Diet in Renal Disease.

* this study is included in the meta-analysis by Proulx NL et al.

GFR is traditionally corrected for body surface area based on standard equations, which assume a fixed ratio of muscle mass to body surface area [60]. Although correction factors can be used to compensate for sex, age [61] and race [62], these equations basically assume a normal distribution of body fat and muscle, whereas patients with cirrhosis may not only have increased weight due to ascitic fluid, but also loss of body fat and muscle mass consequent upon chronic liver disease and protein energy wasting, so adding additional errors to the estimation of GFR.

b) Limitations of Endogenous Markers

a) Factors Affecting Serum Creatinine

Creatinine is an end product of metabolism of creatine in humans. Creatine is released from the liver, is taken up by muscle and non-enzymatically dehydrated to creatinine [28]. Thus, serum creatinine is also dependent upon other extra-renal factors, such as the total pool of body creatine (total muscle mass) [28], physical activity and dietary meat intake, leading to differences in serum creatinine measurements between individuals with the same renal function (same GFR), but of different ages sex, races, body mass index or having concomitant chronic catabolic disease (e.g. malignancy, cirrhosis, inflammation and endocrinopathies [28]. Thus, women typically have lower creatinine values compared to men with the same renal function [63] and the elderly may have overestimation of their renal residual function, compared to younger individuals.

In the UNOS database(64), although women were listed with lower median MELD scores, compared to men (14 vs 15, $p<0.001$), they were more likely to die waiting in the post-MELD era, compared to the pre-MELD one. These findings cannot be explained solely by the difficulty in finding a suitable graft for women due to their smaller size [65, 66]. However, this can be partially explained by considering that the creatinine values in women represent a worse GFR than in men, for the same creatinine value [64, 67]. Thus, we believe that the potential gender bias, we highlighted [67], and reported by others [64], could partially explain a systematic bias, although other factors should be considered [68]. Correcting creatinine by equalising the GFR between men and women resulted in an increase in MELD score by 2 or 3 points in 65% of female LT candidates in our study [67]. Huo S et al [69], confirmed that, compared to females, male patients had a higher MELD (14.5+/-5.5 vs. 13.8+/-5.7) and significantly higher GFR (61.7+/-21.4 vs. 54.7+/-25.6 mL/min, $p=0.0002$) because their creatinine value was higher (1.4+/-0.4 vs. 1.3+/-0.5 mg/dL, $P=0.0002$). In addition, using the methodology from our report [67], they also found that [69] these discrepancies have a significant effect on MELD score calculation and may influence waiting list mortality: a corrected-Cr MELD score, which would prioritize female patients for liver transplantation, may better predict intermediate-term (9- and 12-month) mortality. Thus, a score corrected for female candidates (MELD-gender) was suggested [69]. Similarly, ethnicity may also affect serum creatinine estimations, as larger muscle mass in Afro-Caribbean patients, and phenotypic variations in creatinine production lead to increased GFR for the same creatinine, compared to other ethnic groups, whereas South Asians have lower GFR (lower muscle mass) [37, 51]. An acute deterioration in renal function in patients with acute or chronic liver disease, particularly following acute complications, such as sepsis [3-5], and also following LT, is strongly associated with increased mortality [1, 2] [11]. Under these circumstances, creatinine is an even more unreliable indicator of reduced GFR. Acute renal failure in cirrhotics usually develops on the basis of complications such as variceal bleeding, spontaneous bacterial peritonitis or sepsis, conditions that are related to increased creatinine tubular excretion [28]. The latter, combined with the underestimation of renal dysfunction of creatinine in stable cirrhotic patients, can lead to a great discrepancy between the creatinine and severity of renal dysfunction.

Alternatives for Evaluation of Renal Function (Table 3)

Cystatin C

Serum cystatin C is a low molecular weight protein functioning as an extracellular inhibitor of cysteine proteases [70]. It was originally thought that cystatin C was produced at the same rate by all nucleated cells. Cystatin C is freely filtered by the renal glomeruli and subsequently metabolized in the proximal tubules. Given these features, and its initial reported independence from age, gender and body composition [71]. It was considered a more sensitive indicator of renal function compared to creatinine, in several disease groups including cirrhosis [72] [73]. Consequently several cystatin C based GFR equations have been derived [74]. Despite being more accurate than creatinine based formulas [75] they still lack significant correlation with direct methods of GFR estimation. Indeed, cystatin C has been reported to be affected by a host of factors including inflammation [76] body composition, proteinuria, cardiovascular risk factors [77] [78], infection, thyroid dysfunction, underlying malignancy, smoking and a number of drugs; including corticosteroids, cotrimoxazole, angiotensin converting enzyme inhibitors, and calcineurin inhibitors. Cystatin C has been proposed as a marker of liver disease stage [79] as it correlates with bilirubin, albumin, INR and platelet count and increases with CTP stage [80]. As cirrhosis evolves the increasing cystatin C values may be related to increased production, secondary to active inflammatory and fibrotic processes, or decreased clearance due to reduced renal function. Such involvement has not been addressed in the initial studies and all existing cystatin C equations had been derived from non liver disease populations [81] [82]. Recently two studies evaluated the cystatin C GFR formulas in patients with cirrhosis [83] [52]. In the first study which included 44 patients with cirrhosis [83] the cystatin C formulas were more accurate than the creatinine formulas, but had significantly different values of GFR in comparison to inulin clearance. On the other hand, we showed [52] that serum cystatin C formulas not only significantly overestimated renal clearance compared with ^{51}Cr-EDTA but did not provide a sufficient improvement over serum creatinine formulas in reflecting renal function in 74 patients with cirrhosis. Multivariate analysis showed that the presence of ascites significantly affected serum cystatin C values. Also each cystatin C formula overestimated renal clearance significantly in comparison to ^{51}Cr-EDTA for the subgroup of patients with the measured ^{51}Cr-EDTA GFR of less than 70ml/min/1.73m^2. Thus, since existing cystatin C formulas do not reflect 'true' GFR with great accuracy in cirrhosis, more studies are required to elucidate it's usefulness as a marker of GFR and to develop accurate GFR formulae. In cirrhosis there needs to be good evidence that cystatin C has significant advantages over creatinine to recommend it's use. This is particularly so when the GFR falls below $<$70ml/min/1.73^2 which is known to have an adverse impact on prognosis both before [5] [4] and after LT [2].

Just as there is no gold standard method of creatinine measurement, there are now a number of currently available commercially available cystatin C assays for which also there is no gold standard method. Indeed even using the same assay, different results may be obtained with different platforms, and thus a consensus is needed for standardisation of cystatin C assays.

Neutrophil Gelatinase Associated Lipocalin (NGAL)

Acute tubular necrosis is a life threatening complication in cirrhosis characterized by severe alterations in renal tubular cells caused mainly by hypovolaemia, sepsis or medications. The differential diagnosis of ATN is often particularly challenging. Neutrophil gelatinase associated lipocalin (NGAL) has been recently evaluated as an early marker of tubular dysfunction. Several studies in the general population showed that NGAL increases in urine or plasma at the time of injury to tubular cells and it can be used to aid the differential diagnosis between ATN and volume responsive causes of acute kidney injury, such as pre-renal azotemia. Urinary neutrophil gelatinase-associated lipocalin distinguishes pre-renal from intrinsic renal failure and predicts outcomes, as it not only reflects renal tubular injury but is also a marker of the host systemic inflammatory response. After initial promising reports of superiority to other known kidney biomarkers including creatinine [84] more recent reports have failed to support such initial promising results, especially when tested in patients with pre-existing CKD.

Its usefulness in cirrhosis has been investigated in 241 patients [85]. Both urinary and plasma levels of NGAL were measured. Patients were classified into three groups namely, without ascites, with ascites but without kidney dysfunction and finally with ascites and kidney dysfunction. Patients with kidney dysfunction irrespective of its cause had higher levels of NGAL compared to those without kidney dysfunction with or without the presence of ascites. Urinary NGAL levels were increased significantly in patients with cirrhosis and ATN (median values 417, range 239-2242 μg/g creatinine) compared to those with other causes of acute impairment of kidney function, like HRS (not associated with active infections), pre-renal azotemia due to volume depletion, and CKD. However, plasma levels of NGAL were not helpful in the differential diagnosis of kidney dysfunction. Regarding active infections, urine NGAL levels are significantly increased with urinary tract infections, and plasma NGAL in other infections are no different, compared to patients without infections. Thus, NGAL as a marker, especially in the differential diagnosis between ATN and HRS associated with infections, is problematic as differences were no longer significant. However among patients with ATN there were no significant differences according to the cause (hypovolaemia or infection). Therefore, larger multicentre trials are awaited to determine the role of urinary NGAL, and newer markers of acute kidney injury, such as kidney injury molecule 1 (KIM-1) and urinary Il-18 excretion. It may be that a panel of markers might provide an earlier warning of deterioration in kidney function than changes in serum creatinine, or one biomarker alone.

Financial Disclosure

None.

References

[1] Baliga P, Merion RM, Turcotte JG, Ham JM, Henley KS, Lucey MR, et al. Preoperative risk factor assessment in liver transplantation. *Surgery* 1992 Oct; 112(4):704-710.

[2] Gonwa TA, McBride MA, Anderson K, Mai ML, Wadei H, Ahsan N. Continued Influence of Preoperative Renal Function on Outcome of Orthotopic Liver Transplant (OLTX) in the US: Where Will MELD Lead Us? *Am. J. Transplant.* 2006 Aug 29;6: 2651-2659.

[3] Cardenas A, Gines P, Uriz J, Bessa X, Salmeron JM, Mas A, et al. Renal failure after upper gastrointestinal bleeding in cirrhosis: incidence, clinical course, predictive factors, and short-term prognosis. *Hepatology* 2001 Oct;34(4 Pt 1):671-676.

[4] Fraley DS, Burr R, Bernardini J, Angus D, Kramer DJ, Johnson JP. Impact of acute renal failure on mortality in end-stage liver disease with or without transplantation. *Kidney Int.* 1998 Aug;54(2):518-524.

[5] Terra C, Guevara M, Torre A, Gilabert R, Fernandez J, Martin-Llahi M, et al. Renal failure in patients with cirrhosis and sepsis unrelated to spontaneous bacterial peritonitis: value of MELD score. *Gastroenterology* 2005 Dec;129(6):1944-1953.

[6] Belcher JM, Garcia-Tsao G, Sanyal AJ, Bhogal H, Lim JK, Ansari N, et al. Association of AKI with mortality and complications in hospitalized patients with cirrhosis. *Hepatology* 2012 Mar 27.

[7] Cholongitas E, Calvaruso V, Senzolo M, Patch D, Shaw S, O'Beirne J, Burroughs AK. Rifle classification as predictive factor mortality in patients with cirrhosis admitted to ICU. *Journal Gastroenterol. Hepatol.* 2009 24(10):1639-47.

[8] Park CW, Tsai NT, Wong LL. Implications of worse renal dysfunction and medical comorbidities in patients with NASH undergoing liver transplant evaluation: impact on MELD and more. *Clin. Transplant.* 2011 Nov;25(6):E606-E611.

[9] Houlihan DD, Armstrong MJ, Davidov Y, Hodson J, Nightingale P, Rowe IA, et al. Renal function in patients undergoing transplantation for nonalcoholic steatohepatitis cirrhosis: time to reconsider immunosuppression regimens? *Liver Transpl.* 2011 Nov; 17(11):1292-1298.

[10] Sharma P, Schaubel DE, Guidinger MK, Goodrich NP, Ojo AO, Merion RM. Impact of MELD-based allocation on end-stage renal disease after liver transplantation. *Am. J. Transplant.* 2011 Nov;11(11):2372-2378.

[11] Rodriguez-Peralvareza M, Germani G, Darius T, Lerut J, Tsochatzis E, Burroughs A. Tacrolimus Trough Levels, Rejection and Renal Impairment in Liver Transplantation: A Systematic Review and Metaanalysis. *Am. J. Transplant.* 2012;in press.

[12] Gines P, Guevara M, Arroyo V, Rodes J. Hepatorenal syndrome. *Lancet* 2003 Nov 29; 362(9398):1819-1827.

[13] Sanyal AJ, Boyer T, Garcia-Tsao G, Regenstein F, Rossaro L, Appenrodt B, et al. A randomized, prospective, double-blind, placebo-controlled trial of terlipressin for type 1 hepatorenal syndrome. *Gastroenterology* 2008 May;134(5):1360-1368.

[14] Arroyo V, Terra C, Gines P. New treatments of hepatorenal syndrome. *Semin. Liver Dis.* 2006 Aug;26(3):254-264.

[15] Moreau R, Durand F, Poynard T, Duhamel C, Cervoni JP, Ichai P, et al. Terlipressin in patients with cirrhosis and type 1 hepatorenal syndrome: a retrospective multicenter study. *Gastroenterology* 2002 Apr;122(4):923-930.

[16] Pham PT, Pham PC, Rastogi A, Wilkinson AH. Review article: current management of renal dysfunction in the cirrhotic patient. *Aliment. Pharmacol. Ther.* 2005 Apr 15;21(8):949-961.

[17] Fasolato S, Angeli P, Dallagnese L, Maresio G, Zola E, Mazza E, et al. Renal failure and bacterial infections in patients with cirrhosis: epidemiology and clinical features. *Hepatology* 2007 Jan;45(1):223-229.

[18] Moller S, Henriksen JH. Review article: pathogenesis and pathophysiology of hepatorenal syndrome--is there scope for prevention? *Aliment. Pharmacol. Ther.* 2004 Sep;20 Suppl 3:31-41.

[19] Sort P, Navasa M, Arroyo V, Aldeguer X, Planas R, Ruiz-del-Arbol L, et al. Effect of intravenous albumin on renal impairment and mortality in patients with cirrhosis and spontaneous bacterial peritonitis. *N. Engl. J. Med.* 1999 Aug 5;341(6):403-409.

[20] Wiesner RH. Patient selection in an era of donor liver shortage: current US policy. *Nature Clinical Practice in Gastroenterology and Hepatology* 2005;2(1):24-30.

[21] Pugh R, Murray-lyon I, Dawson J. Transcection of the oesophagus for bleeding oesophageal varices. *Br. J. Surg.* 1973;60:646-649.

[22] Durand F, Valla D. Assessment of the prognosis of cirrhosis: Child-Pugh versus MELD. *J. Hepatol.* 2005;42 Suppl(1):S100-S107.

[23] Trotter JF, Brimhall B, Arjal R, Phillips C. Specific laboratory methodologies achieve higher model for endstage liver disease (MELD) scores for patients listed for liver transplantation. *Liver Transpl.* 2004 Aug;10(8):995-1000.

[24] Porte RJ, Lisman T, Tripodi A, Caldwell SH, Trotter JF. The International Normalized Ratio (INR) in the MELD score: problems and solutions. *Am. J. Transplant.* 2010 Jun;10(6):1349-1353.

[25] Cholongitas E, Marelli L, Kerry A, Senzolo M, Goodier D, Nair D, et al. Different methods of creatinine measurement significantly affect MELD scores. *Liver Transpl.* 2007;13(4):523-529.

[26] Cholongitas E, Germani G, Burroughs AK. Prioritization for liver transplantation. *Nat. Rev. Gastroenterol. Hepatol.* 2010 Dec;7(12):659-668.

[27] Sharma P, Schaubel DE, Sima CS, Merion RM, Lok AS. Re-weighting the model for end-stage liver disease score components. *Gastroenterology* 2008 Nov;135(5): 1575-1581.

[28] Levey AS, Perrone RD, Madias NE. Serum creatinine and renal function. *Annu. Rev. Med.* 1988;39:465-490.

[29] De Santo NG, Capasso G, Anastasio P, Coppola S, Policastro M, Bellini L, et al. Renal functional reserve. *Child Nephrol. Urol.* 1991;11(3):140-145.

[30] Davenport A, Cholongitas E, Xirouchakis E, Burroughs AK. Pitfalls in assessing renal function in patients with cirrhosis--potential inequity for access to treatment of hepatorenal failure and liver transplantation. *Nephrol. Dial Transplant.* 2011 Sep;26(9): 2735-2742.

[31] Fleming JS, Nunan TO. The new BNMS guidelines for measurement of glomerular filtration rate. *Nucl. Med. Commun.* 2004 Aug;25(8):755-757.

[32] Henriksen JH, Brochner-Mortensen J, Malchow-Moller A, Schlichting P. Over-estimation of glomerular filtration rate by single injection [51Cr]EDTA plasma clearance determination in patients with ascites. *Scand. J. Clin. Lab. Invest.* 1980 May; 40(3):279-284.

[33] Wesolowski CA, Ling L, Xirouchakis E, Burniston MT, Puetter RC, Babyn PS, et al. Validation of Tikhonov adaptively regularized gamma variate fitting with 24-h plasma clearance in cirrhotic patients with ascites. *Eur. J. Nucl. Med. Mol. Imaging* 2011 Dec; 38(12):2247-2256.

[34] Lamb EJ, Tomson CR, Roderick PJ. Estimating kidney function in adults using formulae. *Ann. Clin. Biochem.* 2005 Sep;42(Pt 5):321-345.

[35] Hood B, Attman PO, Ahlmen J, Jagenburg R. Renal hemodynamics and limitations of creatinine clearance in determining filtration rate in glomerular disease. *Scand. J. Urol. Nephrol.* 1971;5(2):154-161.

[36] Goldberg TH, Finkelstein MS. Difficulties in estimating glomerular filtration rate in the elderly. *Arch. Intern. Med.* 1987 Aug;147(8):1430-1433.

[37] Lamb EJ, O'Riordan SE, Delaney MP. Kidney function in older people: pathology, assessment and management. *Clin. Chim. Acta* 2003 Aug;334(1-2):25-40.

[38] Proulx NL, Akbari A, Garg AX, Rostom A, Jaffey J, Clark HD. Measured creatinine clearance from timed urine collections substantially overestimates glomerular filtration rate in patients with liver cirrhosis: a systematic review and individual patient meta-analysis. *Nephrol. Dial Transplant.* 2005 Aug;20(8):1617-1622.

[39] Cockcroft DW, Gault MH. Prediction of creatinine clearance from serum creatinine. *Nephron* 1976;16(1):31-41.

[40] Levey AS, Bosch JP, Lewis JB, Greene T, Rogers N, Roth D. A more accurate method to estimate glomerular filtration rate from serum creatinine: a new prediction equation. Modification of Diet in Renal Disease Study Group. *Ann. Intern. Med.* 1999 Mar 16; 130(6):461-470.

[41] Gonwa TA, Jennings L, Mai ML, Stark PC, Levey AS, Klintmalm GB. Estimation of glomerular filtration rates before and after orthotopic liver transplantation: evaluation of current equations. *Liver Transpl.* 2004 Feb;10(2):301-309.

[42] Myers GL, Miller WG, Coresh J, Fleming J, Greenberg N, Greene T, et al. Recommendations for Improving Serum Creatinine Measurement: A Report from the Laboratory Working Group of the National Kidney Disease Education Program. *Clin. Chem.* 2006 Mar 23.

[43] Levey AS, Coresh J, Greene T, Stevens LA, Zhang YL, Hendriksen S, et al. Using standardized serum creatinine values in the modification of diet in renal disease study equation for estimating glomerular filtration rate. *Ann. Intern. Med.* 2006 Aug 15; 145(4):247-254.

[44] Rule AD, Larson TS, Bergstralh EJ, Slezak JM, Jacobsen SJ, Cosio FG. Using serum creatinine to estimate glomerular filtration rate: accuracy in good health and in chronic kidney disease. *Ann. Intern. Med.* 2004 Dec 21;141(12):929-937.

[45] Kletzel M, Pirich L, Haut P, Cohn RA. Comparison of Tc-99 measurement of glomerular filtration rate vs. calculated creatinine clearance to assess renal function pretransplant in pediatric patients undergoing hematopoietic stem cell transplantation. *Pediatr. Transplant.* 2005 Oct;9(5):584-588.

[46] Gaspari F, Ferrari S, Stucchi N, Centemeri E, Carrara F, Pellegrino M, et al. Performance of different prediction equations for estimating renal function in kidney transplantation. *Am. J. Transplant.* 2004 Nov;4(11):1826-1835.

[47] Mariat C, Alamartine E, Barthelemy JC, De Filippis JP, Thibaudin D, Berthoux P, et al. Assessing renal graft function in clinical trials: can tests predicting glomerular filtration rate substitute for a reference method? *Kidney Int.* 2004 Jan;65(1):289-297.

[48] Rognant N Bacchetta J, Dubourg L, Ahmed SN, Radenne S, Dumortier J, Hadj-Aïssa A. What is the best alternative to inulin clearance to estimate GFR in patients with decompensated alcoholic cirrhosis? *Nephrol. Dial Transplant.* 2010; 25(11):3569-75.

[49] Gerhardt T, Poge U, Stoffel-Wagner B, Palmedo H, Sauerbruch T, Woitas RP. Creatinine-based glomerular filtration rate estimation in patients with liver disease: the

new Chronic Kidney Disease Epidemiology Collaboration equation is not better. *Eur. J. Gastroenterol. Hepatol.* 2011 Nov;23(11):969-973.

[50] Hetu PO, Gingras ME, Vinet B. Development and validation of a rapid liquid chromatography isotope dilution tandem mass spectrometry (LC-IDMS/MS) method for serum creatinine. *Clin. Biochem.* 2010;43(13-14).

[51] Perrone RD, Madias NE, Levey AS. Serum creatinine as an index of renal function: new insights into old concepts. *Clin. Chem.* 1992 Oct;38(10):1933-1953.

[52] Xirouchakis E, Marelli L, Cholongitas E, Manousou P, Calvaruso V, Pleguezuelo M, et al. Comparison of cystatin C and creatinine-based glomerular filtration rate formulas with 51Cr-EDTA clearance in patients with cirrhosis. *Clin. J. Am. Soc. Nephrol.* 2011 Jan;6(1):84-92.

[53] Duncan L, Heathcote J, Djurdjev O, Levin A. Screening for renal disease using serum creatinine: who are we missing? *Nephrol. Dial Transplant.* 2001 May;16(5):1042-1046.

[54] Goulding C, Cholongitas E, Nair D, Kerry A, Patch D, Akyol M, et al. Assessment of reproducibility of creatinine measurement and MELD scoring in four liver transplant units in the UK. *Nephrol. Dial Transplant.* 2010 Nov 5;25:960-966.

[55] Vickery S, Stevens PE, Dalton RN, Lente FV, Lamb EJ. Does the ID-MS traceable MDRD equation work and is it suitable for use with compensated Jaffe and enzymatic creatinine assays? *Nephrol. Dial Transplant.* 2006 ;21(9):2439-45.

[56] Tietz NW, Shuey DF, Wekstein DR. Laboratory values in fit aging individuals--sexagenarians through centenarians. *Clin. Chem.* 1992 Jun;38(6):1167-1185.

[57] Sterner G, Frennby B, Mansson S, Nyman U, Van WD, Almen T. Determining 'true' glomerular filtration rate in healthy adults using infusion of inulin and comparing it with values obtained using other clearance techniques or prediction equations. *Scand. J. Urol. Nephrol.* 2008;42(3):278-285.

[58] Furstenberg A, Davenport A. Comparison of multifrequency bioelectrical impedance analysis and dual-energy X-ray absorptiometry assessments in outpatient hemodialysis patients. *Am. J. Kidney Dis.* 2011 Jan;57(1):123-129.

[59] Bjork J, Back SE, Sterner G, Carlson J, Lindstrom V, Bakoush O, et al. Prediction of relative glomerular filtration rate in adults: new improved equations based on Swedish Caucasians and standardized plasma-creatinine assays. *Scand. J. Clin. Lab. Invest.* 2007;67(7):678-695.

[60] Mosteller RD. Simplified calculation of body-surface area. *N. Engl. J. Med.* 1987 Oct 22;317(17):1098.

[61] Haycock GB, Schwartz GJ, Wisotsky DH. Geometric method for measuring body surface area: a height-weight formula validated in infants, children, and adults. *J. Pediatr.* 1978 Jul;93(1):62-66.

[62] Fujimoto S, Watanabe T, Sakamoto A, Yukawa K, Morimoto K. [Studies on the physical surface area of Japanese. 18. Calculation formulas in three stages over all ages]. *Nihon Eiseigaku Zasshi* 1968 Dec;23(5):443-450.

[63] Swedko PJ, Clark HD, Paramsothy K, Akbari A. Serum creatinine is an inadequate screening test for renal failure in elderly patients. *Arch. Intern. Med.* 2003 Feb 10; 163(3):356-360.

[64] Moylan CA, Brady CW, Johnson JL, Smith AD, Tuttle-Newhall JE, Muir AJ. Disparities in liver transplantation before and after introduction of the MELD score. *JAMA* 2008 Nov 26;300(20):2371-2378.

[65] Axelrod DA, Pomfret EA. Race and sex disparities in liver transplantation: progress toward achieving equal access? *JAMA* 2008 Nov 26;300(20):2425-2426.

[66] Lai J. Height Explains the Gender Difference in Wait-list Mortality Under the MELD-Based Liver Allocation System. *Am. J. Transplant.* 2010;in press.

[67] Cholongitas E, Marelli L, Kerry A, Goodier DW, Nair D, Thomas M, et al. Female liver transplant recipients with the same GFR as male recipients have lower MELD scores--a systematic bias. *Am. J. Transplant.* 2007 Mar;7(3):685-692.

[68] Lim Y, Larson T, Benson J, Kamath P, Kremers W, Therneau T, et al. Serum sodium, renal function and survival of patients with end-stage liver disease. *J. Hepatol.* 2010; 52:523-528.

[69] Huo S, Huo T, Lin H, Chi C, Lee P, Tseng F, et al. Is the Corrected-Creatinine Model for End-Stage Liver Disease a Feasible Strategy to Adjust Gender Difference in Organ Allocation for Liver Transplantation? *Transplantation* 2007;84:1406-1412.

[70] Newman DJ. Cystatin C. *Ann. Clin. Biochem.* 2002 Mar;39(Pt 2):89-104.

[71] Filler G, Bokenkamp A, Hofmann W, Le Bricon T, Martinez-Bru C, Grubb A. Cystatin C as a marker of GFR--history, indications, and future research. *Clin. Biochem.* 2005 Jan;38(1):1-8.

[72] Woitas RP, Stoffel-Wagner B, Flommersfeld S, Poege U, Schiedermaier P, Klehr HU, et al. Correlation of serum concentrations of cystatin C and creatinine to inulin clearance in liver cirrhosis. *Clin. Chem.* 2000 May;46(5):712-715.

[73] Orlando R, Mussap M, Plebani M, Piccoli P, De Martin S, Floreani M, et al. Diagnostic value of plasma cystatin C as a glomerular filtration marker in decompensated liver cirrhosis. *Clin. Chem.* 2002 Jun;48(6 Pt 1):850-858.

[74] Grubb A, Nyman U, Bjork J, Lindstrom V, Rippe B, Sterner G, et al. Simple cystatin C-based prediction equations for glomerular filtration rate compared with the modification of diet in renal disease prediction equation for adults and the Schwartz and the Counahan-Barratt prediction equations for children. *Clin. Chem.* 2005 Aug;51(8): 1420-1431.

[75] Zahran A, El-Husseini A, Shoker A. Can cystatin C replace creatinine to estimate glomerular filtration rate? A literature review. *Am. J. Nephrol.* 2007;27(2):197-205.

[76] Evangelopoulos AA, Vallianou NG, Bountziouka V, Katsagoni C, Bathrellou E, Vogiatzakis ED, et al. Association between serum cystatin C, monocytes and other inflammatory markers. *Intern. Med. J.* 2012;42(5):517-22.

[77] Shlipak MG, Weekley CC, Li Y, Hansson LO, Larsson A, Whooley M. Comparison of cardiovascular prognosis by 3 serum cystatin C methods in the Heart and Soul Study. *Clin. Chem.* 2011 May;57(5):737-745.

[78] Singh D, Whooley MA, Ix JH, Ali S, Shlipak MG. Association of cystatin C and estimated GFR with inflammatory biomarkers: the Heart and Soul Study. *Nephrol. Dial Transplant.* 2007 Apr;22(4):1087-1092.

[79] Demirtas S, Bozbas A, Akbay A, Yavuz Y, Karaca L. Diagnostic value of serum cystatin C for evaluation of hepatorenal syndrome. *Clin. Chim. Acta* 2001 Sep 25; 311(2):81-89.

[80] Ustundag Y, Samsar U, Acikgoz S, Cabuk M, Kiran S, Kulah E, et al. Analysis of glomerular filtration rate, serum cystatin C levels, and renal resistive index values in cirrhosis patients. *Clin. Chem. Lab. Med.* 2007;45(7):890-894.

[81] Hoek FJ, Kemperman FA, Krediet RT. A comparison between cystatin C, plasma creatinine and the Cockcroft and Gault formula for the estimation of glomerular filtration rate. *Nephrol. Dial Transplant.* 2003 Oct;18(10):2024-2031.

[82] Larsson A, Malm J, Grubb A, Hansson LO. Calculation of glomerular filtration rate expressed in mL/min from plasma cystatin C values in mg/L. *Scand. J. Clin. Lab. Invest.* 2004;64(1):25-30.

[83] Poge U, Gerhardt T, Stoffel-Wagner B, Klehr HU, Sauerbruch T, Woitas RP. Calculation of glomerular filtration rate based on cystatin C in cirrhotic patients. *Nephrol. Dial Transplant.* 2006 Mar;21(3):660-664.

[84] Nickolas TL, O'Rourke MJ, Yang J, Sise ME, Canetta PA, Barasch N, et al. Sensitivity and specificity of a single emergency department measurement of urinary neutrophil gelatinase-associated lipocalin for diagnosing acute kidney injury. *Ann. Intern. Med.* 2008 Jun 3;148(11):810-819.

[85] Fagundes C, Pepin MN, Guevara M, Barreto R, Casals G, Sola E, et al. Urinary neutrophil gelatinase-associated lipocalin as biomarker in the differential diagnosis of impairment of kidney function in cirrhosis. *J. Hepatol.* 2012 (in press).

[86] Samyn M, Cheeseman P, Bevis L, Taylor R, Samaroo B, Buxton-Thomas M, et al. Cystatin C, an easy and reliable marker for assessment of renal dysfunction in children with liver disease and after liver transplantation. *Liver Transpl.* 2005 Mar;11(3): 344-349.

[87] Skluzacek PA, Szewc RG, Nolan CR, III, Riley DJ, Lee S, Pergola PE. Prediction of GFR in liver transplant candidates. *Am. J. Kidney Dis.* 2003 Dec;42(6):1169-1176.

[88] MacAulay J, Thompson K, Kiberd BA, Barnes DC, Peltekian KM. Serum creatinine in patients with advanced liver disease is of limited value for identification of moderate renal dysfunction: are the equations for estimating renal function better? *Can. J. Gastroenterol.* 2006 Aug;20(8):521-526.

In: Creatinine
Editors: I. H. Perkins and C. M. Chapman

ISBN: 978-1-62257-475-9

Chapter V

Serum Creatinine and Kidney Dysfunction in the Critically Ill. A New Insight for an Old Measure

***Gemma Seller-Perez** *and Manuel E. Herrera-Gutierrez*#**
I. C. U., University Hospital Carlos Haya, Malaga, Spain

Abstract

Glomerular filtration rate (GFR) is an accepted parameter for assessing kidney function. Measurement of clearance of external substances that are freely filtered in the glomerulus but not reabsorbed or excreted in the tubules (inulin or some isotopic agents) is the "gold standard" for GFR, but this method is cumbersome for critical practice and so GFR is usually based in the clearance of endogenous substances, i.e. serum creatinine (Crs).

So, for the critically ill patient, 24 hours creatinine clearance (or shorter intervals) is the method of reference for the estimation of the GFR, although this is often not measured but estimated by equations based on anthropometric data and isolated valued of Crs (i.e. Cockroft-Gault or MDRD equations), event though these were not designed for ICU patients and perform poorly in this setting.

Whatever the method employed, renal evaluation rests in Crs but this is subjected to wide variations dependent on multiple factors, among which we should highlight race, sex, nutritional status, proteins intake and, specially significant in critical care, the over-hydration and the loss of muscle mass. Also the laboratory method used, either the Jaffe or the more recently introduced enzymatic one, introduce variations in Crs.

It is significant that in subjects with normal kidney function, when the Crs amounts to 2 mg/dL, over a fifty per cent of the kidney reserve has been lost. Also it has been proven that small increases in Crs, either absolute or as relative changes over the basal value, has serious repercussion on the prognosis of patients.

But even when it is well accepted that acute kidney injury (AKI) is common in patients in ICU and it conditions a longer stay and an increase on cost, as well as an increase in associated mortality, it has not been until the last decade that really serious efforts have been undertook by

* Ph. D. Intensivist. I. C .U., University Hospital Carlos Haya, Malaga, Spain.
# Ph. D. Associate professor. Intensivist. I. C. U., University Hospital Carlos Haya, Malaga, Spain.

the professionals directly involved in AKI management (nephrologists and intensivists) in order to unify diagnostic criteria and to stratify risk.

In this sense, since the beginning of this century, various approaches such as the SHARF or SIRE initiatives initiated what eventually crystallized in the RIFLE and later in the AKIN systems. Both are based on the evaluation of sequential changes in GFR (estimated either through clearance or Crs) or urine flow.

The experience accumulated with these systems has made evident their usefulness but also some potential problems and areas for improvement.

For one side RIFLE or AKIN have provided a common definition of AKI for those who treat ICU patients and because their sensitivity for detecting AKI have meant a considerable advantage for the clinician (previously we had more than 25 definitions of renal failure) but, on the other side this same fact is a drawback for clinical research because potentially overestimating AKI incidence if we count on the early stages of these systems (R or 1) as kidney failure. Other significant problem is the unavoidable delay before a patient is classified that is perhaps the one to be overcome in the near future.

The Impact of Acute Kidney Injury in the ICU

Acute kidney injury (AKI) can be defined as a decrease of the glomerular filtration rate (GFR) that appears acutely, stays for some time, causes an accumulation of waste products from metabolism and uremic toxins and conditions a mishandling of body fluids and a loss of the ability to maintain homeostasis of electrolytes and acid-base balance.

In the intensive care setting, AKI presents with a high incidence and, once established, has an important impact in the patient (worsening the prognosis) and in the resources (because the costs inherent to the treatments administered and the prolongation of stay) [1, 2].

The reported incidence of AKI in the intensive care units (ICU) shows a wide variability depending of the population analyzed and the criteria employed for its definition but when this is based in the new systems for stratification, as RIFLE [3] or AKIN [4], more than 30% of ICU patients are found to present with AKI, either already present at ICU admission or developing during their stay [5]. For the ICU patient with AKI mortality rate is high and increases according to the degree of renal dysfunction [6, 7].

These figures are a good measure of the magnitude of the problem, and even when the prognosis of AKI regarding functional recovery is good, it has been demonstrated that the development of severe AKI can lead to an increase in long-term mortality [8] with an estimation of the incidence of chronic kidney disease (CKD) after an episode of AKI as high as 7.8 per 100 patients per year [9]. These facts, together with the problems resulting from the limited options in the treatment and the increased resources imposed by its management, make AKI a focus of growing interest among professionals managing critically ill patients [10].

In the ICU an early diagnosis of AKI emerges as a necessity in order to treat this condition as soon as possible and, even more important considering the lack of effective therapies, to optimize the management and prevent in these initial stages of the aggression a secondary renal damage caused by inadequate or potentially harmful interventions (as nephrotoxic drugs or intravenous contrasts). This scenario has put in evidence the necessity of new tools for continuous assessment of kidney function, given that the classical approach of measurements of isolated determinations of serum creatinine (Crs) has proven insufficient because its delayed elevation when a derangement in the glomerular filtration rate (GFR) is ongoing, being precisely in this moment when a timely intervention should be expected to have the highest impact [11].

How to Measure Kidney Function: Glomerular Filtration Rate

It has been assumed that AKI is derived from a misbalance between the oxygen available for kidneys and that really needed to sustain the function of the renal cells. This mismatch results in damage for the epithelial cells in the tubules that, depending of the intensity of the insult, can lead to appearance of apoptosis or necrosis [12-14].

One way to evaluate renal function is studying its capability to maintain an adequate filtration in the glomerulus, i.e. estimation of the GFR. The GFR is a measure of the amount of blood filtered by the glomerulus per unit of time and is expressed in $mL/min/m^2$. Normal values for GFR are approximately over 120 $ml/min/1.73m^2$, but we must keep in mind that this figure is highly dependent in many exogenous factors and continuously adapting to our metabolic necessities, so it is no possible to define exactly what should be considered a normal GFR. Because this capability, there is not a direct relationship between the renal mass and renal functionality until a significant amount of damage has already developed, because until late in the process, the kidneys are able to compensate the loss of renal tissue through a raise in the filtration rate in those nephrons still functioning. However, when a significant damage has developed, kidneys reach a point where the remaining renal parenchyma cannot compensate for the loss of function and from this point on the relation between kidney damage and the GFR becomes lineal and a estimation of GFR can provide as an adequate measure of the degree of kidney damage (Figure 1) [15]. GFR can be estimated by the measurement of the rate of elimination (clearance) of different molecules that are filtered by the glomerulus but not secreted or re-absorbed by the tubule. The most accurate method ("gold standard" for GFR estimation) is that based in the introduction in the blood stream of molecules not produced naturally in the body and cleared exclusively by the kidney that are freely filtered by the glomerulus without being secreted by the tubule.

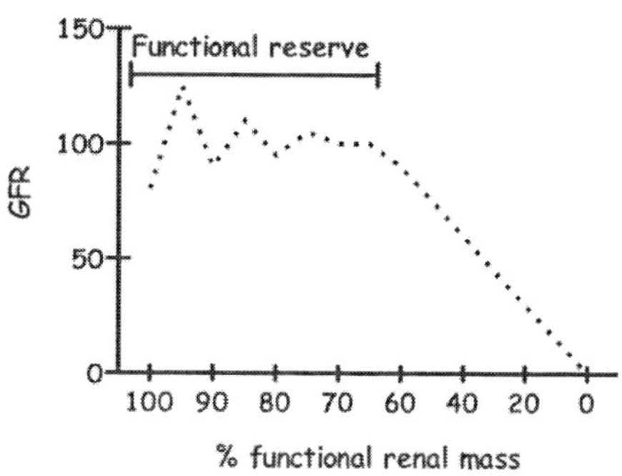

Figure 1. Simulation of the relationship between renal functional mass and glomerular filtration rate (GFR). When enough renal mass is present, GFR changes in response to patient necessities but when damage is severe this "renal reserve" is lost. Adapted from [15].

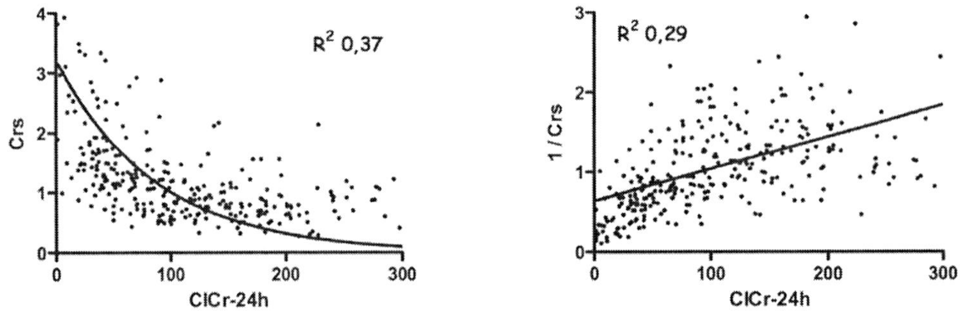

Figure 2. Relationship between serum creatinine and creatinine clearance. Data from the authors, adapted from [31].

Inulin is the most standardized method for GFR estimation but there are other alternatives as is the case for certain isotopic agents. These methods are not useful for clinical practice and the use of endogenous molecules naturally producing in the organism have been proposed as an alternative, mainly Crs.

Serum Creatinine

Crs is an organic protein resulting from the degradation of creatine, synthesized in the liver and stored in the muscle. It is produced and eliminated at a constant rate and is exclusively cleared by the kidneys, being filtered at the glomerulus without significant tubular reabsorption or tubular secretion. These facts make Crs a suitable marker to measure GFR. Its main drawback is based on the fact that changes in Crs does not to follow a linear relationship after changes in GFR, so when facing changes in its concentration we can not can not assume similar changes in the GFR (this relationship becomes linear if we consider the inverse of the Crs value instead) (Figure 2) [16]. The absence of a linear relationship means that for certain intervals in the concentration of Crs, a small increase in its value may be indicating the presence of a large increase in GFR. In addition, being Crs an endogenous molecule, its metabolism is subjected to interpersonal variations depending on different factors, intake and metabolic stress rate being the most prominent but including also others such as muscle mass, gender, age or race [17]. Crs is the parameter universally adopted for the diagnosis of kidney failure all over the world, and this prominent role sometimes shades the fact that its value reflects the functionality of the kidney but not necessarily the presence of actual damage, so when facing an increase in its levels we must not beforehand assume the presence of kidney damage. For a renal dysfunction of pre-renal origin, and despite the significant rise that Crs may experience, treatment and prognosis are totally different from those due to an acute tubular necrosis (ATN) even for the same Crs increment. On the other hand Crs can in certain circumstances maintain its normal concentration in the presence of significant kidney damage (and therefore with decreased GFR) as can be the presence of liver cirrhosis.

As already mentioned, Crs is a functional parameter and its role in the diagnosis of renal injury is closely related to its kinetics and what we can address as "renal reserve"; When a patient initially presenting a normal Crs concentration surpasses 2 mg/dL, he must have lost approximately 50% of the functioning renal mass [18] [15]. Changes in Crs after a serious renal insult depend largely in the the basal function as well, so that 24 hours after a 90% fall in the creatinine clearance (CrCl), the increase of Crs might be up to 246% when kidney function is normal, but only of 174% when the patient already featured a dysfunction in stage 2 of the KDIGO guidelines (Table 1) [19] or as low as 74% when the patient was in stage 4, in all the cases for a virtually identical absolute increase in the Crs (between 1.8 to 2 mg/dL). For this reason, some authors have advocated for a definition of AKI based upon changes of Crs levels for a given period (between 24 and 48 hours) instead of absolute serum levels [20]. Another important aspect to keep in mind is that changes in Crs levels present with a delay of more than 48 hours following a change in GFR. So we can hypothetically face a progressive rise in Crs in spite of a GFR improvement when renal recovery is initiating (Figure 3) [18, 21]. These facts emphasize the importance of not acting only based on isolated determinations of Crs because the result may not reflect the actual function of the kidney. One scenario where this disagreement can become obvious would be in pre-renal AKI, when (as opposed to the ATN) the disproportionate increase in Crs can be reversed quickly to normal with an adequate resuscitation.

Table 1. Classification of chronic kidney disease (19)

Stage	Description	GFR (ml/min/1.73 m^2)
1	Kidney damage with normal or high GFR.	≥ 90
2	Kidney damage with mild decrement of GFR.	60-89
3	Moderate decrement of GFR.	30-59
4	Severe decrement of GFR.	15-29
5	Kidney failure.	< 15 (or dialysis)

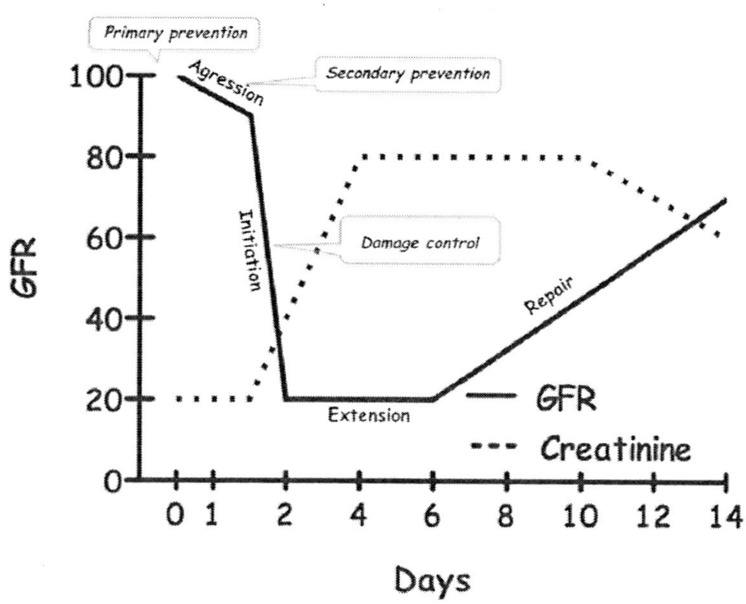

Figure 3. Theoretical relationship between glomerular filtration rate (GFR) and serum creatinine (Crs) in time, with emphasis in the possible impact of timely interventions in the course of kidney injury. Adapted from [18, 21].

Fluids and Crs. Another key point when assessing serial changes in Crs is the repercussion of the balance of fluids. In those situations where aggressive hydration has been necessary and water balance is positive, the relative serum concentration of Crs decreases and therefore induces an error by underestimation of the real value. We must also bear in mind that an aggressive resuscitation may in fact lead to a deterioration of kidney function or development of secondary AKI due among others to the development of visceral edema with increase intra-abdominal pressure and increased pressure in the Bowman's capsule [22, 23].

Discrepancies in the classification of renal dysfunction based on the determination of Crs in over-hydrated patients can be over 18% [24], and some authors have proposed different approaches to overcome this problems, as Macedo et al, that have developed an equation taking into consideration this factor [25].

Crs assay. The scenario for the AKI patient in the ICU is changing in recent years, due in part to changes in what we understand for renal injury but also to the development of new diagnostic methods [26]. The method described by Jaffé for the assay of Crs (based on the use of alkaline picrate) has been the cornerstone for the diagnosis of the renal failure until recently, but this method shows variations for a range from 0.06 to 0.31 mg/dL. Deviations within this range, previously considered safe, are now considered to be of potential prognostic value in our patients [27]. This fact has favored the displacement of this method by the enzymatic assay [28], that avoids also the problems affecting the Jaffé assay because interactions with different substances, especially with bilirubin. The enzymatic assay had been included in the last recommendations of the KDIGO guidelines *http://www.kdigo.org*.

Creatinine Clearance

A more accurate method to estimate GFR is the determination of CrCl, based in a collection of the diuresis during 24 hours and a measure of Crs and the concentration of creatinine in the urine. This method does not suffer the lack of lineal relationship of Crs and GFR and is less affected by the delay in Crs increase after GFR decrement, but shares all the other problems of the Crs already mentioned. Even when this method is the most widely used and is considered the most accurate for the estimation of GFR in clinical practice, its application is in any case burdensome and implies a high workload and the manipulation of high volumes of urine, not being therefore a practical method for the monitoring of renal function in the ICU, where seriated and frequent measurements in a significant number of patients simultaneously is the rule. In addition, the inevitable delay of 24 hours before the result are ready makes it a method unattractive for the critically ill patient.

For these reasons, in routine clinical practice, CrCl measured with diuresis of 24 hours is not operational and different investigators have sought alternatives more adapted to the ICU environment. An approach is the measurement of CrCl with samples of urine collected in shorter intervals of time, making repetitive measures more feasible, urine samples from simultaneous patients easier to handle and (the most critical aspect) without delay for the results. In the initial stages of AKI in the critically ill patient, when GFR falls rapidly, a determination of CrCl that takes 24 hours will encompass major fluctuations of its value (due in some small measure to fluctuations in the levels of Crs, but above all to variations in their urinary excretion) and this problem could be minimized with this short sampling time [29].

Different timings for collection of urine have been validated by some authors, ranging from one hour by Hoste et al. [30], two hours by Herrera-Gutierrez et al (31) or periods from two to twelve hours by Wilson et al [32], finding all of them a close correlation between these measures and the CrCl in urine collected for 24 hours. In these cases, delay until the result is available is sensibly shortened and the problems derived from the manipulation of large urine samples minimized but also implies that the timing for recollection is critical to assure the exactness of the measurement. Relationship between short-time samples and 24 hours collection is even closer when values of CrCl are below 70 ml/Kg/1.73m^2, and external factors as hemodynamic stability, oliguria or diuretic use (all of them frequent in the ICU patient) do not interfere with its validity as demonstrated by Herrera-Gutierrez et al [31], making this an interesting approach for the monitoring of renal function in the critically ill.

In addition, these studies show how, among those patients with Crs in normal or near-normal range (below 1.5 mg/dl) up to 25% already had a significantly diminished 24-hour CrCl (less than 60 ml/min/1.73m^2), and these patients were well detected by shot-time CrCl. These studies also put in evidence that the most widely used equations for estimation of GFR in the ICU (Cockroft-Gault and MDRD) are not adequate in this setting [30, 31].

Short-timed CrCl is not exempt of error, first and foremost because creatinine reabsorption and tubular filtration of creatinine are not taken into account, but the main source of concern arises, as already stated, from the critical role of the exactness of collection timing, because the potential impact of an error measuring the volume is proportionally higher when the time shortens.

CrCl has been considered inappropriate for the evaluation of acute patient because of the rapid changes in GFR that occur in these cases, but it is precisely in this AKI patient, once renal reserve has been exhausted and GFR reaches a linear dependency with the residual renal mass (Figure 1) [15] that any change detected in CrCl should reflect an actual change in the renal function. Under this assumption, a measurement undertaken in a short time frame is with all probability a more accurate reflection of the actual renal function in that precise moment that a measurement that extends for 24 hours.

Equations Based in Isolated Crs Values

An easier and most extended practice is to estimate CrCl with wide populations-designed equations that include an isolated value from a biochemical marker (usually Crs) and anthropometric data of the patient. This approach gives a close estimate avoiding the inconveniences of 24-hour CrCl and has become the standard way to estimate CrCl in the chronic renal patient. Cockroft-Gault (C-G) [33] or MDRD (in the original [34] or simplified version [35]), are the most widely used equations.

These equations have clearly shown their usefulness and have become the standard method of assessment in chronic patient (where kidney function remains relatively stable), but do not have the same validity in the acute patient, where frequent initial changes in renal function are the rule time and where these equations tend to overestimate the actual renal function. However, despite the scarcity of studies addressing the validity of these equations in the acute patient (and specifically in the ICU patient) and the general agreement against its use in this scenario, these equations (especially MDRD) have become the usual tool for estimation of CrCl and guide dosage of drugs requiring adjustment of dose in the presence of renal dysfunction [36, 37] in the ICU.

Despite its potential impact in the clinic practice and patient safety, attempts to validate these equations in the critically ill patient are scarce but the study carried out by the PICARD group [38] shows how these equations (CG or MDRD) over-estimate the degree of renal dysfunction, being the equation described by Jelliffe et al. [39] the one that best reflects CrCl. But when an exact measure is deemed necessary none of these equations replaces a measurement of CrCl [40] (Figure 4). Other biochemical parameters have been used to build predictive equations, such as the Cystatine C (Cys-C), but these should be used even with greater caution in the critically ill patient given the absence of studies that validate their usefulness. In fact the use of equations that combine two markers (Crs and Cys-C) do not offer a significant improvement over those that use only one of them [41, 42]. The specification of the method used for the determination of both markers should be taken once more into account because it can suppose relevant differences in the results [26, 43].

Other Biomarkers

Cys-C is a low molecular weight protein produced by all nucleated cells at a constant rate, being filtered by the glomerulus and reabsorbed and metabolized in the proximal tubule without tubular secretion and only minimal extra-renal elimination. Cys-C has shown promising results as estimator of GFR in patients with stable renal function [44]. More recently Cys-C has also been studied in the critically ill patients showing similar results but a significantly earlier elevation than Crs [45].

Different biomarkers of kidney injury have recently been developed, of special interest for the critically ill patient the NGAL (Neutrophil Gelatinase-Associated Lipocalin), used with promising results for the diagnosis of AKI secondary to cardiac surgery or for the septic patient (in this last pathology with more controversial results). Other biomarkers are the KIM-1 (Kidney Injury Molecule-1) or the interleukins, notably the IL-6 and IL-18, have been evaluated with mixed results [46]. It is still necessary to define the kinetics of these molecules and their relationship to the development of kidney injury [47].

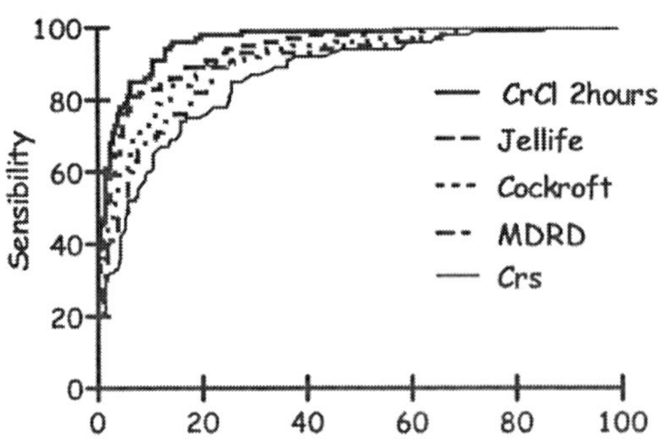

Figure 4. Different methods of estimation of creatinine clearance in the ICU patient and their accurateness to detect acute kidney injury (defined as a creatinine clearance < 60 mL/min/1.73m^2). Data from the authors, adapted from [40].

Another important point to emphasize is that these new biomarkers are not aimed to the assessment of renal function (do not estimate GFR) and therefore can not replace Crs or Cys-C, but by detecting the presence of tubular damage can be complementary them.

Currently, despite the promise of future posed by the new biomarkers, we must continue positioning Crs in the central axis of detection and stratification of kidney dysfunction because it is the best known, is fast and easy to measure and is affordable to any laboratory.

Defining AKI and Stratifying Damage

Diagnosis of AKI, regardless of the definition used, refers to an acute event resulting in an inability to excrete uremic toxins which will therefore accumulate in blood, but we must include in this definition other factors derived from the kidney malfunction, such as the inability to maintain the homeostasis of water, electrolytes, and acid-base, or the inability to synthesize certain substances (even when this last aspect has less significance for acutely ill patients).

From the moment that the aggression occurs until the kidney begins to show alterations and dysfunction becomes obvious, different mechanisms of compensation have been launched that finally produce a decrease in the GFR [48]. In part due to an insufficient knowledge of the changes that occur in these early stages and in part by the lack of sensible methods of diagnosis at the moment of the aggression, we acknowledge the presence of renal failure once this initial phase has already been surpassed, and there is no possibility to implement measures aimed to decrease or even stop the progression of the lesion. This problem is worsened because there is not a clear definition of what we must consider AKI, finding almost as many definitions as works published on this topic and ranging from isolated values of Crs (with different thresholds) to different levels of increment in Crs or even only considering the need for a replacement therapy [49, 50].

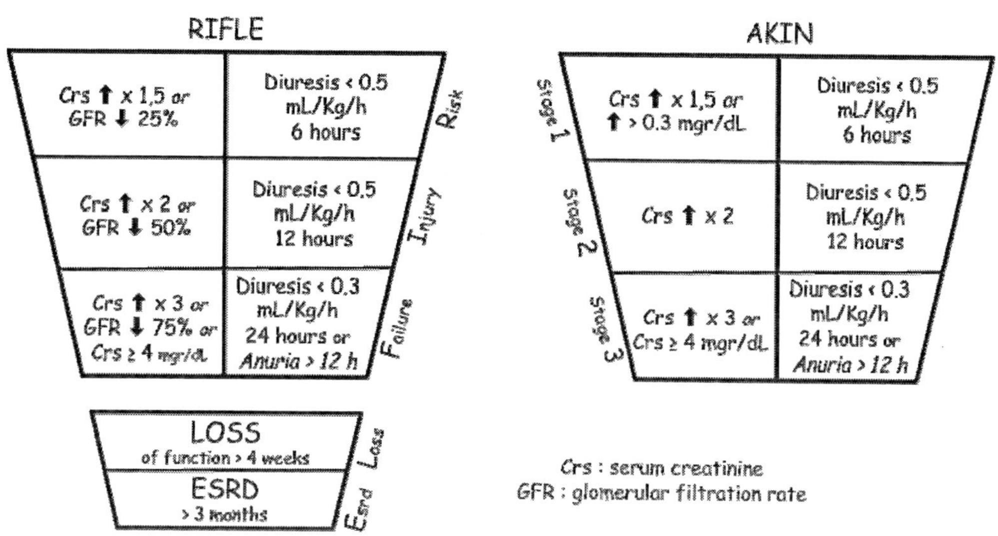

Figure 5. RIFLE and AKIN classification systems [3, 4, 53].

The recent proposal of the concept "Acute Kidney Injury" as a replacement for the classic "Acute Renal Failure" aims to fulfill this deficiency by bundling in the definition these initial phases characterized by little or no clinical expression. The main benefit carried on by this new perspective is the presentation of AKI as a dynamic process that can be measured and classified in terms of intensity of the damage. This change of concept can arguably be considered the most significant advance in the field of critical care nephrology in recent years and has constructed also a common platform for different groups devoted to the study of the AKI in the critical patient [51].

In contrast with the chronic patient, who presents with a (in some way) stable renal function that lets us to stratify the process on the basis of the residual GFR (Kidney Disease Outcomes Quality Initiative (K/DOQI)) (Table 1) [19, 52], in acute cases this stratification is much more difficult to establish precisely because the already mentioned changes in GFR. The definition of two systems aimed to stratify acute kidney dysfunction based on sequential changes of Crs has come to fill this gap for the AKI patient (Figure 5) [3, 4].

RIFLE System, or the Importance of Changes in Creatinine

At the beginning of the last decade some initiatives arose aimed to define what we understand as acute renal dysfunction and to stratify its course based in the severity of the process. In the year 2004, a panel of experts integrated in the Acute Dialysis Quality Initiative (ADQI), developed a system called RIFLE (an acronym for Risk, Injury Failure, Loss and End-stage) [53] based on the determination of sequential changes of GFR (estimate by Crs or CrCl) and changes in urine flow, proposing the basics of what could be a common language with regard to the problem of AKI (Figure 5).

Furthermore (and arguably their more relevant result) this group made a proposal for a new definition of AKI that included the need to maintain the injury in time, to consider AKI as a dynamic process that should not be evaluated with isolated Crs and to include urinary flow as a relevant parameter. The definition proposed by the ADQI group is as follows: "a sharp decrease of GFR, urine volume, or both, which is maintained at least for 24 hours". Another major advantage of this system was its simplicity, advocating for the use of biomarkers universally affordable (Crs and diuresis).

AKIN System, or the Importance of Small Changes in Creatinine

Coincident with the publication of the conclusions of the ADQI initiative, Lassnigg et al demonstrated in a series of patients undergoing cardiac surgery [27] something that was already suspected, the fact that small increases in the concentration of Crs (changes generally accepted as innocent and within the range of error provided by Jaffe method) carried a proportional increase in the mortality of their patients. This fact was subsequently confirmed by these same researchers demonstrating that patients who presented with an elevation greater than 0.3 mg/dL in the first 48 hours of ICU stay were 8 times more likely to die in hospital (odds ratio, 7.9; 95% CI 2.9 - 15.3) and were 5 times more likely to have prolonged hospital stays (OR 5.2; 95% CI, 3.5-7.9) [54, 55]. Even more, the recovery of renal function provide for even a protective effect in these cases [56].

Given the relationship between Crs and GFR [16], we should expect a relationship between percentage of increase in Crs and prognosis but as Coca et al have evidenced in a recent meta-analysis, this relationship presents for both increase in percentage (between 10% and 24%) and changes in absolute numbers of Crs (between 0.3 and 0.4 mg/dL) [57].

In 2007, the AKIN (Acute Kidney Injury Network) Group designed a new stratification system based on the premises of the RIFLE system but incorporating these findings, and including a minimum threshold at which we must consider that kidney injury is present (0.3 mg/dL) [4]. Looking for simplicity and more according to clinical practice, this classification dispenses with the L and E levels of the RIFLE and does not include the CrCl, maintaining the criteria relating to Crs and urine output. Another significant contribution of this system is the definition of a window of 48 hours to assess changes in Crs or diuresis, as well as the admission that any patient undergoing a replacement therapy is in the highest level of the scale (stage 3). It was specifically in this document where the term AKI was proposed to refer to the entire spectrum of kidney damage.

Pitfalls of RIFLE and AKIN

These two systems have been evaluated in large series of UCI patients and are currently consolidated as reference for stratification of AKI in this scenario, but both systems presents some problems that should be discussed [58].

After their introduction in he clinical practice, the high sensitivity for AKI detection that both provide has conditioned a substantial increase in the percentages of incidence of AKI published in contrast to previous studies that were based in more traditional definitions, having in fact increased the incidence detected by the RIFLE system on the order of 2 to 10 times [59]. The first stage of the RIFLE system can be considered the most relevant because it is simple to perform, is sensible and with a low cost, alerting the clinicians at a time when the situation is still reversible through both preventive and therapeutic measures [60], but on the other side, as already discussed, results in a significant increase in the incidence of reported AKI.

Because the way both RIFLE and AKIN systems were designed, we can force the stratification indistinctly by GFR criteria (particularly Crs, shared by both systems) or by urinary flow, opting in theory for the worst recorded parameter (Crs or diuresis), but in the practice this is not the case. Clinical experience shows us that oliguria is a common problem in the critical care patient and, in addition to being an early marker of renal perfusion function, has a direct relationship with the prognosis of our patients [61]. Macedo et al diagnosed AKI in 28% of their patients when applying Crs criteria but when urinary flow was the selected parameter this percentage rose by an additional 32%. In addition, up to 55% of their patients presented at least one episode of oliguria during their stay, and this group of patients carried a higher mortality [62]. Therefore, depending on the estimator employed the results can be significantly different being precisely diuresis more sensible but, even when the control of urinary output is routine practice in ICU, the vast majority of studies performed on the validation of these scores make reference only to Crs, a trend that likely reproduces what is happening in clinical practice as well.

Urinary flow also presents with problems, as those resulting from the possibility of an obstruction to urine flow or the presence of a pre-renal situation, in which case we will diagnose AKI in patients who really do not present this problem. This second situation can be of relevance according to Uchino et al, that demonstrated how 32% of patients developing AKI according to the RIFLE criteria actually presented a pre-renal azotemia and recovered renal function in the first three days of ICU stay [63]. Therefore, following the RIFLE recommendations, before trying to apply the score an adequate resuscitation must has been undertaken, and the patient must be properly hydrated and without diuretics (a condition difficult to fulfill in ICU patients, at least in the initial stages of management) and, following AKIN recommendations, not only the intravascular volume must be restored, but we must exclude the possibility of an obstructive cause of AKI as well.

The analysis of sequential changes in both parameters (Crs and diuresis) can be of aid in differentiating pre-renal dysfunction from established acute tubular necrosis [64] and perhaps in the near future the introduction of a biomarker of tubular damage (such as the NGAL) in the early stages of the dysfunction could be an useful tool to distinguish between them [65], guiding us in our resuscitation efforts.

Regarding Crs, for this parameter to be useful in RIFLE as GFR estimator we must count on a reference value (basal Crs) that in a significant number of patients is missing. Different approaches have been advised to overcome this problem but none has shown as ideal. It has been suggested the adoption of an average GFR of 75 $mL/min/1.73m^2$ in patients without prior known AKI, although this approach has rarely been applied, hardly surprising if we consider that Crs and not the CrCl is he parameter commonly used. Other suggestion would be to apply the lower value of Crs of those known or to introduce the first recorded Crs after admission, but it must be understood that with any of these approaches we will be introducing an important bias, especially relevant in those patients that received an aggressive resuscitation due to the known impact of over-hydration on Crs levels.

The approach more extended is to include an estimate of normal Crs according to age, race and sex, as with the MDRD equation. But in this case, as was the case when using a GFR of 75 mL/min, we are taking for granted a normal kidney function, which not necessarily has to be the case. Finally, we could use a predefined value for all the patients, as 0.8 mg/dL in women and 1 mg/dL in men as advocated by Závada et al. [66]. Although all of these methods are far from ideal, those based on anthropometric data are probably prone to lesser error, but always keeping in mind that categorization will be only successful if basal kidney function is normal and therefore we must avoid this approach in cases with known prior renal dysfunction [67].

Therefore and with reference to the presentation of clinical studies and their results, it is essential to reflect clearly the method used to stratify our patients and the approach taken to estimate basal Crs, since this considerations will have a significant impact on to the results (especially relevant when referring to the R stage of the RIFLE scale). It is advisable to undertake every possible effort in order to get the actual basal value of basal Crs.

Another problem, shared by both systems, is the need for a minimum timeframe to proceed with the classification, which in RIFLE extends up to a week and in AKIN for 48 hours. This inevitable time window will condition an undesirable delay in the detection of AKI.

Yet another problem with RIFLE arises from the possibility to choose indistinctly between CrCl or Crs, even when these values are not linearly related and do not change simultaneous in time; in the early stages of dysfunction Crs maintains a low serum concentration when CrCl is actually falling and in this case the degree of renal dysfunction will be underestimate by Crs compared to CrCl [68].

Another relevant aspect and one that questions the consistency of these systems is the finding of similar outcomes for patients in the AKIN 1 and 2 levels with a significant increment for level 3 and with a similar behavior for RIFLE [69], that could be suggesting the convenience for a reappraisal of the ranges of Crs considered in each level.

We must stress that these systems, despite their limitations, have promoted a significant leap in the clinical approach to AKI, focusing the clinician on the possible existence of an ongoing renal dysfunction, but at the same time, regarding clinical research (and despite the obvious advantage of setting a common language), have introduced a new uncertainty in the epidemiology of renal dysfunction (especially because of the R stage in RIFLE and 1 in AKIN) and advocate for a consensus of what must be considered AKI when applying these scales.

The Best Approach to AKI

A proper definition for AKI should establish the presence or absence of disease, report on its severity and prognosis and, perhaps more important, should be easy to understand and implement [70]. Although these assumptions have been partly met by RIFLE and AKIN, it is likely that in a near future our understanding about AKI and its impact will be modified. Right now AKI definition is in continuous reassessment and indeed the latest recommendations proposed by the KDIGO group call for a new stratification system that resumes the two existing now (RIFLE and AKIN) and collects the best and most practical aspects of both. As Srisawat et al point out [71], beside the functional criteria already in use (Crs, FG and urine flow) new biomarkers of kidney damage will be simultaneously included resulting in a new step in the concept of renal dysfunction. This combined approach could also solve the problem posed by the differentiation between pre-renal AKI and ATN, a serious issue given the difference on the prognosis carried by each one of them and the fact that restoration of the circulating volume in pre-renal AKI could reverse the process [72].

It is important to stress the fact that at least 20% of hospitalized patients develop some degree of renal dysfunction and the prognosis for these patients worsens as the degree of dysfunction increases [73] but, regardless whether they receive or not a replacement therapy, only about 10% of those who survive will eventually be in need for prolonged renal replacement [74]. These figures reinforce the relevance of a timely detection of impending AKI in order to apply secondary preventive measures that limit the progression and increase the chances of recovery of our patients.

Although Crs is a sensible parameter to decide whether a patient's kidney function remains stable, worsens or improves, its role in the diagnosis of early renal dysfunction is more debatable, and in order to evaluate the information it provides we must understand the pathophysiology of acute renal failure and the kinetics of creatinine (be it Crs, measured CrCl or its estimated by equations), and in any case, we must integrate this information in one of the stratification systems currently in force, acknowledging their limitations.

Conclusion

Serum creatinine is and probably will continue being in the near future the key factor in the evaluation of kidney function because it is affordable, reproducible and easy to perform, but the measurement should be based in the enzymatic method instead of the most extended Jaffé method.

Clinicians must be aware of Crs limitations, among others that it is a functional marker and not a marker of injury but also that changes in Crs are delayed after changes in GFR or the fact that fluid management in critically ill patients can seriously difficult the capability of Crs to detect small changes in kidney function.

Equations based in Crs that estimate creatinine clearance are not well suited for the evaluation of kidney function in the ICU setting and should not be used as a guide to drugs dosage.

Recent proposed changes in terminology with a shift from acute renal failure to acute kidney injure reflect in a clear and precise way the new paradigm of acute renal dysfunction as a dynamic and progressive process.

New trends in stratification (ADQI or AKIN) could have a significant impact in clinical practice and solve the problem of diagnosing renal dysfunction, alerting the clinician of the real value of small changes in Crs.

These classification systems possibly over-estimating the epidemiological impact of this problem so a consensus is needed about what should be considered AKI.

Novel biomarkers of kidney damage (in particular of tubular injury) may in the near future have a role in the diagnosis of AKI, once they are included in the classification systems.

References

[1] Uchino S., Kellum J. A., Bellomo R., Doig G. S., Morimatsu H., Morgera S., et al. Acute renal failure in critically ill patients: A multinational, multicenter study. *J. A. M. A.*, 2005; 294:813-8.

[2] Joannidis M., Metnitz P. G. Epidemiology and natural history of acute renal failure in the icu. *Crit. Care Clin.*, 2005; 21:239-49.

[3] Bellomo R., Ronco C., Kellum J. A., Mehta R. L., Palevsky P. Acute renal failure - definition, outcome measures, animal models, fluid therapy and information technology needs: The second international consensus conference of the acute dialysis quality initiative (A. D. Q. I.) group. *Crit. Care*, 2004; 8:R204-12.

[4] Mehta R. L., Kellum J. A., Shah S. V., Molitoris B. A., Ronco C., Warnock D. G., et al. Acute kidney injury network: Report of an initiative to improve outcomes in acute kidney injury. *Crit. Care*, 2007; 11:R31.

[5] Ostermann M., Chang R. W. Acute kidney injury in the intensive care unit according to R. I. F. L. E. *Crit. Care Med.*, 2007; 35:1837-43.

[6] Ricci Z., Cruz D., Ronco C. The rifle criteria and mortality in acute kidney injury: A systematic review. *Kidney Int.*, 2008; 73:538-46.

[7] Hoste E. A., Clermont G., Kersten A., Venkataraman R., Angus D. C., De Bacquer D., et al. Rifle criteria for acute kidney injury are associated with hospital mortality in critically ill patients: A cohort analysis. *Crit. Care*, 2006; 10:R73.

[8] Schiffl H., Fischer R. Five-year outcomes of severe acute kidney injury requiring renal replacement therapy. *Nephrol. Dial. Transplant.*, 2008; 23:2235-41.

[9] Coca S. G., Yusuf B., Shlipak M. G., Garg A. X., Parikh C. R. Long-term risk of mortality and other adverse outcomes after acute kidney injury: A systematic review and meta-analysis. *Am. J. Kidney Dis.*, 2009; 53:961-73.

[10] Murugan R., Kellum J. A. Acute kidney injury: What's the prognosis? *Nat. Rev. Nephrol.*, 2011; 7:209-17.

[11] Dennen P., Douglas I. S., Anderson R. Acute kidney injury in the intensive care unit: An update and primer for the intensivist. *Crit. Care Med.*, 2010; 38:261-75.

[12] Havasi A., Borkan S. C. Apoptosis and acute kidney injury. *Kidney Int.*, 2011; 80:29-40.

[13] Sharfuddin A. A., Molitoris B. A. Pathophysiology of ischemic acute kidney injury. *Nat. Rev. Nephrol.*, 2011; 7:189-200.

[14] Bonventre J. V., Yang L. Cellular pathophysiology of ischemic acute kidney injury. *J. Clin. Invest.*, 2011; 121:4210-21.

[15] Bellomo R., Kellum J. A., Ronco C. Defining acute renal failure: Physiological principles. *Intensive Care Med.*, 2004; 30:33-7.

[16] Stevens L. A., Coresh J., Greene T., Levey A. S. Assessing kidney function--measured and estimated glomerular filtration rate. *N. Engl. J. Med.*, 2006; 354:2473-83.

[17] Beddhu S., Samore M. H., Roberts M. S., Stoddard G. J., Pappas L. M., Cheung A. K. Creatinine production, nutrition, and glomerular filtration rate estimation. *J. Am. Soc. Nephrol.*, 2003; 14:1000-5.

[18] Moran S. M., Myers B. D. Course of acute renal failure studied by a model of creatinine kinetics. *Kidney Int.*, 1985; 27:928-37.

[19] Levey A. S., Eckardt K. U., Tsukamoto Y., Levin A., Coresh J., Rossert J., et al. Definition and classification of chronic kidney disease: A position statement from kidney disease: Improving global outcomes (K. D. I. G. O.). *Kidney Int.*, 2005; 67:2089-100.

[20] Waikar S. S., Bonventre J. V. Creatinine kinetics and the definition of acute kidney injury. *J. Am. Soc. Nephrol.*, 2009; 20:672-9.

[21] Liu K. D. Molecular mechanisms of recovery from acute renal failure. *Crit. Care Med.*, 2003; 31:S572-81.

[22] Prowle J. R., Echeverri J. E., Ligabo E. V., Ronco C., Bellomo R. Fluid balance and acute kidney injury. *Nat. Rev. Nephrol.*, 2010; 6:107-15.

[23] Bouchard J., Mehta R. L. Fluid accumulation and acute kidney injury: Consequence or cause. *Curr. Opin. Crit. Care*, 2009; 15:509-13.

[24] Liu K. D., Thompson B. T., Ancukiewicz M., Steingrub J. S., Douglas I. S., Matthay M. A., et al. Acute kidney injury in patients with acute lung injury: Impact of fluid

accumulation on classification of acute kidney injury and associated outcomes. *Crit. Care Med.*, 2011; 39:2665-71.

[25] Macedo E., Bouchard J., Soroko S. H., Chertow G. M., Himmelfarb J., Ikizler T. A., et al. Fluid accumulation, recognition and staging of acute kidney injury in critically-ill patients. *Crit. Care*, 2010; 14:R82.

[26] Udy A., O'Donoghue S., D'Intini V., Healy H., Lipman J. Point of care measurement of plasma creatinine in critically ill patients with acute kidney injury. *Anaesthesia*, 2009; 64:403-7.

[27] Lassnigg A., Schmidlin D., Mouhieddine M., Bachmann L. M., Druml W., Bauer P., et al. Minimal changes of serum creatinine predict prognosis in patients after cardiothoracic surgery: A prospective cohort study. *J. Am. Soc. Nephrol.*, 2004; 15:1597-605.

[28] Myers G. L., Miller W. G., Coresh J., Fleming J., Greenberg N., Greene T., et al. Recommendations for improving serum creatinine measurement: A report from the laboratory working group of the national kidney disease education program. *Clin. Chem.*, 2006; 52:5-18.

[29] Lameire N., Hoste E. Reflections on the definition, classification, and diagnostic evaluation of acute renal failure. *Curr. Opin. Crit. Care*, 2004; 10:468-75.

[30] Hoste E. A., Damen J., Vanholder R. C., Lameire N. H., Delanghe J. R., Van den Hauwe K., et al. Assessment of renal function in recently admitted critically ill patients with normal serum creatinine. *Nephrol. Dial. Transplant.*, 2005; 20:747-53.

[31] Herrera-Gutiérrez M. E., Seller-Pérez G., Banderas-Bravo E., Muñoz-Bono J., Lebrón-Gallardo M., Fernandez-Ortega J. F. Replacement of 24-h creatinine clearance by 2-h creatinine clearance in intensive care unit patients: A single-center study. *Intensive Care Med.*, 2007; 33:1900-6.

[32] Wilson R. F., Soullier G. The validity of two-hour creatinine clearance studies in critically ill patients. *Crit. Care Med.*, 1980; 8:281-4.

[33] Cockcroft D. W., Gault M. H. Prediction of creatinine clearance from serum creatinine. *Nephron.*, 1976; 16:31-41.

[34] Levey A. S., Bosch J. P., Lewis J. B., Greene T., Rogers N., Roth D. A more accurate method to estimate glomerular filtration rate from serum creatinine: A new prediction equation. Modification of diet in renal disease study group. *Ann. Intern. Med.*, 1999; 130:461-70.

[35] Levey A., Greene T., Kusek J. W., Beck G. L., Group. M. S., A simplified equation to predict glomerular filtration rate from serum creatinine. *J. Am. Soc. Nephrol.*, 2000:155A.

[36] Lameire N., Adam A., Becker C. R., Davidson C., McCullough P. A., Stacul F., et al. Baseline renal function screening. *Am. J. Cardiol.*, 2006; 98:21-6.

[37] Herrera-Gutiérrez M. E., Seller-Pérez G., Maynar-Moliner J., Sánchez-Izquierdo Riera J. A., C. O. F. R. A. D. E. study group. Variability in renal dysfunction defining criteria and detection methods in intensive care units: Are the international consensus criteria used for diagnosing renal dysfunction? *Med. Intensiva*, 2011;10.1016/j.medin. 2011.10.003.

[38] Bouchard J., Macedo E., Soroko S., Chertow G. M., Himmelfarb J., Ikizler T. A., et al. Comparison of methods for estimating glomerular filtration rate in critically ill patients with acute kidney injury. *Nephrol. Dial. Transplant.*, 2010; 25:102-7.

[39] Jelliffe R. Estimation of creatinine clearance in patients with unstable renal function, without a urine specimen. *Am. J. Nephrol.*, 2002; 22:320-4.

[40] Seller-Pérez G., Herrera-Gutiérrez M. E., Banderas-Bravo E., Olalla-Sánchez R., Lozano-Sáez R., Quesada-García G. Concordance in critical patients between the equations designed for the calculation of glomerular filtration rate and 24-hour creatinine clearance. *Med. Intensiva,* 2010; 34:294-302.

[41] Inker L. A., Okparavero A. Cystatin C as a marker of glomerular filtration rate: Prospects and limitations. *Curr. Opin. Nephrol. Hypertens.*, 2011; 20:631-9.

[42] Tidman M., Sjöström P., Jones I. A comparison of gfr estimating formulae based upon s-cystatin C and s-creatinine and a combination of the two. *Nephrol. Dial. Transplant.*, 2008; 23:154-60.

[43] Grubb A., Nyman U., Björk J., Lindström V., Rippe B., Sterner G., et al. Simple cystatin C-based prediction equations for glomerular filtration rate compared with the modification of diet in renal disease prediction equation for adults and the Schwartz and the Counahan-Barratt prediction equations for children. *Clin. Chem.*, 2005; 51:1420-31.

[44] Herget-Rosenthal S., Bokenkamp A., Hofmann W. How to estimate GFR-serum creatinine, serum cystatin c or equations? *Clin. Biochem.*, 2007; 40:153-61.

[45] Nejat M., Pickering J. W., Walker R. J., Endre Z. H. Rapid detection of acute kidney injury by plasma cystatin C in the intensive care unit. *Nephrol. Dial. Transplant.*, 2010; 25:3283-9.

[46] Coca S. G., Yalavarthy R., Concato J., Parikh C. R. Biomarkers for the diagnosis and risk stratification of acute kidney injury: A systematic review. *Kidney Int.*, 2008; 73:1008-16.

[47] Endre Z. H., Pickering J. W., Walker R. J., Devarajan P., Edelstein C. L., Bonventre J. V., et al. Improved performance of urinary biomarkers of acute kidney injury in the critically ill by stratification for injury duration and baseline renal function. *Kidney Int.*, 2011; 79:1119-30.

[48] Lameire N., Van Biesen W., Vanholder R. Acute renal failure. *Lancet,* 2005; 365: 417-30.

[49] Mehta R. L., Chertow G. M. Acute renal failure definitions and classification: Time for change? *J. Am. Soc. Nephrol.*, 2003; 14:2178-87.

[50] Bellomo R., Kellum J., Ronco C. Acute renal failure: Time for consensus. *Intensive Care Med.*, 2001; 27:1685-8.

[51] Himmelfarb J., Ikizler T. A. Acute kidney injury: Changing lexicography, definitions, and epidemiology. *Kidney Int.*, 2007; 71:971-6.

[52] K/DOQI clinical practice guidelines for chronic kidney disease: Evaluation, classification, and stratification. *Am. J. Kidney Dis.*, 2002; 39:S1-266.

[53] Bellomo R., Kellum J. A., Ronco C. Defining and classifying acute renal failure: From advocacy to consensus and validation of the R. I. F. L. E. criteria. *Intensive Care Med.*, 2007; 33:409-13.

[54] Barrantes F., Tian J., Vazquez R., Amoateng-Adjepong Y., Manthous C. A. Acute kidney injury criteria predict outcomes of critically ill patients. *Crit. Care Med.*, 2008; 36:1397-403.

[55] Chertow G. M., Burdick E., Honour M., Bonventre J. V., Bates D. W. Acute kidney injury, mortality, length of stay, and costs in hospitalized patients. *J. Am. Soc. Nephrol.*, 2005; 16:3365-70.

[56] Thakar C. V., Christianson A., Freyberg R., Almenoff P., Render M. L. Incidence and outcomes of acute kidney injury in intensive care units: A veterans administration study. *Crit. Care Med.*, 2009; 37:2552-8.

[57] Coca S. G., Peixoto A. J., Garg A. X., Krumholz H. M., Parikh C. R. The prognostic importance of a small acute decrement in kidney function in hospitalized patients: A systematic review and meta-analysis. *Am. J. Kidney Dis.*, 2007; 50:712-20.

[58] Cruz D. N., Ricci Z., Ronco C. Clinical review: R. I. F. L. E. and A. K. I. N.--time for reappraisal. *Crit. Care*, 2009; 13:211.

[59] Hoste E. A., Kellum J. A. Acute kidney injury: Epidemiology and diagnostic criteria. *Curr. Opin. Crit. Care*, 2006; 12:531-7.

[60] Van Biesen W., Vanholder R., Lameire N. Defining acute renal failure: R. I. F. L. E. and beyond. *Clin. J. Am. Soc. Nephrol.*, 2006; 1:1314-9.

[61] Macedo E., Malhotra R., Claure-Del Granado R., Fedullo P., Mehta R. L. Defining urine output criterion for acute kidney injury in critically ill patients. *Nephrol. Dial. Transplant.*, 2011; 26:509-15.

[62] Macedo E., Malhotra R., Bouchard J., Wynn S. K., Mehta R. L. Oliguria is an early predictor of higher mortality in critically ill patients. *Kidney Int.*, 2011; 80:760-7.

[63] Uchino S., Bellomo R., Bagshaw S. M., Goldsmith D. Transient azotaemia is associated with a high risk of death in hospitalized patients. *Nephrol. Dial. Transplant.*, 2010; 25:1833-9.

[64] Macedo E., Mehta R. L. Prerenal failure: From old concepts to new paradigms. *Curr. Opin. Crit. Care*, 2009; 15:467-73.

[65] Singer E., Elger A., Elitok S., Kettritz R., Nickolas T. L., Barasch J., et al. Urinary neutrophil gelatinase-associated lipocalin distinguishes pre-renal from intrinsic renal failure and predicts outcomes. *Kidney Int.*, 2011; 80:405-14.

[66] Závada J., Hoste E., Cartin-Ceba R., Calzavacca P., Gajic O., Clermont G., et al. A comparison of three methods to estimate baseline creatinine for rifle classification. *Nephrol. Dial. Transplant.*, 2010; 25:3911-8.

[67] Bagshaw S. M., Uchino S., Cruz D., Bellomo R., Morimatsu H., Morgera S., et al. A comparison of observed versus estimated baseline creatinine for determination of R. I. F. L. E. class in patients with acute kidney injury. *Nephrol. Dial. Transplant.*, 2009; 24:2739-44.

[68] Herrera-Gutiérrez M. E., Seller-Pérez G., Banderas-Bravo E., Aragón-Gonzalez C., Olalla-Sánchez R., Lozano-Sáez R. Discrepancies in the RIFLE classification are due to the method used to assess the level of derangement of kidney function. *J. Crit. Care*, 2011; 26:572-6.

[69] Mandelbaum T., Scott D. J., Lee J., Mark R. G., Malhotra A., Waikar S. S., et al. Outcome of critically ill patients with acute kidney injury using the acute kidney injury network criteria. *Crit. Care Med.*, 2011; 39:2659-64.

[70] Ricci Z., Cruz D. N., Ronco C. Classification and staging of acute kidney injury: Beyond the R. I. F. L. E. and A. K. I. N. criteria. *Nat. Rev. Nephrol.*, 2011; 7:201-8.

[71] Srisawat N., Kellum J. A. Acute kidney injury: Definition, epidemiology, and outcome. *Curr. Opin. Crit. Care*, 2011; 17:548-55.

[72] Schrier R. W., Wang W., Poole B., Mitra A. Acute renal failure: Definitions, diagnosis, pathogenesis, and therapy. *J. Clin. Invest.*, 2004; 114:5-14.

[73] Uchino S., Bellomo R., Goldsmith D., Bates S., Ronco C. An assessment of the R. I. F. L. E. criteria for acute renal failure in hospitalized patients. *Crit. Care Med.*, 2006; 34:1913-7.

[74] Morgera S., Schneider M., Neumayer H. H. Long-term outcomes after acute kidney injury. *Crit. Care Med.*, 2008; 36:S193-7.

In: Creatinine
Editors: I. H. Perkins and C. M. Chapman
ISBN: 978-1-62257-475-9

Chapter VI

Serum Creatinine: Its Role as a Biomarker of Renal Function

***Kalyani Perumal*[1,*], *Chijoke Onyenwenyi*[2,†] *and Hemanth Hampole*[2,‡]**
[1]Division of Nephrology, John. H. Stroger Hospital of Cook County, Chicago, IL, US
[2]Department of Internal Medicine, John. H. Stroger Hospital of Cook County, Chicago, IL, US

Abstract

Kidney disease has become a global pandemic in the last decade and it is estimated that more than 2 million people in the United States will require transplantation or dialysis for kidney failure by the year 2030. Chronic kidney disease is defined as an estimated glomerular filtration rate (GFR) of less than 60ml/min/1.73m2 or the presence of kidney damage (detected by abnormalities in urinalysis, imaging or pathology) for 3 months or more. Several studies have shown that kidney disease is an independent predictor for cardiovascular and all-cause mortality. There is also ample evidence to show that early detection and effective treatment may halt or retard the progression of kidney disease. This highlights the importance of raising awareness among health care providers and increases their familiarity with the most commonly used methods of evaluating kidney function.

Serum creatinine is the most commonly used measure for estimating kidney function. It is an amino acid derived from the non-enzymatic breakdown of creatine and creatine phosphate in skeletal muscle. Several factors affect its generation including age, gender, race or ethnic group, body habitus, diet, and malnutrition. It is freely filtered across the glomerulus and is neither metabolized nor reabsorbed by the kidney. It is however secreted by the organic cation secretory pathways in the proximal tubules: thus, the creatinine clearance exceeds the actual GFR. Creatinine is measured in most laboratories in the US using the colorimetric alkaline picrate (Jaffe) method which is prone to analytical errors because it also detects non-creatinine

---

* Primary Author.
† Co Author.
‡ Co Author.

chromogens like acetoacetate. Enzymatic methods for measuring creatinine have been reported to have less interference than the Jaffe method.

Elevations in serum creatinine (SCr) almost always reflects decreased glomerular filtration rate (GFR) especially in the absence of drugs that interfere with its tubular secretion (like cimetidine or trimethoprim) or rhabdomyolysis where there is increased creatinine generation. However the relationship between SCr and GFR is not linear, hence small increases in SCr signify marked reduction in GFR. Because of these limitations of SCr as an index of GFR, several prediction equations are in use for estimating GFR and appear to provide a substantial improvement over the measurement of SCr alone in the clinical assessment of kidney function. The commonly used prediction equations are the Cockcroft-Gault (CG) and Modification of Diet in Renal Disease (MDRD) equations. More recently, the Chronic Kidney Disease Epidemiology Collaboration (CKD-EPI) equation is being increasingly used, particularly in many clinical trials. However, these equations have their own limitations, not least because they also depend on SCr measurements. In addition, these equations were derived in specific populations, so it may be inaccurate when used in different subpopulations.

In conclusion, although measurement of SCr and the GFR estimation equations are imperfect methods for evaluating kidney function (especially in populations without kidney disease); they facilitate early detection, evaluation and management of the renal disease.

Introduction

Kidney disease has emerged as a global pandemic in the last decade. It is estimated that more than 10% of the population have chronic kidney disease in the United States [1]. It is thought that by 2030, more than 2 million people will require transplantation or dialysis due to kidney failure [2]. Chronic kidney disease is defined as glomerular filtration rate of less than 60ml/min/1.73m2 of body surface area, or the presence of kidney damage (detected by abnormalities in urinalysis, imaging or pathology) for 3 or more months [3]. There is increasing evidence that kidney disease is an independent risk factor for all-cause mortality and cardiovascular mortality. Furthermore studies show that an estimated GFR of less than 6oml/min/1.73m2 is associated with a graded increase in the risk of the major adverse outcomes of chronic kidney disease, which are impaired kidney function, progression to kidney failure and premature death caused by cardiovascular disease [4-7].

There is evidence to show that earlier detection and effective treatment of kidney disease may halt or retard the progression of kidney disease, thus improve outcomes. However due to the paucity of symptoms, kidney disease is often unrecognized in the early stages. Thus simple, accurate, standardized tests that can be applied universally are needed to assess kidney function. This chapter will discuss the use of serum creatinine, creatinine clearance and estimation equations using serum creatinine for the evaluation of kidney function. We will also highlight the limitations of these tests and discuss other modalities which are currently being investigated to evaluate kidney function.

Serum Creatinine and Creatinine Clearance

Traditionally, glomerular filtration rate (GFR) is considered the best overall index for assessing renal function. It is usually measured through urinary or plasma clearance of an ideal filtration marker, such as inulin or alternative exogenous markers such iothalamate and iohexol. However, using these measurements is cumbersome, time consuming, and expensive. Therefore, these measurements cannot be routinely applied in clinical practice.

The use of the serum creatinine as an index of GFR is based on three major assumptions: (1) creatinine is an ideal filtration marker whose clearance approximates GFR; (2) creatinine excretion rate is constant among individuals and over time; and (3) measurement of serum creatinine is accurate and reproducible across clinical laboratories.

Creatinine is an aminoacid product derived from the non-enzymatic breakdown of creatine and phosphocreatine in skeletal muscle and from dietary meat intake. In subjects on a stable diet and weight, creatinine is thought to be released in the circulation at a relatively constant rate, and thus has a stable plasma concentration. It is freely filtered across the glomerulus and is neither reabsorbed nor metabolized by the kidneys. It is however secreted by the organic cation secretory pathways in the proximal tubules. As much as 10-20% of the urine creatinine concentration is accounted for by tubular secretion and this percentage rises as kidney function declines [8]. Creatinine values vary depending on age, muscle mass, gender, ethnicity and diet. Serum creatinine values are higher in men because of a higher muscle mass and it is presumed that higher levels in African Americans as compared to the Hispanic population are also due to a higher muscle mass and hence creatinine production. Similarly a recent meat diet may also elevate the serum creatinine.

Creatinine is measured by most laboratories in the US using the kinetic alkaline picrate method. This is a colorimetric assay that also detects non-creatinine chromogens such as acetone, acetoacetate, and ascorbic acid leading to an overestimation of serum creatinine by as much as 15-25% within the reference interval [9]. This error is of course increased when these substances are present in large amounts in the serum (for example in diabetic ketoacidosis) [10-12]. The anti-fungal agent flucytosine and the cephalosporin cefoxitin are other agents that are thought to produce a similar effect. However national standardization of serum creatinine assays to creatinine reference materials has largely abolished this error.

Creatinine can also be measured by enzymatic methods such as the creatinine PAP method (Boehringer Mannheim) and Ektachem (Eastman Kodak Co., Rochester, New York). These methods are thought to be less subject to interferences from non-creatinine chromogens. However there have been reports that dopamine, dobutamine, bilirubin, and monoclonal IgM may interfere with these methods [13-15]. High performance liquid chromatography (HPLC) and isotope dilution mass spectrometry (IDMS) are other methods that have been used to measure creatinine. IDMS is now considered the method of choice for establishing the true concentration of creatinine because of its high specificity. The National Kidney Disease Education Program Laboratory Working Group has recommended recalibration of serum creatinine measurement methods to the IDMS [16].

Serum Creatinine (SCr) and Glomerular Filtration Rate

As mentioned earlier, creatinine production is relatively constant in patients on a stable diet and muscle mass. Glomerular filtration rate (GFR) is defined as the amount of plasma cleared of a substance per unit of time. The GFR is the sum of the filtration rates of all the functioning nephrons. The filtering units of the kidney, the glomeruli, filter about 180 liters of plasma daily (approximately 125ml/min). SCr is commonly used as a marker of GFR. There is a reciprocal relationship between SCr and GFR. The shape of this curve has important clinical implications. An initial small rise in SCr usually reflects a marked decline in GFR (an initial small rise in SCr from 0.8 to 1.0 may represent loss of up to 40ml/min per 1.73m2 of GFR) whereas larger increases in SCr at later stages of renal dysfunction (for example from 4mg/dl to 6mg/dl) may only reflect a loss of about 5ml/min/1.73m2.

Elevated SCr almost always reflects a decrease in GFR (exceptions include the use of medications that retard tubular secretion of creatinine like cimetidine and trimethoprim). As a marker of GFR, SCr levels can only be used with certainty in patients with stable kidney function. For example, in patients with acute renal failure with a decline in GFR, there may not have been enough time for the creatinine to accumulate to reflect the degree of kidney damage.

Limitations with the Use of SCr as a Marker of GFR

Serum creatinine (SCr) is easily measured in most laboratories and is readily reported as a component of the basic metabolic profiles in most hospitals. However there are several limitations to the use of SCr as a marker of GFR.

- Assay variations- as mentioned above, various substances can interfere with the assays used for creatinine measurements [9-15].
- Variations in creatinine production- there is inter- and intra patient variability in creatinine production with time. For example, a recent meal consisting of meat may elevate the SCr. Patients with significant variations in diet (for example vegetarians) or muscle mass (muscle wasting, malnutrition and amputations) may have significant variation in creatinine production. It is well known that serum creatinine rises rapidly in patients with rhabdomyolysis before the onset of acute kidney injury, due to the release of preformed creatine from muscle [17]. In this setting, it is very difficult to ascertain the degree of acute kidney injury as serum creatinine levels may not reflect the actual kidney function.
- Variation in creatinine secretion- as mentioned earlier, drugs such as cimetidine and trimethoprim may decrease tubular secretion of creatinine, thereby leading to an increase in SCr without any change in GFR as measured by exogenous filtration markers like iothalamate or iohexol [18-20]. Also, in the initial stages of kidney dysfunction, a decline in GFR may not lead to an initial increase in SCr because of increased tubular creatinine secretion. Thus, a relatively stable SCr does not always indicate stable GFR. However these tubular secretory sites become saturated as the GFR progressively declines eventually leading to a rise in the SCr [8]. For unclear reasons, tubular secretion of creatinine may increase in patients with the nephrotic syndrome [21].
- Hyperfiltration- Early glomerular injury may not lead to an increase in SCr because of compensatory glomerular hypertrophy and hyperfiltration in normal or less

dysfunctional nephrons [22-24]. In these situations, other markers of kidney injury such as an active urine sediment (dysmorphic red cells /red cell casts) and/or proteinuria may reflect ongoing kidney damage

- Intestinal bacterial excretion- Intestinal creatinine elimination increases in severe kidney dysfunction (usually at GFR<15). It is thought that bacterial overgrowth with increased bacterial creatininase activity may account for this leading to lesser SCr elevations than would be expected for the degree of renal dysfunction [25].

Creatinine Clearance (CCr) and GFR

We mentioned earlier that creatinine is freely filtered across the glomerulus and is not metabolized or reabsorbed. However it is secreted by the proximal renal tubules. If the effect of the secretion is ignored, then all of the filtered creatinine (GFR X SCr) will be excreted (UCr X V) where GFR is the glomerular filtration rate, SCr is the serum creatinine concentration, UCr is the urine creatinine concentration, and V is the urine flow rate or volume.

GFR x SCr =UCr x V. Expressed another way;

GFR = UCr x V/ SCr.

This formula is called the creatinine clearance and tends to overestimate the true GFR by up to 20% depending on the contribution of tubular secretion to urinary creatinine concentration [26]. It was thought in the past that this error was counterbalanced by the errors in measurement of SCr [27]. However this is no longer an issue with standardization of SCr assays to creatinine reference materials.

Creatinine clearance is usually measured by a 24hour urine collection with measurement of SCr done at any point during the collection. Let us use an example:

Let us assume that the following results are obtained in a 60kg male.

SCr = 1.1mg/dl

UCr = 110mg/dl

V =1.2L/day. Then

CCr = (110mg/dl X 1.2L/day)/1.1mg/dl = 120L/day. To convert this to ml/min, we need to multiply by 1000(1000ml =1L) and divide by 1440(24 x 60 minutes in one day). Thus

CCr = (120L/day x 1000)/ 1440 = 83ml/min.

This value should be normalized to a body surface area of $1.73m^2$. Suppose our patient's height is 1.60m and his weight is 70kg, then his BSA is estimated to be $1.62m^2$ by the DuBois equation. Thus our creatinine clearance corrected to a BSA of $1.73m^2$ is

CCr = 83 x 1.73 / 1.62 = 89ml/min approximately

Limitations of creatinine clearance

1) 24 hour urine collections are cumbersome and prone to error. An incomplete urine collection will lead to an underestimate of the creatinine excretion and hence the GFR, whereas an over collection will lead to an overestimate of the creatinine excretion, and hence the GFR. One way of assessing the completeness of collection is by knowing the normal rate of creatinine excretion, which is equal to creatinine production in the steady state. In adults under 50, creatinine excretion should equal 20-25mg/kg lean body weight in men, and 15-20mg/kg lean body weight in females in steady state [28]. Our patient in the above example excreted a total of 1320mg of creatinine, or 22mg/kg body weight which likely represents a complete collection.
2) Creatinine secretion by the renal tubules- the accuracy of using the CCr as a measure of the GFR is limited by the fact that 10-20 percent of urinary creatinine excretion is derived from proximal tubular secretion of creatinine, thus leading to an overestimate of the GFR. This ratio increases as the GFR falls leading to larger errors in GFR estimates in patients with markedly impaired kidney function. The inference is that CCr determined from an accurate 24 hour urine collections represents an upper limit of where the true GFR lies(the true GFR may be as low as 50% of the measured CCr). Some authorities have advocated the use of cimetidine to block tubular secretion of creatinine in an effort to improve the accuracy of the CCr as a marker of GFR [19, 22, 29]. However there is no consensus on the exact dose of cimetidine which provides adequate tubular blockade. Also, there is inter- and intra-patient variability in the response to cimetidine which complicates the interpretation of a cimetidine creatinine clearance.

Equations Using Creatinine to Estimate GFR

Prediction equations for GFR take into account some of the limitations of serum creatinine as a marker of GFR and therefore are valuable when evaluating renal function. The Kidney Disease Outcomes and Quality Initiative (K/DOQI) advocates the use of such estimation equations such as the Cockcroft-Gault (CG) and the Modification of Diet in Renal Disease (MDRD)to estimate the GFR [30]. The Chronic Kidney Disease Epidemiology Collaboration (CKD-EPI) is another recently introduced equation which is still being studied in various subpopulations and is undergoing validation.

Cockcroft-Gault Equation-

The Cockcroft-Gault equation was developed in 1973 with data from 249 hospitalized, predominantly male patients. It provides an estimate of creatinine clearance rather than GFR. As such, it often over estimates GFR as it does not take into account tubular secretion of creatinine [31].

CCr (ml/min) = (140-age) x lean body weight (kg)/ SCr (mg/dl) x72

The formula has to be multiplied by 0.85 to account for the presumed 15% lower body mass in women compared to men. This is based on the assumption that females have 15% less muscle mass than males, which might be inaccurate, given the small sample size of women within the study population. [18, 21] The original formula was not adjusted to body surface area. Adjustment to a body surface area of $1.73m^2$ is thought to improve the accuracy of this equation, especially in patients with decreased kidney function. This equation is the most commonly used in drug pharmacokinetics and to guide drug dosing. However, it is important to remember that this CG formula was determined with serum creatinine obtained using the outdated Jaffe assay and not using currently used methodology [32].

Modification of Diet in Renal Disease (MDRD) Equation

The MDRD equation was derived in 1999 from data from 1628 patients with non-diabetic chronic kidney disease [33]. The original equation used 6 variables and was expressed as

GFR in ml/min per $1.73m^2$ = 170 x SCr $(mg/dl)^{-0.999}$x $age^{-0.176}$ x BUN $(mg/dl)^{-0.170}$ x alb $(g/dl)^{+0.318}$ x 0.762(if female) x1.18 (if black) where SCr is the serum creatinine, BUN is blood urea nitrogen, alb is albumin. The original equation was re-expressed to facilitate calculation of the GFR as

GFR in ml/min per $1.73m^2$ = 186.3 x $SCr^{-1.154}$ x $age^{-0.203}$ x 0.742 (if female) x 1.21 (if black).

The above equation was again re-expressed in 2005 for use with a standardized serum creatinine assay, which yields SCr values that are 5 percent lower.

GFR in ml/min per 1.73m2 = 175 x $SCr^{-1.154}$ x $age^{-0.203}$ x 0.742 (if female) x 1.21 (if black).

This equation can be accessed at:
www.kidney.org/professionals/KLS/gfr calculator.cfm

The MDRD equation was derived from mainly Caucasian subjects with non-diabetic kidney disease. It has however been evaluated in other populations and some of the findings are summarized below

1) The MDRD equation is less accurate in patients with normal kidney function. It tends to underestimate kidney function in people with normal kidney function [34-38].
2) The MDRD equation may be less accurate in obese patients and patients with unusual muscle mass such as amputees [37, 39-40].
3) The MDRD equation may be less accurate in different ethnicities, especially the Asian population [41-45].
4) The MDRD equation may be less accurate in elderly patients, children, pregnant patients, recipients of renal allograft, and patients with other co-morbid conditions [34, 37, 46].

Despite these limitations, estimating GFR using this equation helps in early identification of kidney disease, particularly in high risk subjects like diabetics, which may allow early intervention, therefore improve renal outcomes. However, the caveats must be remembered as automatic reporting of GFR using this equation has become universal practice, which may lead to misdiagnosis of kidney disease in normal individuals. . If applied to low risk populations (e.g. potential kidney donors, healthy adults), it will likely result in high false positive rates. [34, 37-38, 46] This will lead to clinical situations where one might have to perform needless additional costly testing. In addition, this kind of misclassification might lead to significant emotional stress and may also affect employment and insurability.

Chronic Kidney Disease Epidemiology Collaboration CKD-EPI equation

The CKD EPI is a recently introduced equation that was developed to provide a more accurate estimation of GFR in normal subjects or patients with only mildly reduced GFR (47). It is expressed as:

$$eGFR = 141 \times \min(SCr/k,1)^{\alpha} \times \max(SCr/k,1)^{-1.209} \times 0.993^{Age} \times [1.018\ if\ Female] \times [1.159\ if\ Black]$$

where S.Cr is serum creatinine, k is 0.7 for females and 0.9 for males, α is -0.329 for females and -0.411 for males, min indicates the minimum of SCr/K or 1, and max indicates the maximum of SCr/K or 1

GFR calculations using the CKD EPI equation can be accessed online at qxmd.com or mdrd.com.

This equation was derived using pooled data from ten studies and validated using data from another 16 studies. The CKD EPI equation has been shown to be as accurate as the MDRD equation among patients with an estimated GFR of less than 60ml/min per $1.73m^2$ and more accurate in subjects with higher GFR. Among patients with GFR greater than 60ml/min per 1.73m2, the CKD EPI equation was associated with less bias, improved precision and greater accuracy [47]. Recent meta-analysis of data from 1.1 million adults from 25 general population cohorts, 13 CKD cohorts and 7 high risk cohorts showed that using CKD –EPI equation reclassified 24% of individuals to higher GFR category and 0.6% to lower GFR category in general population. This shift to higher GFR category was more evident among young individuals, females and non- blacks. In contrast, older individuals in general population tends to be reclassified to lower GFR category compared to other individuals.

Similarly blacks in CKD cohorts were often regrouped to lower GFR category than non-blacks. Thus, this meta-analysis revealed overall lower prevalence of CKD, especially early stages of CKD when using CKD-EPI equation as compared to MDRD equation in general population. The reclassification to high GFR category was much less in CKD cohorts.

Furthermore, this study showed that CKD-EPI equation is a better predictor of risk with respect to all cause mortality, cardiovascular mortality and end stage renal disease [48]. There is growing evidence that this equation performs better in estimation of GFR particularly in normal individuals and patients with near normal renal function.

Limitations of Estimation Equations

All the estimation equations described above are limited by their reliance on the SCr; thus the limitations in the use of the SCr as a measure of GFR listed in previous sections apply to them. In these situations, it is recommended that measurement of clearance of an exogenous filtration marker such as iothalamate, iohexol, DTPA, or EDTA be used to more accurately evaluate the GFR [49].

Table 1. Comparison of GFR estimation equations

Cockcroft-Gault	MDRD	CKD EPI
(140-age) x lean body weight (kg)/ SCr (mg/dl) x72	175 x $SCr^{-1.154}$ x age $^{-0.203}$ x 0.742 (if female) x 1.21 (if black).	141 x $\min(SCr/k,1)^{\alpha}$ x max $(SCr/k,1)^{-1.209}$ x 0.993^{age} x(1.018 if female) x (1.159 if Black)
Equation derived from population database	Equation derived from population database	Equation derived from population database
Less bias than the MDRD	Greater precision than the Cockcroft-Gault	More precision and accuracy than MDRD, and less bias
	Compared to the CKD EPI in population based studies, it provides lower eGFR and therefore higher prevalence of CKD	Compared with the MDRD in population based studies, it provides higher eGFR and therefore lower prevalence of CKD
Limitations due to use of creatinine	Limitations due to use of creatinine	Limitations due to use of creatinine

Important Clinical Application of Estimation Equations

The current estimation equations appear to provide a substantial improvement over the use of SCr alone in the evaluation of kidney function.

1) Drug dosing- The CG equation has traditionally been used to guide drug dosing because of extensive experience with it. This is consistent with the Food and Drug administration recommendations which were issued prior to the widespread use of the MDRD equation [50]. Recent studies have however shown a high concordance rate for kidney function estimates obtained from the CG equation and the recalibrated MDRD study for drug dosing adjustment [51]. The National Kidney Disease Education Program recommends that either the MDRD or CG equation be used to estimate kidney function for drug dosing [52]. Since these equations are limited by their reliance on the SCr, these equations may be inaccurate in patients with unusual diets or extremes of muscle mass. In such situations, a measured CCr or measured GFR using exogenous filtration markers should ideally be performed.
2) Detection and monitoring of chronic kidney disease- Chronic kidney disease is defined as a persistent reduction in GFR to less than 60ml/min per 1.73m^2. Estimation equations for GFR are commonly used in clinical practice to detect kidney disease. However because of the inaccuracies alluded to earlier, it becomes imperative to look for other markers of kidney damage. Patients with persistent proteinuria or abnormalities in imaging studies or kidney biopsy have CKD regardless of GFR. Repeated measurement of SCr and GFR may also help detect progression of kidney disease, though as mentioned above, there are limitations.

Cystatin C

Because of the problems associated with using SCr and its estimation equations in evaluating kidney function, recently other endogenous compounds have been evaluated to provide a more accurate estimate of GFR. Cystatin C is a non-glycosylated protein which is thought to be produced by all nucleated cells. It is freely filtered at the glomerulus and not reabsorbed. It is however metabolized by the tubular epithelial cells which prevents its use to measure clearance. Serum Cystatin C levels have been purported not to be affected by age, gender, or muscle mass. However recent studies have shown that cystatin C levels are increased in males, individuals with greater muscle mass and with increasing age [53-55]. Cystatin C levels have also been shown to be affected by hypo- and hyperthyroidism and corticosteroid therapy, and C-reactive protein levels [53, 56-57]. There is currently no standard for cystatin c measurements and testing is not available in most laboratories [58].

Serum Cystatin C measurements may correlate better with GFR than serum creatinine, especially in patients with only mild reductions in GFR [59-63]. Estimation equations using Cystatin C have been proposed [64-66]. It is however unclear whether this would improve patient care at this time [67].

Conclusion

Serum creatinine and creatinine based equations used for estimating glomerular filtration rate are valuable for the detection, evaluation and monitoring of patients with chronic kidney disease. Despite the limitations, they provide easy, readily available tool to identify patients with kidney disease, so timely diagnosis and intervention can be done. However, one must remember the caveats in using serum creatinine and its equations when applying to the general population and population subgroups that requires more studies on validation. There are other novel serum biomarkers that are being studied, which may replace serum creatinine as the marker of kidney disease. More accurate markers of kidney function may become available in near future which will help further in early identification of kidney injury, therefore may improve patient outcomes.

References

[1] Coresh J, Astor BC, Greene T, Levy AS. Prevalence of chronic kidney disease and decreased kidney function in the adult US population. Third National Health and Nutrition Examination Survey. *Am. J. Kidney Dis.* 2003;41: 1-12.

[2] Renal Data System. 2005 Annual Data Report. Atlas of end stage renal disease in the United States. Bethesda, Md. National Institute of Diabetes and Digestive *Kidney Diseases* 2005.

[3] National Kidney Foundation. K/DOQI clinical practice guidelines for chronic kidney disease: evaluation, classification and stratification. *Am. J. Kidney Dis.* 2002; 39: suppl 1: s1-s266.

[4] Sarnak M J, Levy AS et al. Kidney disease as a risk factor for development of cardiovascular disease: a statement from the American Heart Association Councils on kidney in Cardiovascular Disease, High Blood Pressure Research, Clinical Cardiology, and Epidemiology and Prevention. *Hypertension* 2003; 42:1050-65.

[5] Go A, Chertow G, et al. Chronic kidney disease and the risks of death, cardiovascular events, and hospitalization. *N. Eng. J. Med.* 2004;351: 1296-304.

[6] Weiner DE, Tighiouart H. Et al. Chronic kidney disease as a risk factor for cardiovascular disease and all cause mortality: a pooled analysis of community-based studies. *J. am. Soc. Nephrol.* 2004; 15:1307-15.

[7] Coresh J, Astor B, et al. Evidence for increased cardiovascular increased risk in patients with chronic kidney disease. *Curr. Opin. Nephrol. Hypertens.* 2004; 13: 73-81.

[8] Shermesh O, Golbetz H, et al. Limitations of creatinine as a filtration marker in glomerulopathic patients. *Kidney Int.* 1985; 28:830.

[9] Perone RD, Madias NE, et al. Serum creatinine as an index of renal function: New insights in old concepts. *Clin. Chem.* 1992; 38:1933-53.

[10] Soldin SJ, Henderson L et al. The effects of bilirubin and ketones on reaction rate methods for the measurement of creatinine. *Clin. Biochem.* 1978; 11:82.

[11] Miller WG, Myers GL et al. Creatinine measurement: state of the art in accuracy and interlaboratory harmonization. *Arch. Pathol. Lab. Med.* 2005; 129:297.

[12] Molitch ME, Rodman E et al. Spurious serum creatinine elevations in ketoacidosis. *Ann. Intern. Med.* 1980; 93:280.

[13] Smith CH, Lanelt M, et al. The Kodak Ektachem 400 Analyzer evaluated for automated enzyme determination of plasma creatinine. *Clin. Chem.* 1983; 29: 1422.

[14] Noble MA, Harper B, et al. Rapid determination of 5 Fluorocytosine levels in blood. *J. Clin. Microbiol.* 1984;20:996.

[15] Herrington D, Drusano GL, et al. False elevation in serum creatinine levels. *JAMA* 1984; 252: 2962.

[16] Myers GL, Miller WG, Coresh J et al. Recommendations for improving serum creatinine measurements: a report from the laboratory working group of the National Kidney Disease Education Program. *Clin. Chem.* 2006; 52: 5-18.

[17] Grossman RA, Hamilton RW et al. Non- traumatic rhabdomyolysis and acute renal failure. *N. Eng. J. Med.* 1974; 291:807.

[18] Berg KJ, Gjellestad A et al. Renal effects of trimethoprim in ciclosporin- and azathioprine- treated kidney-allografted patients. *Nephron* 1989; 53: 218.

[19] Hilbrands LB, Artz MA et al. Cimetidine improves the reliability of creatinine as a marker of glomerular filtration. *Kidney Int.* 1991; 40: 1171.

[20] Rocci ML, Vlasses PH et al. Creatinine serum concentrations and H2 receptor antagonists. *Clin. Nephrol.* 1984; 22:214.

[21] Braten AJ, Vervoot G et al. Serum creatinine as a poor marker of GFR in nephritic syndrome. *Nephrol. Dial Transplant.* 2005; 20: 707.

[22] Van Acker BA, Koomer GC et al. Creatinine clearance during cimetidine administration for measurement of glomerular filtration rate. *Lancet* 1992; 340: 1326.

[23] Petri M, Bockenstedt L, Coleman J, et al. Serial assessment of glomerular filtration rate in lupus nephropathy. *Kidney Int.* 1988; 34: 832.

[24] Chagnac A, Kiberd BA, et al. Outcome of the acute glomerular injury in proliferative lupus nephritis. *J. Clin. Invest.* 1989; 84: 922.

[25] Dunn SR, Gabuzda GM, et al. Induction of creatininase activity in chronic renal failure: timing of creatinine degradation and effect of antibiotics. *Am. J. Kidney Dis.* 1997; 29: 72.

[26] Doolan PD, Alpen EL, Theil GB. A clinical appraisal of the plasma concentration and endogenous clearance of creatinine. *Am. J. Med.* 1962; 32: 65.

[27] Coresh J, Astor BC, et al. Calibration and random variation of the serum creatinine assay as critical elements of using equations to estimate glomerular filtration rate. *Am. J. Kidney Dis.* 2002; 39: 920.

[28] Walser M. Creatinie excretion as a measure of protein nutrition in adults of varying age. *JPEN J. Parenter Enteral. Nutr.* 1987; 11: 73S.

[29] Zaltzman JS, Whiteside C, et al. Accurate measurement of impaired glomerular filtration using single dose cimetidine. *Am. J. Kidney Dis.* 1996; 27:504.

[30] Levy AS, Coresh J, Balk E, et al. National Kidney Foundation practice guidelines for chronic kidney disease; Evaluation, Classification and Stratification. *Ann. Int. Med.* 2003; 139(2): 137-47.

[31] Cockcroft DW, Gault MH. Predication of creatinine clearance from serum creatinine. *Nephron* 1976; 16: 31-41.

[32] Hergert-Rosenthal S, Bokenkamp A, et al. How to estimate GFR- serum creatinine, serum cystatin c or equations? *Clin. Biochem.* 2007; 40: 153-161.

[33] Klahr S, Levy AS, Beck GJ, et al. The effects of dietary protein restriction and blood pressure control on the progression of chronic renal disease. *N. Eng. J. Med.* 1994;330: 877-884.

[34] Poggio ED, Wang X, Greene T, et al. Performance of the modification of diet in renal disease and Cockcroft- Gault study equations in the estimation of GFR in health and chronic kidney disease. *J. Am. Soc. Nephrol.* 2005; 16: 459.

[35] Rule AD, Larson TS, Bergstralh EG, et al. Using serum creatinine to estimate the glomerular filtration rate: accuracy in good health and chronic kidney disease. *Ann. Int. Med.* 2004; 141: 929.

[36] Gonwa TA, Jennings L, Mai ML, et al. Estimation of glomerular filtration rates before and after orthoptic liver transplantation: evaluation of current estimation equations. *Liver Transpl.* 2004; 10: 301.

[37] Froissant M, Rossert J, Jacquot C, et al. Predictive performance of the modification of diet in renal disease and Cockcroft Gault study equations for estimating renal function. *J. Am. Soc. Nephrol.* 2005; 16: 763.

[38] Lin J, Knight EL, Hogan ME, et al. A comparison of prediction equations for estimating glomerular filtration rate in adults without kidney disease. *J. Am. Soc. Nephrol.* 2003; 14: 2573.

[39] Verhave JC, Fesler P, Ribstein J, et al. Estimation of renal function in subjects with normal serum creatinine levels: influence of age and body mass index. *Am. J. Kidney Dis.* 2005; 46: 233.

[40] Cirillo M, Anastasio P, DeSanto NG. Relationship of gender, age, and body mass index to errors in predicted kidney function. *Nephrol. Dial Transplant.* 2005; 20:1791.

[41] Zuo L, Ma YC, Zhon YH, et al. Application of the GFR estimating equations in Chinese patients with chronic kidney disease. *Am. J. Kidney Dis.* 2005; 45: 463.

[42] Mahajan S, Mukhiya GK, Singh R, et al. Assessing glomerular filtration rates in healthy Indian adults: a comparison of prediction equations. *J. Nephrol.* 2005; 18:257.

[43] Jafar TH, Schmid CH, Levy AS. Serum creatinine as a marker of kidney function in South Asians: a study of reduced GFR of adults in Pakistan. *J. Am. Soc. Nephrol.* 2005; 16: 1413.

[44] Ssaki S. Nephrologists Sans Frontieres: Chronic kidney disease in Japan. *Kidney Int.* 2006; 69: 1485.

[45] Agarwal R. Estimating GFR from serum creatinine concentration: pitfalls of GFR estimating equations. *Am. J. Kidney Dis.* 2005; 45: 610.

[46] Vervoot G, Willems HL, Wetzels JFM. Assessment of glomerular filtration rates in healthy subjects and normoalbuminuric diabetic patients: validity of a new (MDRD) prediction equation. *Nephrol. Dial. Transp.* 2002; 17: 1909-13.

[47] Levy AS, Stevens LA, Schmid CH, et al. A new equation to estimate glomerular filtration rate. *Ann. Int. Med.* 2009; 150: 64.

[48] Levy AS, Coresh J, Matsushita K, Mahmoodi BK, Woodward M et al. Comparison of Risk Prediction using the CKD-EPI equation and the MDRD study equation for estimated glomerular filtration rate. *JAMA* 2012;307:1941-1951.

[49] Brandstrom E, Grzegorczyk A, Jacobsen L, et al. GFR measurement with iohexol and 51Cr-EDTA. Acomparison of two favoured markers in Europe. *Nephrol. Dial. Transplant.* 1998; 13: 1176.

[50] Food and Drug administration: Guidance for Industry: Pharmacokinetics in patients with Impaired Renal Function-Study Design, Data Analysis, and the Impact on Dosing. Rockville, MD, US Department of Health and Human Services, May 1998.

[51] Stevens LA, Nolin TD, Richardson MM, et al. Comparison of drug dosing recommendations based on measured GFR and kidney function estimating equations. *Am. J. Kidney Dis*. 2009; 54:33.

[52] http://www,nkdep.nih.fgov/professionals/drug-dosing-information.htm.

[53] Knight EL, Verhave JC, Spiegelman D, et al. Factors influencing serum cystatin C levels other than renal function and the impact on renal function measurement. *Kidney Int*. 2004; 65:1416.

[54] Groesbeck D, Koltgen A, Parekh R, et al. Age, gender and race effects on cystatin C levels in US adolescents. *Clin. J. Am. Soc. Nephrol*. 2008; 3:1777.

[55] Macdonald J, Marcora S, Jibani M, et al. GFR estimation using cystatin C is not independent of body composition. *Am. J. Kidney Dis*. 2006; 48: 712.

[56] Manetti L, Pardini E, Genovesi M, et al. Thyroid function differently affects serum cystatin C and creatinine concentrations. *J. Endocrinol. Invest*. 2005; 28: 346.

[57] Stevens LA, Schmid CH, Greene T, et al. Factors other glomerular filtration rate affect serum cystatin C levels. *Kidney Int*. 2009;75:652.

[58] Mussap M, Plebani M. Biochemistry and clinical role of human cystatin C. *Crit. Rev. Clin. Lab. Sci*. 2004; 41: 467.

[59] Newman DJ, Thakker H, Edwards RG, et al. Serum cystatin C measured by automated immunoassay: a more sensitive marker of changes in GFR than serum creatinine. *Kidney Int*. 1995; 47:312.

[60] Coll E, Botey A, Alvarez L, et al. Serum cystatin C as a new marker for non-invasive estimation of glomerular filtration rate and as a marker for early renal impairment. *Am. J. Kidney Dis*. 2000; 36:29.

[61] Fliser D, Ritz E. Serum cystatin C concentration as a marker of renal dysfunction in the elderly. *Am. J. Kidney Dis*. 2001; 37: 79.

[62] Hoek FJ, Kemperman FA, Krediet RT. A comparison between cystatin C, plasma creatinine and the Cockcroft Gault formula for the estimation of glomerular filtration rate. *Nephrol. Dial. Transplant*. 2003; 18:2024.

[63] Dharnidharka VR, Kwon C, Stevens G. Serum cystatin C is superior to serum creatinine as a marker of kidney function: a meta-analysis. *Am. J. Kidney Dis*. 2002; 40:221.

[64] Grubb A, Nyman U et al. Simple cystatin C based prediction equations for glomerular filtration rate compared with the modification of diet in renal disease prediction equation for adults and the Schwartz and Counahan-Barratt prediction equations for children. *Clin. Chem*. 2005; 51:1420.

[65] Sjostrom P, Tidman M, Jones I. Determination of the production rate, and non-renal clearance of cystatin C and estimation of glomerular filtration rate from the serum concentration of cystatin C in humans. *Scand. J. Clin. Lab. Invest*. 2005; 65: 111.

[66] Grubb A, Bjork J, Lindstrom V, et al. A cystatin C based formula without anthropometric variables estimates glomerular filtration rates better than creatinine clearance using the Cockcroft Gault formula. *Scand. J. Clin. Lab. Invest*. 2005; 65: 153.

[67] DeinumJ, Derkx FH. Cystatin C for estimation of glomerular filtration rate? *Lancet* 2000; 356: 1624.

In: Creatinine
Editors: I. H. Perkins and C. M. Chapman
ISBN: 978-1-62257-475-9

Chapter VII

Role of Creatinine in Renal Disease

Athanasia K. Papazafiropoulou, Marina S. Kardara and Stavros I. Pappas*
3rd Department of Internal Medicine and Center of Diabetes,
General Hospital of Nikaia "Ag. Panteleimon",Piraeus, Greece

Abstract

Creatinine, a muscle waste product, is widely interpreted as a measure of renal function. However, the serum level reflects not only renal excretion, but also the generation, intake, and metabolism of creatinine. In stable normal or reduced renal function they are determined by the rate of creatinine production and the endogenous creatinine clearance, and, during changing renal function, also by the apparent volume of distribution of creatinine. The rate of creatinine production is proportional to body weight, and it decreases with age and is slower in females than in males. Elevated creatinine levels suggest the differential diagnosis of renal failure. History and a complete physical examination are important. An ultrasound scan is particularly useful for eliminating an obstructive cause while complementary blood tests and imaging studies might be useful. We reviewed the principles of physiology, metabolism of creatinine, and its diagnostic uses and role in renal disease.

Introduction

Creatinine was discovered in 1847 by Liebig [1] who obtained creatinine by heating creatine with mineral acids. In 1885 Horbaczewski first synthesized creatinine [2] and in 1894 Paulmann showed that creatine was methylguanidoacetic acid and that creatinine was its internal anhydride [3]. Creatinine except for serum and erythrocytes is also present in sweat, bile, gastrointestinal fluids [4] and in the cerebrospinal fluid [5]. The amount of creatinine in

* Correspondence:A. Papazafiropoulou, MD PhD, 3rd Department of Internal Medicine and Center of Diabetes, General Hospital of Nikaia "Ag. Panteleimon" - Piraeus, Greece, 3 D.Mantouvalou Street, GR-184 54 Nikaia, Greece, Tel : +30 213 207 2662, Fax : +30 213 207 6404, Email: pathan@ath.forthnet.gr.

urine is related to muscle mass than with body weight, and higher creatinine levels are seeing in healthy men than in women [6]. In addition, obese individuals have lower creatinine levels than lean individuals [7]. The urinary output of creatinine varies little with diet and is independent of diuresis [8] while physical exercise appears to increase its level slightly.

Glomerular Filtration Rate

Because small amounts of creatinine are secreted by the tubules, creatinine clearance values are not an exact estimate of the glomerular filtration rate (GFR). GFR is estimated clinically from serum concentrations of creatinine [9]. However, serum creatinine should not be used alone to estimate GFR because it is affected by age, sex, race, body size, diet, certain drugs, and laboratory analytical methods [10, 11].

More accurate estimations of GFR can be obtained with equations that combine the effects from factors that affect serum creatinine other than GFR [12]. The currently recommended estimating equation was developed from the Modification of Diet in Renal Disease (MDRD) Study [13] and is based on GFR values measured by iothalamate clearance in 1628 adults and subsequently validated in another 1775 adults in the African American Study of Kidney Disease [14]. The "four-variable" MDRD Study equation (Eq. 1) uses age, sex, race (African-American vs. non–African-American), and serum creatinine (sCr) [15]:

$$\text{GFR } [\text{mL/min/}(1.73\text{ m}^2)] = 186 \times (\text{sCr})^{-1.154} \times (\text{age})^{-0.203} \times (0.742 \text{ if female}) \times (1.210 \text{ if African-American})$$

The MDRD Study equation does not require a body weight variable because it normalizes GFR for a standard body surface area of 1.73 m^2. The MDRD Study equation has been demonstrated to be useful for chronic kindey disease patients and performs similarly in diabetic vs nondiabetic individuals [16], but its use is unclear for healthy individuals and is not recommended for hospitalized patients [17].

Creatinine Production and Metabolism

Liver is the place where synthesis of creatine, the precursor of creatinine, takes place. Creatine, after its release into the circulation, is actively taken up by muscle and other tissues. Muscle contains -98% of the total body creatine pool, of which 60-70% exists as phosphocreatine, and the rest as free creatine [18]. Creatine is filtered and reabsorbed by the kidney, and urinary creatine excretion is less than 100 mg/24h [19].

The most important determinant of creatinine production is total muscle mass [20]. Age and sex affect creatinine production rates because of their impact on muscle mass. It is known that muscle mass declines with advancing age [21]. In addition, the larger muscle mass of men accounts for the greater creatinine production and renal excretion than in women [22]. Associated with decreased creatinine production, are muscle-wasting conditions such as chronic glucocorticoid therapy [23], hyperthyroidism [24], progressive muscular dystrophy

[25], myotonia atrophica [24], amyotrophic lateral sclerosis [24], poliomyelitis [26], paraplegia and quadriplegia [27], and dermatomyositis and polymyositis [24].

Creatine is largely ingested in meat; uncooked lean beef contains 3.5-5 mg of creatine per gram [28, 29]. Although each gram of uncooked lean beef contains only 0.2-0.4 mg of preformed creatiine, as much as 18-65% of the creatine in meat is converted to creatinine during cooking; this conversion depends on the temperature and cooking time [28, 29].

Creatinine Measurement

Creatinine can be measured readily in serum, plasma, or urine [30]. The standard method for measurement of creatinine uses the Jaffe reaction [31], in which creatinine reacts directly with picrate ion under alkaline conditions to form an equimolar complex whose red-orange color is easily detected and quantified [32]. The advantages of methods using the Jaffe reaction are their simplicity and the wide clinical acceptance gained over almost 80 years of use. The major disadvantage of these methods is that in normal subjects as much as 20% of the color reaction in serum or plasma arises from substances other than creatinine [33-37]. These positive interferences can be classified into two categories: substances such as glucose, ascorbate, and uric acid, which slowly reduce the alkaline picrate; and substances such as acetoacetate, pyruvate, other ketoacids, and protein, which react with alkaline picrate to form colored complexes.

The presence of these non creatinine chromogens results in an apparent creatinine value that is 20% higher than the true value. Although such overestimation does not usually impact on clinical decision-making, in ketoacidosis increased concentrations of acetoacetate may substantially increase the concentration of serum creatiine measured by this technique [38]. Certain cephalosporins may also contribute to the colorimetric reaction [39, 40]. As a general rule, noncreatinine chromogens do not interfere significantly with measurements in urine. Another drawback of the Jaffe reaction is negative interference from high concentrations of bilirubin or other compounds in the serum of jaundiced patients.

Various methods developed to measure creatinine include separation of creatinine from non creatinine chromogens by enzymatic digestion or adsorption of creatinine with porous aluminum silicate clays (Fuller's earth, Lloyd's reagent) coupled with the Jaffe reaction, kinetic alkaline picrate assays (the AutoAnalyzer method) [41-43], high-pressure liquid chromatography [44, 45], ion-exchange chromatography [46], mass fragmentography [47], and several enzymatic methods [38, 48].

Clinical Applications

Aging

Aging is associated with alterations in renal function and creatinine metabolism. Renal pathological features in patients over 60 years old include arterial medial sclerosis and global glomerular sclerosis [49, 50], that are related to generalized arteriosclerosis and, the higher blood pressure observed in older populations, and a lifetime of excessive intake of dietary protein [50-52].

GFR normally decrease with aging. Cross-sectional studies in healthy men show that the average decline in the GFR is 10 mL/min per 1.73 m^2 per decade after 30 years old [53]. The average GFR declines from 130 to 80 mL/min per 1.73 m^2 as the subject age from 30 to 80 years.

It is of great importance to notify that a normal concentration of serum creatinine in elderly subjects does not indicate the same extent of renal function as in younger individuals. Awareness of the normal decrease in the GFR in elderly subjects is important in order to reduce the dosage of drugs that are excreted by glomerular filtration, even if the serum creatinine concentration is normal [53].

In patients with renal disease the aging-associated decline in creatinine production may significantly blunt an increase of the serum creatinine, despite a marked reduction in the GFR and creatinine clearance [53].

Pregnancy

GFR and kidney size increase markedly during pregnancy because of the changed hormonal milieu and the increased metabolic demands associated with pregnancy. Measurements of inulin clearance at the end of the first trimester demonstrate a 50% increase in the GFR [54, 55]. Outpatient or ambulatory 24-h creatinine clearance is increased by 20% from the non pregnant state by the fourth week after conception and by 30-40% at the end of the first trimester [56]. This increase is sustained throughout the second trimester [56]. Similar increments in the GFR and creatinine clearance during pregnancy are also obtained in women with mild preexisting renal disease [57] or after renal transplantation [58].

The consequence of increased GFR and creatinine clearance in the presence of unchanged creatinine generation is a marked decrease in the concentration of serum creatinine. The implication of this decrease in serum creatinine during uncomplicated pregnancy is that serum creatinine values usually considered to be normal for the non pregnant state may in fact represent a serious decrement in renal function during pregnancy [59].

Diabetes Mellitus

The metabolic and microvascular complications of diabetes mellitus are associated with multiple effects on renal function and creatinine metabolism. Studies of subjects with recent onset (usually <6 years) of type 1 diabetes who are maintained on insulin therapy demonstrate that the GFR is increased by as much as 25% to 50% over that in normal subjects [60, 61]. The difficulty in detecting the onset of type 2 diabetes prevents a precise description of the range of GFRs in such subjects.

The mechanism of the increased GFR in diabetes is complex and various causes have been proposed, including hyperglycemia per se, volume expansion secondary to hyperglycemia, increased secretion of atrial natriuretic peptide, increased production of vasodilatory prostaglandins, increased concentrations of growth hormone and glucagon, and insulinopenia [62, 63]. Maintenance of glycemic control with conventional subcutaneous insulin therapy reduces the GFR, but only to values that still exceed normal [64]. Even with excellent glycemic control, the GFR does not return completely to normal [61].

Long-standing diabetes mellitus is associated with the development of renal failure in 30-50% of type 1 subjects and in 5% of type 2 subjects [65, 66]. Pathological features include diffuse and nodular gbmerulosclerosis associated with sclerosis of afferent and efferent arterioles. Detecting the early decrease in renal function in diabetic nephropathy by means of the serum creatinine concentration is difficult. As in other forms of chronic renal disease, the serum creatinine concentration is insensitive for detecting decreased GFRS in diabetic nephropathy [67, 68].

Drug Administration

Cimetidine

Early clinical observations revealed that cimetidine in doses of 1.6 g day could increase plasma creatinine concentrations by an average of 15% in patients with normal renal function [69, 70]. Later studies showed that in high single doses, 300 mg i.v. or 800 mg orally, cimetidine could cause a decrease in the clearances of endogenous as well as exogenous creatinine of 20±30% in healthy volunteers [71, 72]. Cimetidine and creatinine are both secreted in the proximal renal tubule by the secretory mechanisms for organic ions [73]. Cimetidine is supposed to possess a higher affinity for the carrier at the luminal membrane of the proximal tubules than does creatinine [74]. Thus, these compounds will compete with each other for tubular secretion [75]. Ranitidine and famotidine, which have similar pharmacokinetic characteristics to cimetidine [76], are known to inhibit tubular secretion of some drugs, such as triamterene, procainamide and cisplatin [77, 78]. However, they do not alter creatinine elimination when administered in therapeutic doses [79].

Trimethoprim

Trimethoprim in therapeutic doses can cause an increase in plasma creatinine concentration of 15±30% and a decrease in creatinine clearance of 20±25% without alterations in GFR [80, 81]. This effect is more pronounced in patients with chronic renal failure [82]. The effect of trimethoprim, which is an organic base, on the renal creatinine handling is explained in the same way as the effect of cimetidine, i.e. competitive inhibition of the renal tubular secretion. Besides this effect, trimethoprim can also cause hyperkalaemia [83, 84]. Cotrimoxazole and trimethoprim can also induce real renal toxicity: acute tubular necrosis and acute interstitial nephritis are reported [85, 86].

Salicylates

In some conditions (salt depletion, advanced age, liver cirrhosis, renal diseases and renal failure), salicylates can induce a rise in plasma creatinine concentration as a result of decreased renal plasma flow and GFR [87, 88]. This result is cited as an example of anionic substances capable of inhibiting creatinine tubular secretion [89].

Other Drugs (Phenacemide, Corticosteroids, Vitamin D Derivatives)

These drugs are also reported to affect plasma creatinine concentration, although the studies are less well documented and the mechanisms not, or only partly, clarified. The anticonvulsant drug phenacemide caused an increase in plasma creatinine that was completely reversible after the drug was stopped [90, 91]. Acute and chronic administrations of corticosteroids are known to increase GFR in experimental animals [92] as well as in humans [93]. Paradoxically, plasma creatinine concentration does not fall, but increases by 10% [94]. The cause of the rise in plasma creatinine is supposed to be the catabolic state with protein degeneration and loss of muscle tissue induced by the steroid treatment [94].

Treatment with calcitriol or alfacalcidol can also cause a rise in plasma creatinine and/or a decrease in creatinine clearance [95-97]. The mechanisms by which vitamin D enhances plasma creatinine concentration are unclear, but might be decreased tubular secretion and/or enhanced creatinine production.

Acute Renal Failure

Acute renal failure is defined as a rapid deterioration in renal function, resulting in the accumulation of nitrogenous waste products, including creatinine.

The mechanism of reduction in GFR in acute renal failure is dependent on the nature of the primary insult, most commonly acute tubular necrosis, caused by renal ischemia or exposure to nephrotoxins [98].

The rate of increase of serum creatinine depend on the severity and time course of resolution of renal injury, rate of generation of creatinine, volume of distribution of creatinine, and extrarenal creatinine elimination. In principle, if the renal function stabilizes, the serum creatinine concentration will reach a plateau at a value where renal creatinine excretion equals the difference between production and extrarenal elimination of creatinine [99].

When renal function then rises toward normal values, the serum creatinine concentration will start to fall, but only when renal creatinine excretion exceeds the difference between creatinine production and extrarenal elimination.

However, because of numerous alterations in acute renal failure, serum creatinine concentration is unuseful in estimating the degree of renal function. First, the GFR may fall to a value so low that dialysis is necessary before the steady-state increased concentration of serum creatinine is reached.

Only after sufficient time has elapsed will the serum creatinine increase to a value usually associated with severe renal failure. Second, the GFR is not constant during acute renal failure. Third, a large increase in total body water, increases the volume in which creatinine is distributed and therefore may blunt or even eliminate the increase in the serum creatinine concentration from acute renal failure [100].

Chronic Renal Disease

Chronic renal disease is characterized by a progressive decline in renal function, eventually culminating in renal failure. The cause of the reduced GFR is a decrease in either glomerular capillary surface area or hydraulic permeability [51]. Many factors contribute to these hemodynamic alterations, including high dietary protein intake, stimulation of the renin-angiotensin system, and augmented synthesis of vasodilatory prostaglandins [101]. Numerous clinical trials have been undertaken to assess whether the progression of renal disease in humans can be delayed by low-protein diets and inhibition of angiotensin converting enzyme, showing beneficial effects [102-105], expect for one study [103].

Later in the course of renal insufficiency, decreases in creatinine generation and an increase in extrarenal creatinine metabolism blunt the increase in serum creatinine despite further decreases in the GFR. Thus, the serum creatinine concentration does not accurately reflect the extent of renal function during the course of progressive renal disease. An increase in serum creatinine generally may be taken as an indication of further deterioration in the GFR; a stable creatinine concentration, however, does not indicate that renal structure and function are stable. The rate of decline of the reciprocal of the serum creatinine concentration has been observed to be relatively constant in patients who progress to severe renal insufficiency [106-108].

Diagnosis of Renal Disease

Patient's History

In taking the history of a patient with kidney disease, the clinician should attempt to determine when the onset of proteinuria and hypertension occurred and whether previous serum creatinine tests have been performed. Patients should also be questioned regarding voiding symptoms, such as hesitancy, decreased stream strength, or intermittent large and small voiding amounts, because these symptoms suggest obstructive uropathy.

Every patient with an elevated serum creatinine level should be asked if they have a history of diabetes, arthritis, or medication exposure. Almost all NSAIDs and antibiotics, have been reported to cause renal failure [109]. Previous use of chemotherapeutic agents, such as gemcitabine and cisplatin, [109] or history of gastroesophageal reflux disease and proton pump inhibitor use [110] should be identified. Recent radiographic studies using radiocontrast agents [111] should also be considered when attempting to identify possible causes of an elevated serum creatinine level.

Diagnostic Examination

First, the clinician should test for prerenal azotemia, lying and standing blood pressure and pulse should be recorded. Funduscopic examination for findings of hypertension and diabetic changes should be performed [112]. During an examination specific to a diagnosis of increasing serum creatinine levels, the clinician should also check for evidence of volume overload (rales, third heart sound, lower-extremity edema), joint effusions or erythema, and splinter hemorrhages, as well as palpate for distended bladder above the symphysis pubis.

Laboratory Testing

Consider testing for creatinine phosphokinase and aldolase levels to determine that the elevated serum creatinine level retains its validity as a marker of renal function and does not reflect increased creatinine production (eg, rhabdomyolysis).

The standard work-up also includes a physician-performed urinalysis; measurement of levels of serum creatinine (usually with a full electrolyte panel), creatinine, and serum cholesterol (nephrotic syndrome); and a 24-hour urinary protein excretion test.

To determine whether systemic illness is the cause of renal disease, an antineutrophil cytoplasmic antibody panel, serum and urine protein electrophoresis, and fat aspiration for amyloidosis may be performed, as should serologic tests to determine C3 and C4 complement levels and to check for the presence of antinuclear antibody, rheumatoid factor, antiglomerular basement membrane antibody, and cryoglobulins. Although commonly performed, these tests only rarely reveal a systemic disease thought to be present without the serologic evidence, and even positive serologic findings do not obviate the need for renal biopsy [113]. However, positive serologic findings may make physicians more comfortable in recommending a renal biopsy. Although most renal biopsies are without incident, 50% of the patient's GFR could be lost if refractory bleeding requires nephrectomy.

Radiography

Renal ultrasonography with arterial Doppler studies is the single most important test for evaluating all patients with an elevated creatinine level.

First and most importantly, it is the least invasive method for identifying obstructive uropathy, the most reversible form of renal failure.

Second, it provides information on renal size. If the kidneys are smaller than 7 to 8 cm, then the likelihood of a reversible form of renal failure is extremely low. Large kidneys (>12-13 cm) have a specific differential diagnosis, including reversible conditions such as acute glomerulonephritis, infiltrative diseases of the kidney (leukemia, lymphoma, Hodgkin disease, multiple myeloma, and amyloidosis), and conditions without reversibility such as diabetic nephropathy, polycystic kidney disease, and obstruction. The Doppler component helps identify patients with bilateral renal artery stenosis, whose renal function would benefit from successful angioplasty.

Conclusion

Creatinine is a well established marker of renal function that should be used with causion in clinical practice since its serum concentrations depends on various factors. Factors, like aging, diabetes mellitus, several drugs, renal disease, even pregnancy, have great impact in its level. More sophisticate methods, like MDRD formula, have now replace creatinine's value in daily clinical practice.

References

[1] Liebig J, Kreatin und Kreatinin, Bestandtheile des Hams der Menschen. *J. Prakt. Chem.,* 1847; 40: 288-292.

[2] Horbaczewskl J. Neue synthese des Kreatins. Weiner Med. Jahrbdcher, p459, 1885; cited from Jahresber. *Their. Chem.*, 1885; 15: 86-87.

[3] Paulmann W. Beitrage zur Kenntniss des Sarkosins. *Arch. Pharm.,* 1894; 232: 601-639.

[4] Schumann R. Uber das Vorkommen von Kreatinin und Kreatin im menschlichen Schweibe. *Z. Ges. Exp. Med.,* 1931; 79: 145-152.

[5] Myers VC, Fine M S. Comparative distribution of urea, creatinine, uric acid and sugar in blood and spinal fluid. *J. Biol. Chem.,* 1919; 37: 239-244.

[6] Clark LC, Thompson HL, Beck EI, Jacobson W. Excretion of creatine and creatinine by children. *Am. J. Dis. Child.,* 1951; 81: 774-783.

[7] Garn SM, Clark LCJr. Creatinine weight coefficient as measurement of obesity. *J. Appi. Physiol.,* 1955; 8: 135-138.

[8] Wang E. Clinical and experimental investigations on creatine metabolism. *Acta. Med. Scand. Suppl.,* 1939; 105: 1-338.

[9] Levey AS. Measurement of renal function in chronic renal disease. *Kidney Int.,* 1990; 38: 167–184.

[10] Shemesh O, Golbety H, Kriss JP, Myers BD. Limitations of creatinine as a filtration marker in glomerulopathic patients. *Kidney Int.,* 1985; 28: 830–838.

[11] Perrone RD, Madias NE, Levey AS. Serum creatinine as an indexof renal function: new insights into old concepts. *Clin. Chem.,* 1992; 38: 1933–1953.

[12] Stevens LA, Levey AS. Clinical implications for estimating equations for GFR. *Ann. Intern. Med.,* 2004; 141: 959–961.

[13] Levey AS, Bosch JP, Lewis JB, Greene T, Rogers N, Roth D, et al. A more accurate method to estimate glomerular filtration rate from serum creatinine: a new prediction equation. *Ann. Intern. Med.,* 1999; 130: 461–470.

[14] Lewis J, Agodoa L, Cheek D, Greene T, Middleton J, O'Connor D, et al. African-American Study of Hypertension and Kidney Disease. Comparison of cross-sectional renal function measurements in African Americans with hypertensive nephrosclerosis and of primary formulas to estimate glomerular filtration rate. *Am. J. Kidney Dis.,* 2001; 38: 744–753.

[15] Levey AS, Greene T, Kusek JW, Beck GJ, Group MS. A simplified equation to predict glomerular filtration rate from serum creatinine [Abstract]. *J. Am. Soc. Nephrol.,* 2000; 11: A0828.

[16] Poggio ED, Wang X, Greene T, Van Lente F, Hall PM. Performance of the modification of diet in renal disease and Cockcroft-Gault equations in the estimation of GFR in health and in chronic kidney disease. *J. Am. Soc. Nephrol.,* 2005; 16: 459–466.

[17] Poggio ED, Nef PC, Wang X, Greene T, Van Lente F, Dennis VW, et al. Performance of the Cockcroft-Gault and modification of diet in renal disease equations in estimating GFR in ill hospitalized patients. *Am. J. Kidney Dis.,* 2005; 46: 242–252.

[18] Geigy scientific tables, 7th ed. Basle, *Ciba-Geigy Ltd.,* 1971: 572,665.

[19] Fitch CD, Sinton DW. A study of creatine metabolism in diseases causing muscle wasting. *J. Clin. Invest.,* 1964; 43: 444-452.

[20] Heymsfield SB, McManus C, Smith J, Stevens V, Nixon DW. Anthropometric measurement of muscle mass: revised equations for calculating bone-free arm muscle area. *Am. J. Clin. Nutr.,* 1982; 36: 680-690.
[21] Tomlinson BE, Walton JN, Rebeiz JJ. The effects of aging or cachexia upon skeletal muscle-a histopathological study. *J. Neurol. Sci.,* 1969; 9: 321-346.
[22] Cockcroft DW, Gault MH. Prediction of creatinine clearance from serum creatinine. *Nephron,* 1976; 16:31-41.
[23] Horber FI', Scheidegger J, Frey FJ. Overestimation of renal function in glucocorticosteroid-treated patients. *Eur. J. Clin. Pharmacal.,* 1985; 28: 537-541.
[24] Friedman RB, Anderson RE, Entine SM, Hirshberg SB. Effect of diseases on clinical laboratory tests. *Clix. Chem.,* 1980; 26: 1D-476D.
[25] Hoagland CL, Gilder H, Shank RE. The synthesis, storage, and excretion of creatine, creatinine, and glycocyamine in progressive muscular dystrophy and the effects of certain hormones on these processes. *J. Exp. Med.,* 1945; 81: 423-438.
[26] Whedon GD, Shore E. Metabolic studies in paralytic acute anterior poliomyelitis. L Alterations in nitrogen and creatine metabolism. *J. Clin. Invest.,* 1957; 36: 942-.965.
[27] Mohler JL, Barton SD, Blouin BA, Cowen DL, Flanigan RC. The evaluation of creatinine clearance in spinal cord injury patients. *J. Urol.,* 1986; 136: 366-369.
[28] Macy RL Jr, Naumann HD, Bailey ME. Water-soluble flavor and odor precursors of meat. 5. Influence of heating on acid extractable nonnucleotide chemical constituents of beef, lamb and pork. *J. Food Sci.,* 1970; 35: 83-87.
[29] Camara AA, Arnk D, Reimer A, Newburgh LH. The 24 hourly endogenous creatinine clearance as a clinical measure of the functional state of the kidneys. *J. Lab. Clin. Med.,* 1951; 37: 743-763.
[30] Kubasik NP, Lisuzzo CW, Same DG, Sine DG, DSouza JP. Multilayered film analysis: evaluation of ammonia and creatimne slides. *Clin. Biochem.,* 1984; 17: 15-18.
[31] Ueber den Niederschlag welchen Pikrinsaure in normalen Ham erzeugt mid uber eine neue Reaction des Kreatinins. *Z .Physiol. Chem.,* 1886; 10: 391-400.
[32] Bonsnes RW, Taussky HA. On the colorimetric determination of creatinine by the Jaffe reaction. *J. Biol. Chem.,* 1945; 158: 581-591.
[33] Mandell EE, Jones FL. Studies in nonprotein nitrogen. EL Evaluation of methods measuring creatimne. *J. Lab. Clin. Med.,* 1953; 41: 323-334.
[34] Doolan PD, Alpen EL, Theil GB. A clinical appraisal of the plasma concentration and endogeneous clearance of creatinine. *Am. J. Med.,* 1962; 32: 65-79.
[35] Young DS, Pestaner LC, Gibberman V. Effects of drugs on clinical laboratory tests. *Clin. Chem.,* 1975; 21: 1D-432D.
[36] Rock RC, Walker WG, Jennings CD. Nitrogen metabolites and renal function. In: Tietz NW, ed. Textbook of clinical chemistry. Philadelphia: *Saunders,* 1986: 1254-316.
[37] Murray RL. Creatiine. In: Peace Ad, Kaplan LA, eds. Methods in clinical chemistry, St. Louis: *Mosby,* 1987:10-17.
[38] Gerard SK, Khayam-Bashi H. Characterization of creatinine error in ketotic patients. A prospective comparison of alkaline picrate methods with an enzymatic method. *Am. J. Clin. Pathol.,* 1985; 84: 659-664.
[39] Kroll MH, Hagengruber C, Elm RJ. Reaction of picrate with creatiine and cepha antibiotics. *Clin. Chem.,* 1984; 30: 1664-1666.

[40] Kroll MH, Koch TR, Drusano GL, Warren JW. Lack of interference with creatimne assays by four cephalosporin-like antibiotics. *Am. J. Clin. Pathol.,* 1984; 82: 214-216.

[41] Technicon Method N-ha. Estimation of creatinine, Auto-Analyzer N methodology. Chauncy, NY: *Technicon Instruments Corporation,* 1963.

[42] Bowers LD. Kinetic serum creatinine assays I. The role of various factors in determining specificity. *Clin. Chem.,* 1980; 26: 551-554.

[43] Bowers LS, Wong ET. Kinetic serum creatimne assays II. A critical evaluation and review. *Clin. Chem.,* 1980; 26: 555-561.

[44] Lim CK, Richmond W, Robinson DP, Brown SS. Toward a definitive assay of creatinine in serum and urine: separation by high-performance liquid chromatography. *J. Chromatogr.,* 1978; 145: 41-49.

[45] Chiou WL, Gadalla MAF, Peng GW. Simple, rapid and micro high-pressure liquid chromatographic determination of endogenous creatinine in plasma, serum, and urine. *J. Pharm. Sci.,* 1978; 67: 182-187.

[46] Weatherburn MW, Trotman RBB, Jackson SH. Specific method for serum creatinine determination based on ion exchange chromatography and an automated alkaline picrate reaction-a proposed reference method. *Clix. Biochem.,* 1978; 11: 159-166.

[47] Bjorkhem I, Blomstrand H, Ohman G. Mass fragmentography of creatimne proposed as a reference method. *Clin. Chem.,* 1977; 23: 2114-2121.

[48] Ektachem Crea Method. Creatimne analysis. Health Sciences Markets Division, Publication MP2-34. Rochester, NY: *Eastman Kodak,* 1983.

[49] Ogden DA. Consequences of renal donation in man. *Am. J. Kidney Dis.,* 1983; 2: 501-511.

[50] Anderson, Brenner BM. Effects of aging on the renal glomerulus. *Am. J. Med.,* 1986; 80: 435-442.

[51] Brenner BM, Meyer TW, Hostetter TH. Dietary protein intake and the progressive nature of kidney disease: the role of hemodynamically mediated glomerular injury in the pathogenesis of progressive glomerular sclerosis in aging, renal ablation, and intrinsic renal disease. *N. Engl. J. Med.,* 1982; 307: 652-659.

[52] Diamond JR, Karnovsky Md. Focal and segmental glomerulosclerosis: analogies to atherosclerosis. *Kidney hit.,* 1988; 33: 917-924.

[53] Watkin DM, Shock NW. Agewise standard value for CIn, CPAH and TmPAH in adult males [Abstract]. *J. Clin. Invest.,* 1955; 34: 969.

[54] Davison JM, Dunlop W. Renal hemodynamics and tubular function in normal human pregnancy. *Kidney hit.,* 1980; 18: 152-161.

[55] Dunlop W. Serial changes in renal hemodynamics during normal human pregnancy. *Br. J. Obstet. Gynaecol.,* 1984; 88: 1-9.

[56] Davison JM, Noble MCB. Serial changes in 24 hour creatinine clearance during normal menstrual cycles and the first trimester of pregnancy. *Br. J. Obstet. Gynaecol.,* 1981; 88: 10-17.

[57] Katz Al, Davison JM, Hayslett JP, Singson E, Lindheimer MD. Pregnancy in women with kidney disease. *Kidney Int.,* 1980; 18: 192-206.

[58] Davison JM. The effect of pregnancy on kidney function in renal allograft recipients. *Kidney Int.,* 1985; 27: 74-79.

[59] Sims EAR, Krantz KE. Serial studies of renal function during pregnancy and the puerperium in normal women. *J. Clix. Invest.,* 1958; 37: 1764-1774.

[60] Christiansen JS, Gammelgaard J, Tronier B, Svendsen PA, Parving H-H. Kidney function and size in diabetics before and during initial insulin treatment. *Kidney Int.,* 1982; 21: 683-688.

[61] Wiseman Md, Saunders Ad, Keen H, Viberti G. Effect of blood glucose control on increased glomer-ular filtration rate and kidney size in insulin-dependent diabetes. *N. Engl. J. Med.,* 1985; 312: 617-621.

[62] Zatz H, Brenner BM. Pathogenesis of diabetic microangiopathy. The hemodynamic view. *Am. J. Med.,* 1986; 80: 443-453.

[63] Bank N. Mechanisms of diabetic hyperfiltration. *Kidney hit.,* 1991; 40: 792-807.

[64] Mogensen CE, Anderson MJF. Increased kidney size and glomerular filtration rate in untreated juvemle diabetes: normalization by insulin-treatment. *Diabetologia,* 1975; 11: 221-224.

[65] Krolewski AS, Warram JH, Christlieb AR, Busick Ed, Kahn CR. The changing natural history of nephropathy in the type 1 diabetes. *Am. J. Med.,* 1985; 78: 785-794.

[66] Balodimos MC. Diabetic nephropathy. In: Marble A, White PA, Bradley RF, Krau LP, eds. Joslin's diabetes mellitus, 11th ed. Philadelphia: *Lea and Febeger,* 1971: 526-561.

[67] Viberti GC, Bilous HW, Mackintosh D, Keen H. Monitoring glomerular function in diabetic nephropathy. A prospective study. *Am. J. Med.,* 1983; 74: 256-264.

[68] Parving H-H, Smidt UM, Friisberg B, Bonnevie-Nielsen V, Anderson AR. A prospective study of glomerular filtration rate and arterial blood pressure in insulin dependent diabetics with diabetic nephropathy. *Diabetologia,* 1981; 20: 457-461.

[69] Haggie SJ, Fermont DC, Wyllie JH. Treatment of duodenal ulcer with cimetidine. *Lancet,* 1976; i: 983-984.

[70] Blackwood WS, Maudgal DP, Pickard RG, Lawrence D, Northfield TC. Cimetidine in duodenal ulcer. *Lancet,* 1976; ii: 174-176.

[71] Burgess E, Blair A, Krichman K, Cutler RE. Inhibition of renal creatinine secretion by cimetidine in humans. *Renal. Physiol.,* 1982; 5: 27-30.

[72] Zaltzman JS, Whiteside C, Cattran DC, Lopez FM, Logan AG. Accurate measurement of impaired glomerular filtration rate using single-dose oral cimetidine. *Am. J. Kidney Dis.,* 1996; 27: 504-511.

[73] van Acker BAC, Koomen GCM, Koopman MG, de Waart DR, Arisz L. Creatinine clearance during cimetidine administration for measurement of glomerular filtration rate. *Lancet,* 1992; 340: 1326-1329.

[74] van Ginneken CAM, Russel FGM. Saturable pharmacokinetics in the renal excretion of drugs. *Clin. Pharmacokinetics.,* 1989; 16: 38-54.

[75] Gisclon LG, Giacomini KM. Inhibition of cimetidine transport by creatinine in luminal membrane vesicles prepared from rabbit kidney. *Drug Metab. Dispos.,* 1988; 16: 331-332.

[76] Brunton L. Agents for control of gastric acidity and treatment of peptic ulcers. In: Hardman J, Limbird L, eds. Goodman and Gilman's The Pharmacological Basis of Therapeutics, 9th edn. New York: *McGraw-Hill,* 1996; 901-917.

[77] Muirhead MR, Somodyi AA. Effect of H-2 antagonists on the differential secretion of triamterene and its sulfate conjugate metabolite by the isolated professed rat kidney. *Drug Metab. Dispos.,* 1991; 19: 312-316.

[78] Somogyi A, Bochner F. Dose and concentration dependent effect of ranitidine on procainamide disposition and renal clearance in man. *Br. J. Clin. Pharmacol.,* 1984; 18: 175-181.

[79] Pachon J, Lorber MI, Bia MJ. Effects of H2-receptor antagonists on renal function in cyclosporine-treated renal transplant patients. *Transplantation,* 1989; 47: 254-259.

[80] Roy MT, First MR, Myre SA, Cacini W. Effect of trimethoprim and sulphamethoxazole on serum creatinine in normal subjects. *Ther. Drug Monit.,* 1982; 4: 77-79.

[81] Kastrup J, Petersen P, Bartram R, Hansen JM. The effect of trimethoprim on serum creatinine. *Br. J. Urol.,* 1985; 57: 265-268.

[82] Myre SA, McCann J, First MR, Cluxton RJ. Effects of trimethoprim on serum creatinine in healthy and chronic renal failure volunteers. *Ther. Drug Monit.,* 1987; 9: 161-165.

[83] Bugge JF. Severe hyperkalaemia induced by trimethoprim in combination with an angiotensin-converting enzyme inhibitor in a patient with transplanted lungs. *J. Intern. Med.,* 1996; 240: 249-251.

[84] Smith GW, Cohen SB. Hyperkalaemia and non oliguric renal failure associated with trimethoprim. *Br. Med. J.,* 1994; 308: 454.

[85] Rudra T, Webb DB, Evans AG. Acute tubular necrosis following cotrimoxazole therapy. *Nephron,* 1989; 53: 85-86.

[86] Chandra M, Chandra P, McVicar M, Susia M, Teichberg S. Rapid onset of cotrimoxazol induced interstitial nephritis. *Int. J. Pediatr. Nephrol.,* 1985; 6: 289-292.

[87] d'Agati V. Does aspirin cause acute or chronic renal failure in experimental animals and in humans? (Review). *Am. J. Kidney. Dis.,* 1996; 28(suppl. 3): S24-29.

[88] Rasmussen S, Petersen J, Nielsen L, Christensen P, Hilden T. Effect of acetylsalicylic acid on renal function in systemic lupus erythematosus. *J. Clin. Pharmacol.,* 1982; 23: 505-508.

[89] Sica DA, Schoolwerth AC. Renal handling of organic anions and cations and renal excretion of uric acid. In: Brenner B, ed. Brenner and Rector's The kidney, 5th edn. Philadelphia: *WB Saunders,* 1996; 607-626.

[90] Duggan E, Hoffman L, Baska R, Lea K, Hellerstein S. Elevated serum creatinine levels in three patients treated with phenacemide. *Drug Intel. Clin. Phar.,* 1986; 20: 225-228.

[91] Cahen R, Martin A, Francois B, Baltassat P, Louisot P. Creatinine metabolism impairment by an anticonvulsant drug, phenacemide. *Ann. Pharmacother,* 1994; 28: 49-51.

[92] Maddox D, Brenner B. Glomerular filtration. In: Brenner B, ed. Brenner and Rector's The kidney, 5th edn. Philadelphia: *WB Saunders,* 1996; 286-333.

[93] George CRP. Non-specific enhancement of glomerular filtration by corticosteroids. *Lancet,* 1974; ii: 728-729.

[94] van Acker BAC, Prummel MF, Weber JA, Wiersinga WM, Arisz L. Effect of prednisone on renal function in man. *Nephron,* 1993; 65: 254-259.

[95] Gallagher JC. Metabolic effects of synthetic calcitriol (Rocaltrol) in the treatment of postmenopausal osteoporosis. Metabolism: *Clin. Exp.,* 1990; 39: 27-29.

[96] Christiansen C, Rodbro P, Christensen MS, Hartnach B, Transbol I. Deterioration of renal function during treatment of chronic renal failure with 1,25-dihydroxycholecalciferol. *Lancet,* 1978; ii: 700-703.

[97] Lund B, Sorensen OH, Lund B. 1a-hydroxycholecalciferol and renal function. *Lancet,* 1978; ii: 731.

[98] Rudnick ME, Bastl CP, Elfinbein lB. Narins HG. The differential diagnosis of acute renal failure. In: Brenner BM, Lazarus JM, eds. Acute renal failure. Philadelphia: *WB Saunders,* 1983: 176-222.

[99] Kassirer JP. Clinical evaluation of kidney function-glomerular function. *N. Engl. J. Med.,* 1971; 285: 385-389.

[100] Moran SM, Myers HD. Course of acute renal failure studied by a model of creatinine kinetics. *Kidney Int.,* 1985; 27: 928-937.

[101] Harris RC, Meyer TW, Scholey JW, Brenner BM. Nephron adaptation to renal injury. In: Brenner BM, Rector FC Jr. eds. The kidney. Philadelphia: *WB Saunders,* 1991: 1871-1908.

[102] Rosman JB, tar Wee PM, Meijer 5, Piers-Becht TPM, Sluiter WJ, Donker AdM. Prospective randomized trial of early dietary protein restriction in chronic renal failure. *Lancet,* 1984; ii: 1291-1296.

[103] Ihle BE, Becker GJ, Whitworth JA, Charlwood HA, Kincaid-Smith PS. The effect of protein restriction on the progression of renal insufficiency. *N. Engl. J. Med.,* 1989; 321: 1773-1777.

[104] Barsotti G, Giannoni A, Morelli E, et al. The decline of renal function slowed by very low phosphorus intake in chronic renal patients following a low nitrogen diet. *Clin. Nephrol.,* 1984; 21: 54-59.

[105] Locatelli F, Alberti D, Graziani G, et al. Prospective randomized, multicentre trial effect of protein restriction on progression of chronic renal insufficiency. *Lancet,* 1991; 337: 1299-1304.

[106] Gretz N, Mans F, Strauch M. Predictability of the progression of chronic renal failure. *Kidney Int.,* 1983; 24: S2-5.

[107] Arbus GS, Bacneyie GS. Method for predicting when children with progressive renal disease may reach serum creatinine levels. *Pediatrics,* 1981; 67 :871-873.

[108] Reimold EW. Chronic progressive renal failure; rate of progression monitored by change of serum creatinine. *Am. J. Dis. Child.,* 1981; 135: 1039-1043.

[109] Perazella MA. Drug-induced renal failure: update on new medications and unique mechanisms of nephrotoxicity. *Am. J. Med. Sci.,* 2003 ;325: 349-362.

[110] Brewster UC, Perazella MA. Acute kidney injury following proton pump inhibitor therapy. *Kidney Int.,* 2007; 71: 589-593

[111] Liss P, Persson PB, Hansell P, Lagerqvist B. Renal failure in 57 925 patients undergoing coronary procedures using iso-osmolar or low-osmolar contrast media. *Kidney Int.,* 2006; 70: 1811-1817.

[112] Welch Allyn Product Catalogue Web site. Eye, Ear, Nose and Throat.www. welchallyn.com/apps/products/product_category.jsp?catcode Accessed July 25, 2012.

[113] Howard AD, Moore J Jr, Gouge SF, et al. Routine serologic tests in the differential diagnosis of the adult nephrotic syndrome. *Am. J. Kidney Dis.,* 1990; 15: 24-30.

In: Creatinine
Editors: I. H. Perkins and C. M. Chapman

ISBN: 978-1-62257-475-9

Chapter VIII

Creatinine: Diagnostic Uses and Role in Kidney Disease in Neonates, Infants and Children

Vasileios I. Giapros * ***and Styliani K. Andronikou***
Neonatal Intensive Care Unit, Child Health Department,
University of Ioannina, Greece

Abstract

The renal excretion of creatinine is very similar to that of inulin and creatinine has been extensively used for estimation of the glomerular function rate (GFR) in adults and children by calculating the clearance of creatinine. GFR is considered the best index of renal function and while it can be measured directly by clearance studies of exogenous markers, such as inulin, these procedures are costly and time consuming. GFR estimation based on endogenous creatinine correlates well with inulin clearance, but necessitates precise urine collection which is not feasible in infants and young children. Estimated GFR, based on plasma creatinine level (PCr) and body length, is a key method for estimating renal function and identifying patients with chronic kidney disease (CKD). Several formulas have been used for estimating GFR, using mainly PCr, body length or height, and a constant. The new Schwartz formula (2009) is in current use, but others have been recently studied.

Serial measurement of PCr is also a useful bedside index of kidney function, especially during the neonatal period. PCr is high at birth, reflecting maternal levels, decreases during the first weeks of life in parallel with an increase in GFR, reaches trough values by the end of the first month then increases gradually during childhood. Its level is inversely correlated with both gestational age and postnatal age. PCr is estimated using several methods, including modified Jaffe methods, enzymatic methods, high-performance liquid chromatography, isotope dilution mass spectrometry (IDMS) and gas chromatography. Commercially available methods for creatinine measurement have limitations and there are differences in results among methods due to lack of assay standardization and the non specificity of the alkaline picrate method used in most

* Address Correspondence to: Vasileios Giapros, University Hospital of Ioannina, P.O. Box 1186, Ioannina 451 10, Greece, Tel: #302651007544, FAX: #302651007032, Email:vgiapros@cc.uoi.gr.

laboratories. Recent international efforts have been made to improve creatinine standardization by assuring traceability to a reference system.

1. Production of Creatinine

Creatinine, the internal anhydrite of creatine was first named by Liebing in 1847 [Liebing J, 1847]. It has a molecular weight of 112 daltons. Creatinine consists a waste product of the metabolism is not reutilized by the body and is exclusively excreted by the kidney. Creatinine is formed by the spontaneous non enzymatic and irreversible conversion of both creatine and creatine phosphate at a relatively constant rate averaging 1.7% per day [Heymsfield SB et al, 1983]. Since 90-98% of total body creatine is in muscle, the main determinant of the rate of creatinine production is muscle mass. Dietary creatine and creatinine from meat can contribute to a less degree to creatinine excretion. Creatinine is excreted through the kidneys in quantities proportional to serum content.

2. Clinical Significance of Creatinine

The renal excretion of creatinine is very similar to that of inulin in humans and several animal species. Creatinine has been extensively used in estimating glomerular function either by calculating clearance of creatinine, or by measuring the serum level of the substance. Furthermore several formulas are used for estimating glomerular filtration rate (GFR) mainly by plasma creatinine (PCr), body length or height and some constant. Its use as an index of renal function it is extended from the neonatal period onwards [Dalton N and Haycock G, 1993].

3. Methods of Estimating PCr

Commonly used creatinine assay methodologies include: alkaline picrate methods (e.g., classic Jaffe method] and modified Jaffe methods, enzymatic methods, high-performance liquid chromatography, isotope dilution mass spectrometry (IDMS), gas chromatography, and liquid chromatography [Ambrose RT et al 1983, Stevens LA et al 2006, Mazzachi BC et al 2000, Junge W et al 2004, Rumbelow BD et al 2000]. Many factors may produce inherent errors in these assay methodologies, including patient-based factors (dietary factors, hydration, serum glucose level, blood pressure and illness), variations in GFR measurements and errors in PCr measurement due to the presence of substances that interfere and assay methodology inaccuracies. With the commonly used classic and modified Jaffe methods, up to 20% of the color reaction may be due to the presence of noncreatinine chromagens in the serum sample, thereby overestimating PCr and underestimating the creatinine clearance (CLCr). This error is most significant within the normal reference range of PCr values. Other commonly used assays, such as the kinetic alkaline picrate assay, also report a serum creatinine value higher than actual underestimating CLCr most significantly within the upper range of normal for creatinine values—values that define early-onset chronic kidney disease

(CKD) [Dalton N and Haycock G, 1993]. A National Kidney Disease Education Program (NKDEP) laboratory working group (USA), formed for the purpose of reevaluating serum creatinine assay performance worldwide, determined that various serum creatinine assays are suboptimal for use as a relible predictor of a patient's actual PCr value. The group concluded that all current equations for estimating GFR in adult populations, including the MDRD equations and the Cockcroft–Gault equation, are less accurate in patients with normal and slightly increased PCr. The NKDEP's Creatinine Standardization Program, in conjunction with the Food and Drug Administration, is encouraging all manufacturers of creatinine assay kits to recalibrate routine PCr methods to be traceable to an isotope dilution mass spectrometry (IDMS) standard. The serum/plasma creatinine standardization initiative has been successful and nearly all methods from manufacturers selling measurement systems in North America and other regions are now selling products with calibration traceable to an IDMS reference measurement procedure [Panteghini M, 2006,Miller WG 2009, Miller WG 2005].

The usefulness of PCr measurements for the identification of renal function is affected by sex, age, race, diet, and muscle mass. Moreover, the analytical quality of the test is usually compromised due to the nonspecificity of the Jaffe method used in most laboratories as have already described previously. The published studies on PCr reference intervals in adults using enzymatic assays traceable to the reference method are scarce and have been recently reviewed by Cerioti et al [Ceriotti et al, 2008]. The reference intervals for PCr, mg/dL, of those enzymatic assays were 0.67-1.18 for men and 0.51-0.95 for women [Junge W 2004]. The pediatric reference intervals for PCr concentrations were for preterm neonates (mg/dl) 0-21 days 0.32-0.98, term neonates 0-14 days 0.31-0.92, 2 months-<1 year 0.16-0.39, 1-3 years 0.17-0.35, 2-5 years 0.26-0.42,5-7 years 0.29-0.48, 7-9 years 0.34-0.55, 9-11 years 0.32-0.64 11-13 years 0.42-0.71 and 13-15 0.46-0.81 [Schlebusch H et al, 2002]. Other recent studies provide normal PCr levels in several neonatal, pediatric and adolescence groups [Chavers BM et al, 2011, Boer DP et al, 2010]. It has been shown that the subtraction of 18–25 mol/L[0.20-0.28 mg/dl] [Junge W et al, 2004, Mårtensson A et al, 2004] to eliminate protein-related unspecific interference on alkaline picrate assays significantly improves the correlation of these assays with enzymatic ones. In this situation, the obtained reference intervals are very similar to those of the enzymatic methods. However, on individual samples, especially at the low PCr concentrations found in children, large differences can be seen. The use of assays being more specific for PCr, such as those based on some enzymatic procedures, may provide more reliable estimated GFR values. Care must be taken when using enzymatic methods with icteric samples in neonates because a negative bias can occur [Owen LJ et al, 2007].

4. Glomerular Filtration Rate (GFR)

Glomerular filtration is one of the most important functions of the kidney, where part of plasma is filtered through the glomerulus. GFR is dependent on the amount of plasma that is filtered in the glomerulus, which is affected by the systemic blood pressure and the total renal vascular resistance. Factors that participate in the filtration process include the hydrostatic pressure in the glomerular capillaries, the hydraulic permeability of the glomerulus and the surface available for filtration [Spitzer A 1971]. Factors countering GFR are the forces of mean colloidosmotic pressure in the capillaries and the hydrostatic pressure of the Bowman's capsule [Spitzer A 1971, Ichikawa I 1979, Corey H 1992, Jose P 1992]. GFR is low at birth in fullterm neonates and even lower in preterm neonates, especially in those with a gestational age below 28 weeks. At every stage of development GFR is dependent on the filtration of each single nephron multiplied by the total nephron number. At completion of anatomical development, which takes place at 34-36 weeks of gestational age, each kidney contains 400,000 to 2,000,000 nephrons. Nephrons differ with respect to their maturity and functionality. The more mature nephrons are those developed in the medullar region of the kidney and these comprise only about 20% of the total nephron number. The nephrons that develop in the outer cortical zone comprise about 80%, and are immature at birth [Spitzer A et al, 1971, Ichikawa I et al, 1979, Corey H et al, 1992, Jose P et al, 1992]. This model of development, the so-called centrifugal model, is of clinical significance because it is related to the pathophysiology of nephrotoxicity at this age. Specifically, the immature nephrons in the outer cortex are not affected by nephrotoxic agents such as gentamicin, and glomerular function is preserved during the first days of life. As nephrons of the outer cortex mature during the first few weeks after birth, the GFR gradually increases. In the fullterm neonate the GFR has been estimated to be 12ml/min/m2 [Fawer CL et al, 1979]. In the preterm infant GFR is even lower and its value is inversely related to gestational age. GFR increases after birth in all neonates and is positively correlated with both gestational age and postnatal age. This postnatal increase in GFR appears to be related to an increase in systematic blood pressure and a decrease in total kidney vascular resistance [Spitzer A 1971, Ichikawa I 1979, Corey H 1992, Jose P 1992].

4.1. Calculation of GFR

The calculation of GFR is based on the principle of the renal clearance of a substance. Clearance of a substance, Cx, is the filtered plasma volume that is cleared from this substance during a specific time unit: Cx=Ux. V/ Px where Ux and Px are the concentrations of the substance in urine and plasma, respectively, and V the urine rate in the time unit.

A substance appropriate for use as a GFR estimator needs to have certain special properties, namely to be filtered freely in the capillaries of the glomerulus, and to be neither produced nor metabolized by the kidney.

Clearance of inulin is regarded as the gold standard for estimation of GFR [Alinei R, Guignard JP, 1987]. Inulin is an exogenous fructose polysaccharide. The renal excretion of inulin is mediated exclusively by glomerular filtration and its clearance is the most accurate index of GFR. Creatinine, in addition to being filtered through the glomerulus, is secreted in part by the tubular cells. On the other hand, the measured PCr is higher than the true creatinine concentration because of the presence of noncreatinine chromogens that interfere with the colorimetric analysis of creatinine (Jaffe reaction) [Guignard JP et al, 1992, Stonestreet B et al, 1978]. There are also experimental data showing that the kidneys of the most immature neonates (<28 weeks GA) not only secret but also reabsorb creatinine [Guignard JP et al, 1999]. This immature reaction affects the PCr level in this population, leading to high PCr levels during the first few days after birth. Overestimation of GFR by creatinine clearance is observed almost exclusively in patients with impaired renal function and low GFR. In these cases the contribution of secreted creatinine may influence the estimated GFR, which is thus not a true reflection of the actual GFR.

During the neonatal period precisely timed urine collections are very difficult to obtain. Urine loss from adhered bags and contamination with feces make urine collections inaccurate during this period. For the above reasons, several techniques have been implemented to estimate GFR in neonates, which use inulin or creatinine but eliminate the need for precise urine collection. Among these, the techniques of stable inulin infusion without urine collection and the method of simple inulin injection or the curve of disappearance of plasma inulin have been used [Alinei R, Guignard JP 1987, Fawer CL et al 1979]. Creatinine measurement has been used to estimate GFR, employing the formula GFR= Kx L/PCr, where L is the body length (crown to heel length) and K is a constant with values of 0.33 for premature and 0.45 for fullterm infants [Counahan R et al 1976, Zacchello G et al, 1982, Alinei R , Guignard JP 1987], but this method has been criticized [Alinei R, Guignard JP, 1987]. These indirect methods of estimating GFR are discussed in detail in next chapters.

5. Plasma Creatinine (PCr) - Clinical Usefulness

PCr expresses the equilibrium between the production of creatinine by the body muscles and its excretion by the kidney. The only source of production of creatinine is the metabolism of creatinine and phosphocreatinine of the total muscle mass. When the total muscle mass remains stable creatinine production and its level in the plasma also remain stable. Creatinine is freely filtered through the glomerulus and its excretion takes place exclusively by the kidney. The stable level of PCr and the exclusive excretion of creatinine by the kidney justify the choice of this substance as a reliable index of kidney function and especially as an estimator of GFR. Measurement of PCr, and especially serial measurements, has been proposed as a reliable index of renal function, especially during the neonatal period where precise urine collections are not feasible [Seikaly M et al, 1992, Arant B 1984, Rudd P et al, 1983, Feldman H, Guignard JP 1982, Parkin A, 1989]. Under stable conditions of renal function, GFR is inversely correlated with PCr. Repeated measurements of PCr are needed in cases with low GFR, because even small increases in PCr may reflect a significant further decrease in GFR. A special characteristic of the neonatal period is the gradual decrease in PCr as postnatal age increases. For this reason in this period the diagnosis of nephrotoxicity is based not only on increase in PCr but also on the inability of the kidneys to effect a gradual reduction in PCr [Arant B 1984]. During the neonatal period PCr changes according to gestational age and the day of life, being higher in more premature neonates on the first days of life [Sertel H et al, 1973, Feldman H et al, 1982]. In order to interpret PCr levels during this period, knowledge of the physiological fluctuations of PCr is needed.

At birth the PCr is high in both fullterm and preterm neonates. Characteristically the more immature preterm neonates have higher levelsof PCr [Bueva A, Guignard JP,1994], which actually represent maternal creatinine that crosses the placenta and is excreted by the neonatal kidneys. In the more immature neonates GFR is very low and consequently the PCr may be very high. In this subgroup of preterm neonates, creatinine appears also to be reabsorbed by the immature renal tubules and this phenomenon leads to even higher PCr levels (i.e., 1.1-1.6 mg/dl) [Matos P et al, 1998, Henderson M et al, 1998]. In fullterm neonates the creatinine of maternal origin is eliminated promptly by the more mature neonatal kidney while in preterm neonates elimination takes place gradually as the kidneys mature [Guignard JP et al 1999].

After elimination of the maternal creatinine fraction a new equilibrium is created and the changes in PCr reflect precisely both the velocity of kidney maturation and the increase in GFR. A rapid decrease in PCr is observed in the first weeks after birth in the fullterm neonate, reaching values as low as 0.2-0.3 mg/dl by the end of the first month of life [Jose P et al, 1992]. The fall of PCr in the preterm neonate takes place more gradually.Wide variation in PCr levels have been shown among preterm neonates, even in those of the same gestational age and the same postnatal age. This phenomenon is attributable to the individualization of maturation of nephrons among the preterm neonates [Sonntag J et al, 1996, Gordjani N et al, 1988]. This observation implies the need for repeated measurements of PCr for the precise estimation of renal function during the neonatal period. PCr continues to serve as a simple bedside index of renal function and renal failure throughout infancy and childhood. Precisely timed urine collections for calculating creatinine clearance are feasible during childhood. At this age nephrotoxicity is heralded by an increase in PCr over a predetermined level (i.e., PCr> 1.2-1.5 mg/dl) or an increase of more than 0.4-0.5 mg/dl over the original values. The respective 'nephrotoxic' values for the neonatal period have not yet been defined and renal damage during this period may occur even in cases with a PCr level well within the 'normal' range. During the neonatal period factors such as administration of aminoglycosides or vancomycin, perinatal asphyxia, jaundice, hypotension, small for gestational age status and sepsis may act synergically in affecting renal function [Theocharis et al, 2011, Giapros et al, 1995, Andronikou et al, 1996, Giapros et al, 2003, Giapros et al 2007]. PCr is affected early in the course of nephrotoxicity and PCr levels may remain elevated for 1-2 days after restoration of renal function. PCr levels may guide the physician throughout childhood in adjustment of the dosages and administration intervals of potentially nephrotoxic drugs such as aminoglycosides, vancomycin, amphotericin B, etc.

6. Estimation of GFR by Using a Creatinine Based Formula

The best index of renal function is considered to be the rate that blood is filtered at the glomerulus, or glomerular filtration rate (GFR). Chronic kidney disease (CKD) can then be precisely defined as a GFR <60 mL/min/1.73m2 for subjects older than 3 months, independently of the cause [National Kidney Foundation, 2002, Peak M et al 2006]. While the GFR can be measured directly by clearance studies of exogenous markers, such as inulin, iohexol, or Cr51-EDTA, these procedures are costly and time consuming. Furthermore they cannot be applying in neonates, infants and young children. Even to measure the clearance of endogenous creatinine, requires both serum and an accurately timed urine collection, so efforts have been directed at more convenient estimates of GFR without the need for urine collections [Peak M et al, 2006].

Estimated GFR (eGFR) is a key method for identifying patients with CKD. In adults, eGFR calculated using the Modification of Diet in Renal Disease (MDRD) Study equation provides a more clinically useful measure of kidney function than PCr alone. This equation takes into account several factors including age, gender, and race. [GFR (mL/min/1.73 m^2) = 175 x $(S_{cr})^{-1.154}$ x $(Age)^{-0.203}$ x (0.742 if female) x (1.212 if African American)]. There are several reasons for using in adults this equation to estimate GFR, including: *the normal serum creatinine reference interval does not necessarily reflect a normal GFR, the MDRD Study equation is the most thoroughly validated equation and is currently superior to other methods of approximating GFR (i.e.* Cockcroft-Gault method) [Poggio ED et al, 2005, Coresh J et al, 2006]

The Chronic Kidney Disease Epidemiology Collaboration CKD-EPI equation is a new equation, published in 2009, to estimate glomerular filtration rate (GFR) from serum creatinine, age, sex, and race for adults age ≥ 18 years [Levey AS et al, 2009]. This equation is still being validated and, while offering some improvement for eGFR between 60 and 120 mL/min/1.73 m^2, it is not clear that implementing CKD-EPI in place of the MDRD equation would alter clinical detection or management of patients with CKD. These equations although very useful in estimating GFR in adults are not appropriate for neonatal or pediatric populations where different formulas have been used since early seventies and have updated recently. In general agreement the Schwartz equations that are discussed latter in this chapter should be used to estimate GFR for infants, toddlers, children, and teens under age 18 [Schwartz G et al, 2009].

It has been shown that endogenous creatinine clearance provides an adequate estimation of glomerular filtration rate in preterm neonates [Zachello et al, 1982]. Tubular secretion of creatinine and plasma chromogens, including bilirubin, interferes with the accuracy but not with the reliability of endogenous creatinine clearance [Zachello et al, 1982]. As precise urine collections are difficult to be obtained during the first 3 years of life some formulae based on PCr and body length have been proposed. Schwartz et al in 1976 reported that an accurate estimate of GFR could be obtained for the simple determination of plasma creatinine and body length [Schwartz G et al, 1976]. An empirical formula derived by Schwartz in a study on infants aged at least 6 months has been extensively applied: GFR=(ml/min/1.73m2) =0.55+1 (cm) PCr(mg/dl). Similar conclusions were reported in 1976 by Counahan et al who used a different constant [Counahan R et al, 1976]. The discrepancy between the constant of Counahan and that of Schwartz 0.43 and 0.55 respectively is explained as follows. For Scwhartz the PCr is represented by a total value while for Counahan the PCr is the real value which does not include the non creatinine chromogens. In 1977 other investigators confirmed Counahan data but in children over 1 year of life. Latter on Zaccello et al confirmed the use of Schwartz formula in preterm and fullterm neonates [Zacchello G et al 1982]. They found a close relationship (r=0.87) between creatinine clearance estimated with precise urine collection and GFR estimated by using the formula. They concluded that the simplicity of Schwartz's formula permits easy monitoring of renal function especially in neonatal asphyxia in which the risk of developing renal failure is great. The mean value of K calculated in 118 low birth weight infants with a corrected age of 25 to 105 weeks was 0.33 plus or minus 0.01. It rose to 0.45 in fullterm infants up to 18 months [Schwartz G et al, 1987]. In both groups a large scatter of values for K was observed which authors attributed to variability in body composition, differences in diet or creatinine excretion errors in collection of urine or inaccuracies in the measurement of creatinine [Schwartz G et al, 1987].

In spite to these limitations this formula has been used extensively in infants and children in several clinical conditions until recently where a new formula has been implemented [Schwartz G et al, 2009]. The accuracy of the K=L/Pcr formula as an estimate of GFR during the neonatal period has been questioned in some studies especially by Guignard's group [Alinei R, Guignard JP 1987, Arant 1984]. In a study in infants younger than 1 year of age the K value varied from 0.17 to 0.82 even thought it was derived from the standard inulin clearance. Factor K was found to vary markedly with the state of hydration. Moreover the regression line relating the clearance estimated from the formula with the results obtained from the standard inulin clearance differed significantly from the identity line [Alinei R, Guignard JP, 1987]. In general the KxL/PCr formula may be more informative clinically than the PCr alone because plasma creatinine in addition to renal function is dependent of muscle mass. Nevertheless the formula is currently used extensively especially in older children. In studies aiming to define pathophysiological mechanisms the use of formula must be applied with caution.

In 2009 Schwartz et al introduced a new more sophisticated formula based on PCr and taking into consideration body length in its basic form but also cystatin C, BUN level and gender in the more analytic form [Schwartz G et al 2009]. This new formula in both types seems to correlate well with standard methods. In their recent study Schwartz et al compared this formula against GFR estimated by using iohexol plasma disappearance as a gold standard in measuring GFR. Iohexol is used as a safe, nonionic, low-osmolar contrast agent of molecular weight 821 Da (Omnipaque). It is not secreted, metabolized, or reabsorbed by the kidney, and has 2% plasma protein binding and nearly negligible extra-renal clearance [Krutzen E et al, 1990].

An overestimation of GFR has been postulated by using the old formula attributable to the change in creatinine methods since the development of the original formula. The more recent enzymatic creatinine method referred above, results in lower determinations compared with the older Jaffe method, even when the latter was improved with a dialysis step and elimination of interfering samples. A more accurate estimate of GFR is crucial to the follow up of children with CKD as well as other renal pathologies. The new equation in its full form is as follows:

$$GFR\ (ml/min\ per\ 1.73\ m^2) = 39.1[height\ (m)/Scr\ (mg/dl)]^{0.516} \times [1.8/cystatin\ C(mg/L)^{0.294}[30/BUN\ (mg/dl)^{0.169}[1.099]^{male}\_[height\ (m)/1.4]^{0.188}$$

The simplified form is:

0.413*(height/serum creatinine), consists a bedside calculation and provides a good approximation to the estimated GFR formula.

The analysis of all of the variables in the CKD population showed that height/PCr still provides the best correlation. Whereas the reciprocal of cystatin C showed a somewhat weaker correlation with iGFR the addition of both cystatin C and BUN to the height/PCr equation substantially improved the estimated GFR. When all three variables were incorporated into a gender based equation with an added coefficient for height alone there was further improvement to level quite comparable to the best equations developed for adults [Schwartz G et al, 2009].

The new formulas proposed by Schwartz to estimate GFR using easily obtained biochemical markers have been developed in a group of children with mild to moderate CKD. A number of limitations preclude rapid generalization of this formula to the general pediatric population for estimation of GFR. Additional studies of children with higher GFR are needed to validate these formulas for use in screening all children for CKD. Other authors have also recently introduced equations to estimate GFR in children [Andersen T et al, 2012, Pottel H et al, 2012, Pottel H et al, 2010]. It is of note that creatinine based formulas used in adult populations as those derived from Cockcroft-Gault and the Modification of Diet in Renal Disease (MDRD) are not useful for children [Pierrat A et al, 2003].

Currently, the best equation for estimating glomerular filtration rate (GFR) from serum creatinine in children is the Bedside Isotope Dilution Mass Spectrometry (IDMS)-traceable Schwartz equation. The IDMS-traceable version of the Schwartz equation is used because at this time all laboratories should be using creatinine methods calibrated to be IDMS traceable. Using the original Schwartz equation with a creatinine value from a method with calibration traceable to IDMS will overestimate.

Conclusion

Creatinine has been extensively used in estimating glomerular function (GFR) either by calculating clearance of creatinine, or by measuring the serum level of the substance or by using several formulas of estimated GFR. It remains an important parameter of glomerular function in neonates, infants and children. During the neonatal period PCr changes according to gestational and postnatal age and these variations must be taken into account when renal function is estimated during this period of life. The new formulas proposed by Schwartz and other researchers the last few years have added precision in estimating GFR in children with CKD and other kidney diseases. There has been an international effort to improve creatinine standardization by assuring traceability to a reference system. These efforts highlighted limitations of commercially available methods for creatinine measurement as well as the differences in results among methods resulting from a lack of assay standardization.

References

[1] Alinei R, Guignard JP. Assessement of glomerular filtration rate in infants. *Helv Paediatr Acta* 1987; 42: 253-262.

[2] Ambrose RT, Ketchum DF, Smith JW: Creatinine determined by "high-performance" liquid chromatography. *Clin Chem* 1983 29: 256–259.

[3] Andersen TB, Jødal L, Boegsted M, Erlandsen EJ, Morsing A, Frøkiær J, Brøchner-Mortensen J.GFR prediction from cystatin C and creatinine in children: effect of including body cell mass. *Am J Kidney Dis*. 2012 ; 59:50-57.

[4] Andronikou S, Giapros V, Cholevas V, Papadopoulou ZI. Effect of aminoglycosides therapy on renal function in fullterm infants. *Pediatr Nephrol* 1996; 10: 766-768.

[5] Arant B. Estimating glomerular filtration rate in infants. *J Pediatr* 1984; 104: 890-893.

[6] Boer DP, de Rijke YB, Hop WC, Cransberg K, Dorresteijn EM. Reference values for serum creatinine in children younger than 1 year of age. *Pediatr Nephrol* 2010; 25:2107-2113.

[7] Bueva A , Guignard JP. Renal function in preterm neonates. *Pediatr Res* 1994; 36: 572-577.

[8] Ceriotti F, Boyd JC, Klein G, Henny J, Queraltó J, Kairisto V, Panteghini M; IFCC Committee on Reference Intervals and Decision Limits (C-RIDL). Reference intervals for serum creatinine concentrations: assessment of available data for global application. *Clin Chem* 2008 ; 54:559-566.

[9] Chavers BM, Rheault MN, Foley RN. Kidney function reference values in US adolescents: National Health And Nutrition Examination Survey 1999-2008. *Clin J Am Soc Nephrol* 2011 ;6:1956-1962

[10] Coresh J, Stevens LA. Kidney function estimating equations: where do we stand? *Current Opinion in Nephrology and Hypertension*. 2006; 15:276–284.

[11] Corey H and Spitzer A. Renal blood flow and glomerular filtration rate during development. In: Edelmann S (ed). Pediatric Kidney Diseases. Boston: Little Brown and Co, 1992; pp: 49-77.

[12] Counahan R, Chandler C, Charali S, Kirkwood B, Rose F, Barratt TM. Estimation of glomerular filtration rate from plasma creatinine concentration in children. *Arch Dis Child* 1976; 51: 875-878.

[13] Dalton N, Haycock G. Laboratory investigation IN Holliday M, Barratt M, Avner A eds Pediatric Nephrology 3rd edition Williams & Wilkins Baltimore 1993 pp 397-420.

[14] Fawer CL, Torrado A, Guignard JP. Maturation of renal function in full-term and premature neonates. *Helv Paediatr* Acta 1979; 34: 11-21.

[15] Feldman H, Guignard JP. Plasma creatinine in the first month of life. *Arch Dis Child* 1982; 57: 123-126.

[16] Giapros V, Papadimitriou P, Challa A, Andronikou S. The effect of intrauterine growth retardation on renal function in the first 2 months of life. *Nephrol Dial Transplant* 2007; 22: 97-103.

[17] Giapros V, Andronikou S, Cholevas V, Papadopoulou ZI. Renal function and effect of aminoglycoside therapy during the first ten days of life. *Pediatr Nephrol* 2003;18: 46-52.

[18] Giapros V, Andronikou S, Cholevas V, Papadopoulou ZI. Renal function in premature infants during aminoglycosides therapy. *Pediatr Nephrol* 1995; 9: 163-166.

[19] Gordjani N, Barghard R, Leititis J, Brondis M. Serum creatinine and creatinine clearance in healthy neonates and prematures during the first 10 days of life. *Eur J Pediatr* 1988; 148: 143-145.

[20] Guignard JP and Drukker A. Why do newborn infants have a high plasma creatinine. *Pediatrics* 1999; 103: 49-53.

[21] Guignard JP. Measurment of glomerular filtration rate in neonates in (eds) Polin R and Fox W: Fetal and neonatal physiology Philadelphia W.B. Saunders co 1992 pp 1205-1211.

[22] Henderson M, Brownlee K, Turner A, Brocklebank J. Serial changes in plasma creatinine in the first week of life in premature babies. *Pediatr Nephrol* 1998; 12: 90.

[23] Heymsfield SB, Arteaga C, McManus C, Smith J, Moffitt s. Measurement of muscle mass in humans. Validity of 24 hour urinary creatinine method. *Am J Clin Nutr* 1983;37: 478-494.

[24] Ichikawa I, Maddox D, Brenner B. Maturational development of glomerular ultrafiltration in the rat. *Am J Physiol* 1979; 236: 465-471.

[25] Jose P, Haramati A, Fildes R. Postnatal maturation of renal blood flow. In: (eds) Polin R and Fox W: Fetal and neonatal physiology Philadelphia W.B. Saunders co 1992 pp 1196-1200.

[26] Junge W, Wilke B, Halabi A, Klein G. Determination of reference intervals for serum creatinine, creatinine excretion and creatinine clearance with an enzymatic and a modified Jaffe method. *Clin Chim Acta* 2004; 344:137-148.

[27] Krutzen E, Back SE, Nilsson-Ehle P: Determination of glomerular filtration rate using iohexol clearance and capillary sampling. *Scand J Clin Lab Invest* 1990;50: 279–283.

[28] Levey AS , Stevens LA, Schmid CH, Zhang YL, Castro AF, 3rd, Feldman HI, et al. A new equation to estimate glomerular filtration rate. *Ann Intern Med.* 2009;150:604-612.

[29] Liebing J. Kreatin und kreatinin Bestandheile des Harns der Menschen *J Pract Chem* 1847;40: 288-292.

[30] Mårtensson A, Rustad P, Lund H, Ossowicki H. Creatininium reference intervals for corrected methods. *Scand J Clin Lab Invest* 2004;64:439–442.

[31] Matos P, Duarte-Silva M, Drukker A, Guignard JP. Creatinine reabsorption by the newborn rabbit kidney. *Pediatr Res* 1998; 44: 639-641.

[32] Mazzachi BC, Peake MJ, Ehrhardt V. Reference range and method comparison studies for enzymatic and Jaffe creatinine assays in plasma and serum and early morning urine. *Clin Lab* 2000;46:53-55.

[33] Miller WG. Estimating glomerular filtration rate. *Clin Chem Lab Med* 2009;47:1017-1019.

[34] Miller WG, Myers GL, Ashwood ER, Killeen AA, Wang E, Thienpont L, Siekmann L. Creatinine measurement: state of the art in accuracy and interlaboratory harmonization. *Arch Pathol Lab Med* 2005; 129:297–304.

[35] National Kidney Foundation. K/DOQI clinical practice guidelines for chronic kidney disease: evaluation, classification and stratification. Kidney Disease Outcome Quality Initiative. *Am J Kidney Dis* 2002; 39: S1-S246.

[36] Owen LJ, Keevil BG. Does bilirubin cause interference in Roche creatinine methods? *Clin Chem* 2007;53:370 –371.

[37] Panteghini M, Myers GL, Miller WG, Greenberg N. The importance of metrological traceability on the validity of creatinine measurement as an index of renal function. *Clin Chem Lab Med* 2006;44 :1287–1292.

[38] Parkin A, Smith H, Brocklebun J. Which routine test for kidney function. *Arch Dis Child* 1989; 64: 1261-1263.

[39] Peak M, Whiting M. Measurement of Serum Creatinine – Current Status and Future Goals *Clin Biochem Rev* 2006; 27: 173-184.

[40] Pierrat A, Gravier E, Saunders C, Caira M-V, Ait-Djafer Z, Legras B, Mallie′ J-P: Predicting GFR in children and adults: A comparison of the Cockcroft-Gault, Schwartz, and Modification of Diet in Renal Disease formulas. *Kidney Int* 2003;64: 1425–1436.

[41] Poggio ED, Wang X, Greene T, Van Lente F, Hall PM. Performance of the modification of diet in renal disease and Cockcroft-Gault equations in the estimation of GFR in health and in chronic kidney disease. *Journal of the American Society of Nephrology* 2005;16:459–466.

[42] Pottel H, Hoste L, Martens F. A simple height-independent equation for estimating glomerular filtration rate in children. *Pediatr Nephrol* 2012 Jan 18.

[43] Pottel H, Mottaghy FM, Zaman Z, Martens F. On the relationship between glomerular filtration rate and serum creatinine in children. *Pediatr Nephrol* 2010;25:927-934.

[44] Rudd P, Hughes E, Placzek M, Hodes DT. Reference ranges for plasma creatinine during the first month of life. *Arch Dis Child* 1983; 58: 212-215.

[45] Rumbelow BD, Peake MJ, Ehrhardt V. Do enzymatic and Jaffe creatinine assays produce comparable results for pre and post dialysis specimens from patients with chronic renal failure? *Clin Lab* 2000;46:589-90.

[46] Schlebusch H, Liappis N, Kalina E, Klein G. High sensitive CRP and creatinine: reference intervals from infancy to childhood. *J Lab Med* 2002;26:341–6.

[47] Schwartz G, Haycock G, Edelman C, Spitzer A. A simple estimate of glomerular filtration rate in children derived from body length and plasma creatinine. *J Pediatr* 1976; 58:259

[48] Schwartz GJ, Brion LP, Spitzer A: The use of plasma creatinine concentration for estimating glomerular filtration rate in infants, children, and adolescents. *Pediatr Clin North Am* 1987; 34: 571–590.

[49] Seikaly M and Arant B. Development of renal hemodynamics: glomerular filtration and renal blood flow. *Clinic Perinatol* 1992; 19: 1-14.

[50] Sertel H and Scopes J. Rates of creatinine clearance in babies less than one week of age. *Arch Dis Child* 1973; 48: 717-720.

[51] Sonntag J, Pronkel B, Waltz S. Serum creatinine concentration, urinary creatinine excretion and creatinine clearance during the first 9 weeks in preterm infants with a birth weight bellow 1500 gr. *Eur J Pediatr* 1996; 155: 815-819.

[52] Spitzer A, Edelmann C. Maturational changes in pressure gradients for glomerular filtration. *Am J Physiol* 1971; 221: 1431-1435.

[53] Stevens LA, Coresh J, Greene T, Levey AS. Assessing kidney function – measured and estimated glomerular filtration rate. *N Engl J Med* 2006; 354:2473-483.

[54] Stonestreet B, Bell E, Oh W. Validity of endogenous creatinine clearance in low birth weight infants. *Pediatr Res* 1978; 37: 1012-1014.

[55] Theocharis P, Giapros V, Tsampoura Z, Basioti M, Andronikou S. Renal glomerular and tubular function in neonates with perinatal problems. *J Matern Fetal Neonatal Med* 2011; 24:1 42-147.

[56] Zacchello G, Bondio M, Sala O, Largaiolli G, Vedaldi R. Simple estimate of creatinine clearance from plasma creatinine in neonates. *Arch Dis Child* 1982; 57: 297-300.

In: Creatinine
Editors: I. H. Perkins and C. M. Chapman

ISBN: 978-1-62257-475-9

Chapter IX

Serum Creatinine and Estimation of Kidney Function

***Sebastjan Bevc*[1,*]*, Robert Ekart*[2] *and Radovan Hojs*[1]**
[1]Clinic of Internal Medicine, Department of Nephrology,
University Medical Centre Maribor, Slovenia
[2]Clinic of Internal Medicine, Department of Dialysis,
University Medical Centre Maribor, Slovenia

Abstract

Chronic kidney disease (CKD) is an important public health problem. CKD is defined as kidney damage or glomerular filtration rate (GFR) less than 60 ml/min/1.73m^2 for 3 months or more, irrespective of cause. CKD is classified into stages according to the level of GFR. Therefore, estimation of the GFR is essential for the evaluation of patients with CKD. GFR allows us to detect early impairment of renal function, prevent further deterioration and complications, to correct the dosage of drugs cleared by the kidney so as to avoid potential drug toxicity and to help us to manage CKD patients.

Over the last decades several different markers for estimation of GFR have been proposed. The ideal marker of GFR should be an endogenous molecule, which, being produced at a constant rate, is cleared solely by the kidneys via free glomerulari filtration, without being either secreted by tubular cells or reabsorbed into peritubular circulation. The "gold standard" for estimation of GFR is clearance of exogenous substances such as inulin, iohexol, ^{51}CrEDTA, ^{99m}TcDTPA or ^{125}I-iothalamate. These techniques are time-consuming, labour-intensive, expensive and require administration of substances, that make them incompatible with routine monitoring. During the last decades, in clinical practice as in most studies, serum creatinine concentration has become the most commonly used marker to estimate GFR. Creatinine is completely filtered across the glomerular membrane and is neither reabsorbed nor metabolized in kidneys and is

* Correspondence: Assist. Prof. Sebastjan Bevc, MD, PhD., Univerzitetni klinični center Maribor, Klinika za interno medicino, Oddelek za nefrologijo, Ljubljanska 5, 2000 Maribor, Slovenia. Tel: + 386 2 321 2871, Fax: + 386 2 3312 393. E-mail: sebastjanbevc@yahoo.com, sebastjan.bevc@ukc-mb.si.

partially secreted into proximal tubule. Tubular secretion causes the increase of creatinine clearance by 10 – 20%. Creatinine is usually measured by the Jaffé reaction (the kinetic method without deproteinisation- isotope dilution mass spectrometry traceable creatinine assay), based on a complex formation between alkaline picrate and creatinine. According to this method, other non-creatinine cromogens are present in serum, which are not found in urine. Thus creatinine concentration is overestimated in serum and the calculated clearance is underestimated (by 10 to 20%). In individuals with normal renal function both irregularities are abolished and creatinine clearance is very close to the inulin clearance. Other factors, including age, gender, race, body size, muscle mass and food intake (meat in diet), also affect the serum creatinine concentration. Creatinine clearance gives a better estimation of GFR than serum creatinine concentration, but it requires the inconvenience of urine collections. The current Kidney Disease Outcomes Quality Initiative (K/DOQI) guidelines emphasize the need to assess kidney function using predictive equations rather than just serum creatinine. Various creatinine-based equations have been developed in an attempt to improve the estimation of GFR from serum creatinine. Recently, serum cystatin C and cystatin C-based formulas were proposed as a new endogenous marker of GFR.

All the above-mentioned topics will be closely analyzed and described in the details in the chapter.

Introduction

Chronic kidney disease (CKD) is an important public health problem. CKD is defined as kidney damage or glomerular filtration rate (GFR) less than 60 $ml/min/1.73m^2$ for 3 months or more, irrespective of cause. CKD is classified into stages according to the level of GFR. Therefore, estimation of the GFR is essential for the evaluation of patients with CKD. GFR allows us to detect early impairment of renal function, prevent further deterioration and complications, to correct the dosage of drugs cleared by the kidney so as to avoid potential drug toxicity and to help us to manage CKD patients.

Over the last decades several different markers for estimation of GFR have been proposed. The ideal marker of GFR should be an endogenous molecule, which, being produced at a constant rate, is cleared solely by the kidneys via free glomerular filtration, without being either secreted by tubular cells or reabsorbed into peritubular circulation. The "gold standard" for estimation of GFR is clearance of exogenous substances such as inulin, iohexol, ^{51}CrEDTA, ^{99m}TcDTPA or ^{125}I-iothalamate. These techniques are time-consuming, labour-intensive, expensive and require administration of substances, that make them incompatible with routine monitoring. During the last decades, in clinical practice as in most studies, serum creatinine concentration has become the most commonly used marker to estimate GFR.

Creatinine Production

Creatinine is a metabolic product of creatine and phosphocreatine, which are both found almost exclusively in muscle. Creatinine production is proportional to muscle mass and varies little from day to day (for less than 10%), but production can change over longer periods of time if there are changes in muscle mass. Age and gender are known to attribute to differences of muscle mass. Although diet ordinarily accounts for only a small proportion of overall creatinine excretion, it can be another source of variability in serum creatinine levels. Creatine from ingested meat is converted to creatinine and can be the source of up to 30% of total creatinine excretion. Thus, variability in meat intake contributes to variability in serum creatinine levels too. The conversion of creatine to creatinine can occur with cooking. Since creatinine is readily absorbed from the gastrointestinal tract, ingesting cooked meat can lead to a rapid increase in serum creatinine levels [1, 2].

Creatinine is a small molecule (mw 113 Daltons), does not bind to plasma proteins, and is freely filtered across the glomerular membrane. Creatinine is neither reabsorbed nor metabolized in the kidneys, but is partially secreted into proximal tubule. Tubular secretion can cause the increase of creatinine clearance by 10 – 20% [1, 3]. Secretion is a saturable process that probably occurs via the organic cation pathway and is blocked by some commonly used medications including cimetidine, trimethoprim, amiloryd, pyrimethamine and dapsone. If tubular secretion of creatinine were constant, differences in serum creatinine and renal clearance could still reflect differences in GFR. However, the secretion of creatinine varies substantially both in the same individuals over time and between different individuals. As plasma concentrations increase, tubular secretion of serum creatinine increases, leading to an overestimation of GFR in patients with moderate to severe chronic kidney disease [1-3]. Serum creatinine is also insensitive for detecting small decreases in GFR because of the nonlinear relationship between plasma concentration and GFR. Calculation of creatinine clearance, by determining its concentration in timed urine collections and simultaneously in blood, correlates with gold standard exogenous methods better than serum creatinine. Unfortunately collection of timed urine is cumbersome and prone to error in the outpatient setting [4].

Measurement of Serum Creatinine

The methods most widely used to measure serum creatinine are alkaline picrate methods, enzymatic or partially enzymatic assays, and High-Performance Liquid Chromatography (HPLC) methods. Recently, Isotope-Dilution Mass Spectrometry (IDMS) high-order reference methods have been developed for assignment of reference materials and implemented in routine serum creatinine calibration methods [5].

The alkaline picrate methods or Jaffe reaction, first proposed by Folin in 1904, have been used with various modifications since [6]. Several modifications, including optimization of kinetic assays, have been made to improve method specificity and minimize susceptibility to interfering substances. Moreover, a number of normal plasma constituents can interfere with creatinine measurement. Glucose, fructose, pyruvate, acetoacetate, uric acid, ascorbic acid, and plasma proteins can all cause the Jaffe colorimetric assay to yield falsely high creatinine values. The low levels of these substances generally do not interfere with the Jaffe assay of creatinine in urine. Normally, interfering chromogens increase the creatinine result by about 20%, but in some disease states the interference can be much greater (diabetic ketoacidosis, use of cephalosporin antibiotics) [1, 7]. In patients with chronic kidney disease, serum creatinine increases and non-creatinine chromogens contribute proportionally less to the total reaction. Several modifications in the classic Jaffe assay have been designed to remove interfering chromogens before analysis, including deproteinization with specific adsorption of creatinine. These methods have largely been replaced by less costly and more convenient autoanalyzer techniques.

Autoanalyzer methods utilize the Jaffe reaction, but separate creatinine from non-creatinine chromogens by the rate of color development, thus avoiding most of the interference seen with the standard Jaffe method. However, very high serum bilirubin levels could still falsely lower creatinine levels [1].

Inorganic chemical–based methods that have been developed as alternatives to the alkaline picrate methods have not been widely implemented clinically because they have not demonstrated improved performance compared with the various adaptations of the Jaffe method. The only alternative methods that have been widely adopted for routine clinical laboratory use are enzymatic creatinine methods [1, 8]. Although the enzymatic methods have been reported to have generally less interference than the Jaffe methods, there have been reports of various substances or medications that do interfere (dopamine, 5-fluorocystine, bilirubine, metamizol) [9-12].

Pseudohypercreatininemia due to positive interference in enzymatic creatinine measurements caused by monoclonal IgM in patients with Waldenstroms macroglobulinemia was also described [13]. The third, HPLC procedures was reported as fairly sensitive and analytically specific method for measuring serum creatinine. Moreover, in the past years many different methods for the analysis of creatinine have been described, including cation-exchange, normal-phase, reversed-phase, and reversed-phase ion-pair chromatography [5, 14]. Sample deproteinization improved the specificity of creatinine measurement by HPLC by removing many protein-bound endogenous and exogenous compounds without altering the quantification of creatinine [5].

Furthermore, interference studies have demonstrated that HPLC methods have greater analytical specificity than conventional methods [5]. The HPLC methods were recognized as an excellent designated comparison method for in-house use by manufacturers. Understanding of the importance of reliable serum creatinine measurements in GFR estimation and of factors that may affect creatinine measurement is critical to ongoing global public health efforts to increase the diagnosis and treatment of patients with CKD by laboratorians worldwide. The National Kidney Disease Education Program (NKDEP) Laboratory Working Group, in collaboration with international professional organizations, has developed standardization and improved accuracy of serum creatinine measurements in clinical laboratories worldwide. With the recent introduction of the reporting of estimated GFR, inter-laboratory agreement of serum creatinine results has become an important international priority.

Expert professional bodies have recommended that all creatinine methods should become traceable to a reference method based on isotope dilution-mass spectrometry (IDMS) on reference material (SRM 967). Furthermore, the International Organization for Standardization (ISO) has developed a written standard that details a pathway for establishing traceability of clinical laboratory measurement results [15-17].

Diagnostic Use and Role in Renal Disease

Serum creatinine is the most widely used indirect measure of GFR, its popularity is attributable to convenience and low cost. GFR is defined as the volume of plasma that can be completely cleared of a particular substance by the kidneys in a unit of time [18]. Unfortunately, the correct interpretation of serum creatinine in the clinical practice is problematic. Interpretation is limited due to the influence of the number of non-renal factors including the muscle mass and age of the individual as well as the actual method of measurement. Failure to consider variation in creatinine production due to differences in muscle mass most frequently leads to misinterpretation of serum creatinine levels. This confusion may be compounded by the use of standard normal ranges for creatinine levels that appear on routine laboratory reports. A serum creatinine that falls in the "normal" range may indicate a normal GFR in a young, healthy individual. However, the same serum creatinine in an elderly individual could indicate a twofold reduction in GFR due to a comparable reduction in muscle mass [1, 19]. Sometimes muscle mass can decline over a short period of time. The significant declines in creatinine excretion were seen in renal transplant patients, especially those who had chronic declines in allograft function [20]. The decline in creatinine excretion was likely due to decreases in muscle mass from multiple causes, including the effects of therapy with corticosteroids [19, 20]. As a result of this therapy changes in serum creatinine underestimate the amount of decline in renal function. Tubular secretion of serum creatinine may be important, especially in patients with reduced renal function, and may lead to overestimation of renal function [1]. Furthermore, the potential for interference from plasma constituents and medications requires the clinician to know what assay is being used to measure serum creatinine and should be aware of the precision of the assay. Precision is commonly measured by the coefficient of variation, which is the mean of replicate samples divided by the standard deviation. There have been many attempts to mathematically transform or correct serum creatinine so that it may more accurately reflect GFR. Under ideal conditions, GFR, as measured by a marker such as serum creatinine, should be equal to the inverse of the creatinine multiplied by a constant rate of creatinine excretion. Thus, in an ideal situation changes in inverse creatinine should be directly proportional to changes in GFR. However, changes in creatinine production, extrarenal elimination, and tubular secretion of creatinine can all create errors in the use of inverse creatinine to measure changes in GFR. Indeed, none of the shortcomings of using serum creatinine as a marker of GFR are avoided by using inverse creatinine [1, 19]. Creatinine clearance measurement using 24-h urine collection is also used to estimate the GFR, but the reliability of this method depends very much on accurate and complete urine collection. Variations in creatinine production due to age- and sex-related differences in muscle mass have been measured and have been incorporated in various serum creatinine-based equations (formulas) to improve the ability of serum creatinine to estimate GFR. The current Kidney Disease Outcomes Quality Initiative (K/DOQI) guidelines emphasize the need to assess kidney function using predictive equations rather than just serum creatinine [21]. Two widely used formulas are the Cockcroft-Gault formula and the abbreviated Modification of Diet in Renal Disease (MDRD) formula [22]. It is known that Cockcroft and Gault formula reduces the variability of serum creatinine estimation of glomerular filtration measured in a population of men and women of different ages [23]. However, the formula does not take into account differences in creatinine production between individuals of the same age and sex or even in the same individual over time. The formula systematically overestimates GFR in individuals who are obese or edematous [1, 24]. Moreover, it does not take into account extrarenal elimination, tubular handling, or inaccuracies in the laboratory measurement of creatinine that each contribute to error in the serum creatinine estimation of GFR [1, 25]. The fact is that GFR has probably never been measured with more accuracy in a large population of patients than in the Modification of Diet in Renal Disease study [26]. In this study the isotopically measured GFR determination was used to derive a MDRD formula for estimating GFR using only readily measurable clinical variables [26]. Significantly, they derived the formula on a randomly selected subset of patients from the whole population and then tested the formula in the remainder of the population. A formula that used only plasma chemistries and patient characteristics was able to predict 90.3% of the variability in isotopically measured GFR [1, 26]. All these formulas are also limited by lack of validation in the full range of the GFR to which they are applied [27]. To minimize some of these limitations, such are imprecision and systematic underestimation of measured GFR with MDRD formula, the new Chronic Kidney Disease Epidemiology Collaboration equation (CKD-EPI formula) was developed [28]. Common features of these equations are reliance on serum creatinine and demographic and anthropometric data, and the accuracy of these formulas is still debated [22, 26, 28]. Recently, NKDEP recommended reporting GFR values above 60 ml/min/1.73m^2 not as an exact number but simply as > 60 ml/min/1.73m^2, and contrary for the values of 60 ml/min/1.73m^2 and below the exact numerical estimate should be reported [21]. For clinicians the GFR below 60 ml/min/1.73m^2 is very important. The values indicate the presence of CKD and represent an increased risk of impaired kidney function, progression to kidney failure and premature death caused by cardiovascular events of patients with CKD [29]. Furthermore, it cannot be assumed that formulas to predict renal function derived from data from one patient population will be valid when applied to another population. Individuals on vegetarian diet, consuming creatinine supplements, with unusual weight (extreme obesity, amputation), with unusual muscle mass, or pregnant women were not included in the study populations that were used to generate these formulas [1]. Additionally, the formulas are not accurate enough for some individuals with normal or near normal kidney function [30]. Thus, it is important to test the accuracy of the formulas in each patient population that may reasonably be expected to differ from the population that was used to derive the formula. In particular, investigators should test the accuracy of the formula in populations with characteristics that can be expected to affect the variables in the formula that differ from the characteristics of the population used to derive the formula [1]. Because of all mentioned disadvantages of serum creatinine and serum creatinine-based formulas regarding estimation of renal function, new marker of GFR like serum cystatin C was proposed. Cystatin C, protease inhibitor with a low molecular weight, is produced at a constant rate by all nucleated cells. It is freely filtered across the glomerular membrane and is reabsorbed and metabolized in the proximal tubule [31]. The generation of cystatin C appears to be less variable from person to person than that of creatinine. Serum cystatin C does not depend on muscle mass, sex and age [32]. Inflammation, fever and/or outside agents do not affect the serum cystatin C concentration [31]. There is contradictory data considering the possible influence of malignant diseases on the serum concentration of cystatin C, however, most authors are of the opinion that malignant processes do not influence the serum cystatin C concentration [31, 33]. Cystatin C concentration is a better indicator of GFR than serum creatinine concentration in patients with spine injury, liver cirrhosis, diabetes, mild to moderate impaired kidney function and in elderly patients [34-36]. Over the last few years some cystatin C-based equations (cystatin C formulas) have also been developed to estimate the GFR from serum cystatin C concentration and been compared to creatinine-based formulas [37-43]. The results of published studies suggest that the serum cystatin C-based prediction equations, which require just one variable (serum cystatin C concentration), achieved a diagnostic performance that is at least as good as the creatinine formulas, including very sophisticated serum creatinine-based equation that uses both serum creatinine and cystatin C (CKD-EPI creatinine & cystatin formula) [38, 39, 44-46].

Conclusion

Despite all known disadvantages, serum creatinine concentration remains the most commonly used marker to estimate GFR in clinical practice as in most studies. The current guidelines emphasize the need to assess kidney function using predictive simple or sophisticated equations or new markers of GFR, rather than just serum creatinine. Until an alternative filtration marker replaces serum creatinine the methods traceable to IDMS must be used for measurement of creatinine.

References

[1] Israni AK, Kasiske BL. Laboratory assessment of kidney disease: clearance, urinalysis, and kidney biopsy. In: Brenner BM (ed), Brenner and Rectors. The Kidney. 8th edition. Philadelphia: Saunders, 2008: 724-56.

[2] Laterza OF, Price CP, Scott MG. Cystatin C: An improved estimator of glomerular filtration rate? *Clin. Chem.* 2002; 48: 699-707.

[3] Levey AS, Berg RL, Gassmann JJ, Hall PM, Walker WG. Creatinine filtration, secretion and excretion during progressive renal disease. *Kidney Int.* 1989; 36 (Suppl 27): S73-80).

[4] Perrone RD, Madias NE, Levey AS. Serum creatinine as an index of renal function: new insights into old concepts. *Clin. Chem.* 1992; 38: 1933-53.

[5] Myers GL, Miller WG, Coresh J, et al. Recommendations for improving serum creatinine measurement: A report from the Laboratory Working Group of the National Kidney Disease Education Program. *Clin. Chem.* 2006; 52: 5-18.

[6] Delange JR, Speeckaert MM. Creatinine determination according to Jaffe-what does it stand for? *NDT Plus* 2011; 4: 83-86.

[7] Young DS. Effects of Drugs on Clinical Laboratory Tests, 3rd ed. Washington, DC; American Association of Clinical Chemistry Press, 1990: 3-128.

[8] Toffaleti J, Blosser N, Hall T, et al. An automated dry-slid enzymatic method evaluated for measurement of creatinine in serum. *Clin. Chem.* 1983; 29: 684-87.

[9] Karon BS, Daly TM, Scott MG. Mechanisms of dopamine and dobutamine interference in biochemical tests that use peroxide and peroxidase to generate chromophore. *Clin. Chem.* 1998; 44: 155-60.

[10] Mitchell RT, Marshall LH, Lefkowitz LB, Stratton CW. Falsely elevated serum creatinine levels secondary to the presence of 5-fluorocytosine. *Am. J. Clin. Pathol.* 1985; 84: 251-3.

[11] Schoenmakers CH, Kuller T, Lindemans J, Blijenberg BG. Automated enzymatic methods for creatinine measurement with special attention to bilirubin interference. *Eur. J. Clin. Chem. Clin. Biochem.* 1993; 31: 861-8.

[12] Bagnoud MA, Reymond JP. Interference of metamizol (dipyrone) on the determination of creatinine with the kodak dry chemistry slide comparison with the enzymatic method from Boehringer. *Eur. J. Clin. Chem. Clin. Biochem.* 1993; 31: 753-7.

[13] Hummel KM, von Ahsen N, Kuhn RB, Kaboth U, Grunewald RW, Oellerich M, et al. Pseudohypercreatininemia due to positive interference in enzymatic creatinine measurements caused by monoclonal IGM in patients with Waldenstrom's macroglobulinemia [Letter]. *Nephron* 2000; 86: 188-9.

[14] Kågedal B, Olsson B. Determination of creatinine in serum by high-performance liquid chromatography: a comparison of three ion-exchange methods. *J. Chromatogr.* 1990; 527: 21-30.

[15] International Organization for Standardization. ISO guide 17511. In vitro diagnostic medical devices—measurement of quantities in biological samples—metrological traceability of values assigned to calibrators and control materials. Geneva, Switzerland: ISO, 2003.

[16] MDRD study equation for estimating GFR with IDMS traceable (gold standard) serum creatinine values (abstract). *J. Am. Soc. Nephrol.* 2005; 16: 69A.

[17] www.nkdep.nih.gov.

[18] Heymsfield SB, Arteaga C, Maccanus C, Smith J, Moffitt S. Measurement of muscle mass in humans: validity of the 24-hour urinary creatinine method. *Am. J. Clin. Nutr.* 1983; 37: 478-94.

[19] Silkensen JR, Kasiske BL. Laboratory assessment of renal disease: clearance, urinalysis, and kidney biopsy. In: Brenner BM (ed), Brenner and Rectors. The Kidney. 7th edition. Philadelphia: Saunders, 2004: 1107-1150.

[20] Kasiske BL. Creatinine excretion after renal transplantation. *Transplantation* 1989; 48: 424-28.

[21] National Kidney Foundation: K/DOQI Clinical practice guideline to define chronic kidney disease: evaluation, classification and stratification. *Am. J. Kidney Dis.* 2002; 39 (Suppl 1): S1-S266.

[22] Froissart M, Rossert J, Jacquot C et al. Predictive performance of the Modification of Diet in Renal disease and Cockcroft-Gault equations for estimating renal function. *J. Am. Soc. Nephrol.* 2005; 16: 763-73.

[23] Cockroft DW, Gault MH. Prediction of creatinine clearence from serum creatinine. *Nephron* 1976; 16: 31-41.

[24] Rolin HA, III, Hall PM, Wei R. Inaccuracy of estimated creatinine clearance for prediction of iothalamate glomerular filtration rate. *Am. J. Kidney Dis.* 1984; 4: 48-54.

[25] Coresh J, Toto RD, Kirk KA, et al. Creatinine clearance as a measure of GFR in screenees for the African-American study of kidney disease and hypertension pilot study. *Am. J. Kidney Dis.* 1998; 32: 32-42.

[26] Levey AS, Bosch JP, Lewis JB, Greene T, Rogers N, Roth D. A more accurate method to estimate glomerular filtration rate from serum creatinine: a new prediction equation. Modification of Diet in Renal Disease Study Group. *Ann. Intern. Med.* 1999; 130: 461-70.

[27] Poggio ED, Wang X, Greene T et al. Performance of the Modification of Diet in Renal disease and Cockcroft-Gault equations in the estimation of GFR in health and in chronic kidney disease. *J. Am. Soc. Nephrol.* 2005; 16: 459-66.

[28] Levey AS, Stevens LA, Schmid CH et al. A new equation to estimate glomerular filtration rate; CKD-EPI (Chronic Kidney Disease Epidemiology Collaboration). *Ann. Intern. Med.* 2009; 150(9): 604-12.

[29] Go AS, Chertow GM, Fan D, McCulloch CE, McCulloch CE, Hsu CY. Chronic kidney disease and the risk of death, cardiovascular events, and hospitalisation. *N. Engl. J. Med.* 2004; 351: 1296-1305.

[30] Lin J, Knight EL, Hogan ML, Singh AK. A comparation of prediction equations for estimating glomerular filtration rate in adults without kidney disease. *J. Am. Soc. Nephrol.* 2003; 14: 2571-80.

[31] Randers E, Erlandsen EJ. Serum cystatin C as an endogenous marker of renal function: a review. *Clin. Chem. Lab. Med.* 1999; 37: 389-95.

[32] Coll E, Botey A, Alvarez L, Poch E, Quintó L, Saurina A, Vera M, Piera C, Darnell A. Serum cystatin C as a new marker for noninvasive estimation of glomerular filtration rate and as a marker for early renal impairment. *Am. J. Kidney* Dis. 2000; 36: 29-34.

[33] Finney H, Williams AH, Price CP. Serum cystatin C in patients with myeloma. *Clin. Chim. Acta* 2001; 309: 1-6.

[34] Dharnidharka VR, Kwon C, Stevens G. Serum cystatin C is superior to serum creatinine as a marker of kidney function: A meta-analysis. *Am. J. Kidney Dis.* 2002; 40: 221-26.

[35] Hojs R, Bevc S, Antolinc B, Gorenjak M, Puklavec L. Serum cystatin C as an endogenous marker of renal function in the elderly. *Int. J. Clin. Pharm.* 2004; 24: 49-54.

[36] Hojs R, Bevc S, Ekart R, Gorenjak M, Puklavec L. Serum cystatin C as an endogenous marker of renal function in patients with mild to moderate impaired kidney function. *Nephrol. Dial Transplant.* 2006; 21: 1855-62.

[37] Grubb A, Nyman U, Bjorak J, Lindström V, Rippe B, Sterner G, Christensson A. Simple cystatin C based prediction equations for glomerular rate compared with modification of diet in renal disease prediction equation for adults and the Schwartz and the Counhan-Barratt prediction equations for children. *Clinical Chemistry* 2005; 51: 1420-31.

[38] Hoek FJ, Kemperman FA, Krediet RT. A comparison between cystatin C, plasma creatinine and the Cockcroft and Gault formula for the estimation of glomerular filtration rate. *Nephrol. Dial Transplan.* 2003; 18: 2024-31.

[39] Larsson A, Malm J, Grubb A, Hansson LO. Calculation of glomerular filtration rate expressed in ml/min from plasma cystatin C values in mg/l. *Scand. J. Clin. Lab. Invest.* 2004; 64: 25-30.

[40] MacIsaac RJ, Tsalamndris C, Thomas MC, Premaratne E, Panagiotopoulos S, Smith TJ et al. Estimating glomerular filtration rate in diabetes: a comparison of cystatin C and creatinine-based methods. *Diabetologia*. 2006; 49: 1686-89.

[41] Rule AD, Bregstraalh EJ, Slezak JM, Bergert J, Larson TS. Glomerular filtration rate estimated by cystatin C among different clinical presentations. *Kidney Int*. 2006; 69: 399-405.

[42] Hojs R, Bevc S, Ekart R, Gorenjak M, Puklavec L. Serum cystatin C-based equation compared to serum creatinine-based equations for estimation of glomerular filtration rate in patients with chronic kidney disease. *Clin. Nephol.* 2008; 70: 10-17.

[43] Hojs R, Bevc S, Ekart R, Gorenjak M, Puklavec L. Serum cystatin C formulas for prediction of glomerular filtration rate in patients with chronic kidney disease. *Nephon Clin. Pract.* 2009; 114(2):118-26.

[44] Tidman M, Sjostrom P, Jones I. A comparison of GFR estimating formulae based upon s-cystatin C and s-creatinine and combination of the two. *Nephrol. Dial Transplant*. 2008; 23: 154-60.

[45] Hojs R, Bevc S, Ekart R, Gorenjak M, Puklavec L. Kidney function estimating equations in patients with chronic kidney disease. *Int. J. Clin. Pract.* 2011: 65: 458-64.

[46] Bevc S, Hojs R, Ekart R, Gorenjak M, Puklavec L. Simple cystatin C formula compared to sophisticated CKD-EPI formulas for estimation of glomerular filtration rate in the elderly. *Therap. Apher. Dial.* 2011; 15: 261-68.

In: Creatinine
Editors: I. H. Perkins and C. M. Chapman
ISBN: 978-1-62257-475-9

Chapter X

Creatinine Transport

Azza Ali Kamel El-Sheikh
Pharmacology Department, Faculty of Medicine, Minia University, Egypt

Abstract

Creatinine is a guanidino metabolic product of muscular creatine phosphate, produced in constant level relative to body muscular mass, thus its renal clearance is used as a marker of kidney function. Renal creatinine handling includes glomerular filtration and active proximal tubular secretion. Pathological conditions as severe renal failure cause reduction in glomerular filtration of creatinine, such that total creatinine excreted is dependent on active tubular secretion. The latter involves proximal tubule directional transport by basolateral uptake via organic cation transporter (OCT) 2, followed by apical efflux into the urine via multidrug and toxin extrusion (MATE) 1 and MATE2-k transporter proteins. Other transporters, as OCT3, have been suggested to contribute to creatinine active renal secretion. A number of factors may alter creatinine renal secretion.

Genetic polymorphisms of transporters involved in active renal efflux of creatinine may impair its secretion. Furthermore, drugs as cimetidine, trimethoprim and levofloxacin may affect renal creatinine excretion. Gender-based differences in creatinine transport have also been implicated. Extra-renal transport of creatinine, as its cerebral clearance via OCT3 efflux protein in the blood-cerebrospinal fluid barrier, contributes to creatinine tissue distribution. Translational research faces difficulty in interpreting mechanisms of creatinine renal handling from animal experiments due to inter-species variation. Still, human pharmacogenomic and molecular studies may provide insights that can be applied to clinical situations.

Introduction

Creatinine is a small water-soluble nitrogenous molecule of 113 Dalton mass (BMJ Evidence Centre, 2011). Chemically, creatinine (Figure 1) is 2-amino-1,5-dihydro-1-methyl-4H-imidazol-4-one, with the chemical formula $C_4H_7N_3O$.

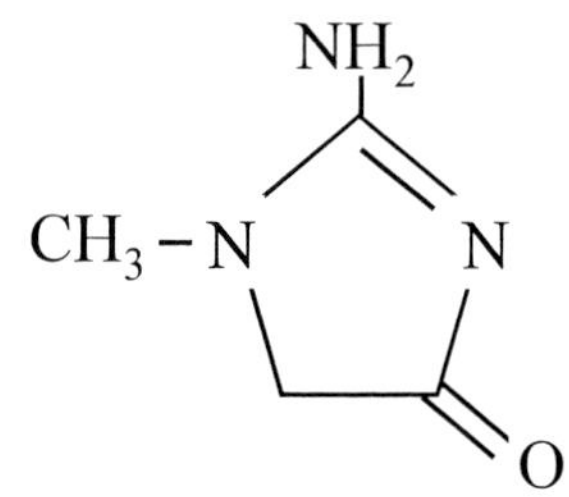

Figure 1. Chemical structure of creatinine.

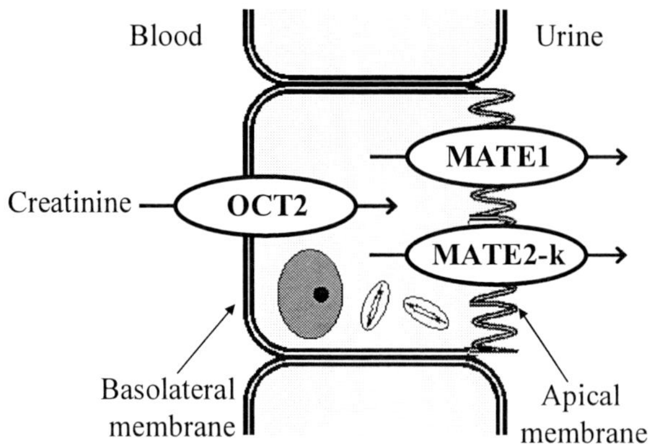

Figure 2. Schematic figure of renal proximal tubule cell showing transporters involved in creatinine active secretion. Oval structures depict transporter proteins and the arrows depict direction of transport. OCT; Organic Cation Transporter, MATE; Multidrug and Toxin Extrusion Transporter.

Historically, Borsook and Dubnoff were the first to report that creatinine is formed by loss of phosphate from phosphocreatine, and considered this as a spontaneous reaction taking place in mammalian body (Rosengart, 1944). Currently, it is known that creatine is initially subjected to reversible phosphorylation by creatine kinase enzyme, forming phosphocreatine. This intermediate step stores high energy phosphate for restoring ATP levels, in cases of body high energy demand. This is followed by the irreversible conversion of phophocreatine into creatinine, with liberation of phosphate. This process occurs at a relatively constant rate, which is directly proportionate to the body muscular mass. Total musclar creatine is around 125 mmol/kg dry mass. Daily, 2% of our body creatine is converted to creatinine, generating constant creatinine in the range of 20-25 mg/kg/day and 15-20 mg/kg/day in males and females, respectively.

The formed creatinine is eliminated via renal route mainly through glomerular filtration, and is neither reabsorbed nor metabolized by the kidney. At normal kidney function, proximal tubular efflux accounts for around 15% of urinary creatinine level (Shemesh *et al.*, 1985). This unique elimination property made serum creatinine one of the most acceptable markers of kidney function. Still, blood creatinine levels may only be increased after marked deterioration of renal function. As a result, it is useless in detecting early-stage kidney impairment. Furthermore, rate of creatinine excretion is different between sexes and is remarkably reduced in extremes of age. Creatinine clearance test is thus a more accurate estimate of renal functionality reflecting glomerular filtration rate (Rose and Post, 2001), as it correlates serum to urinary creatinine levels with respect to individual age, sex and ethnicity (Barr *et al.*, 2005).

Renal Creatinine Handling

Creatinine is freely filtered through the renal glomeruli, which accounts for the majority of urinary excretion during normal kidney function. During acute kidney damage, serum creatinine rises about 2 mg/day and may exceed 5 mg/day in cases with severe rhabdomyolysis, manifesting with massive breakdown of skeletal muscle. Patients with acute rapidly progressing glomerulonephritis, in which about 50% of renal function may be impaired within weeks, show considerable increment in serum creatinine. With the loss of nephron functionality and the progress of renal failure, creatinine passive glomerular filtration is minimal and active proximal tubular secretion becomes the main creatinine renal excretory pathway. Renal proximal tubular secretion involves directional transport of creatinine (Urakami *et al.*, 2005). Firstly, an uptake step from the blood to the proximal tubule cells via electrogenic organic transporters present in the basolateral membrane. Secondly, an extrusion step where creatinine is actively secreted from the proximal tubule cells into the urine by transporters present in the apical membrane (Figure 2). The latter is an active and rate-limiting step in creatinine secretion, mediated by electroneutral OC/H^+ exchange. So far, few renal transporters have been shown to contribute in creatinine renal active secretion.

1. Creatinine Renal Proximal Tubule Basolateral Uptake

Organic Cation Transporter 2

Organic cation transporter (OCT) 2 has been recently confirmed as one of the human transporters involved in creatinine active uptake from the blood to the renal proximal tubule cells through the basolateral membrane (Ciarimboli *et al.*, 2012). OCT2 protein belongs to the solute carrier (*SLC*) family of transporters and is encoded by the gene *SLC22A2*, which was previously characterized as the potential sensitive organic cation uptake transporter of the basolateral membrane. In the kidney, it is subcellularly localized solely in the basolateral membrane of proximal tubule cells, mainly in S_2 and S_3 segments. Hormonal therapy or pathological plasma testosterone or estradiol changes regulate OCT2 expression levels through modulation of nuclear transcription, mRNA stability and/or protein synthesis (Urakami *et al.*, 2000;Shu *et al.*, 2001). OCT2 transport of organic cations into tubule cells is mediated by facilitated transport mechanism and is membrane-potential sensitive (Fujita *et al.*, 2006). OCT2 mediates creatinine transport with michaelis constant (Km) of 4 mM, suggesting low affinity of OCT2 to creatinine (Urakami *et al.*, 2004). In addition to creatinine renal basolateral uptake, OCT2 accept a number of medically prescribed drugs and dietary supplements as substrates including metformin, phenformin, amantadine, memantine, cimetidine, choline, and quinine. Others interact with OCT2 without being transported by the protein and acts as inhibitors of the transport, including cocaine, desipramine, imipramine, grepafloxacin, mepiperphenidol, nafamostat mesilate, nicotine, phenoxybenzamine, procainamide, quinidine, trimethoprim, and verapamil (Fujita *et al.*, 2006).

Other Renal Creatinine Uptake Transporters

Creatinine has been suggested as a substrate of OCT3 (Hayer-Zillgen *et al.*, 2002; Tachikawa *et al.*, 2008; Hosoya and Tachikawa, 2011), although still to be confirmed. OCT3 transporter is encoded by the gene *SLC22A3*. Preliminary subcellular localization studies suggested that OCT3 is expressed in the basolateral membrane of the renal proximal tubule cells (Glube and Langguth, 2008). The expression of OCT2 compared to that of OCT3 in proximal tubule cells was reported to be in the ratio of 1 to 0.03 (Holle *et al.*, 2011), suggesting that OCT2 has more prominent role in creatinine renal uptake. Interestingly, despite that creatinine is cationic; the organic anion transporter (OAT) 3, encoded by *SLC22A8* gene, has been suggested to accept it as a substrate in oat3$^{-/-}$ mice (Vallon *et al.*, 2012), contributing to its renal elimination. Similarly, taurine transporter (TauT), encoded by *SLC6A6* gene, was also suggested as a basolateral transporter accepting creatinine as substrate, as urinary creatinine was significantly lower in taut$^{-/-}$ than taut$^{+/+}$ mice (Huang *et al.*, 2006). It is possible that this is a mere species difference between human and mice (see below).

2. Creatinine Renal Proximal Tubule Apical Efflux

Multidrug and Toxin Extrusion Transporter Proteins

Apical efflux of creatinine from the proximal tubule cells into the urine through the brush-border membrane is thought to be via the multidrug and toxin extrusion (MATE) 1 transporter and its kidney-specific isoform; MATE2-k transporter protein (Tanihara *et al.*, 2007).

MATE1 and MATE2-k are encoded by *SLC47A1* and *SLC47A2*, respectively. MATE2-k is a functional isoform of human MATE2, coding for a 566-amino acid protein. Both transporters are predominantly expressed in human renal proximal tubule, and are subcellularly localized in the luminal brush border membrane (Nies *et al.*, 2011). Human MATE1 is also expressed in liver, skeletal muscle, adrenal gland and testis. Interestingly, despite immunolocalization of MATE1 apically in the kidney, the protein is expressed in the canalicular (basolateral) membrane of hepatocytes. MATEs are electro-neutral, sodium-independent cation efflux transporters that operate using an oppositely directed proton gradient as driving force.

Thus the translocation of organic cations across the membranes may occur in both directions, depending on the proton gradient direction. Apical MATE1 and MATE2-K proteins have similar substrate and inhibitor specificities. Such specificity overlaps with that of the renal basolateral OCTs, thus comprising the directional pathway of their common substrates.

In addition to creatinine, MATE1 and MATE2-k accept other endogenous compounds as substrates, including guanidine, thiamine, and also the organic anion estrone sulfate, in addition to more than 30 clinically used drugs as metformin, cimetidine, oxaliplatin, acyclovir and fexofenadine (Nies *et al.*, 2011).

Other Renal Creatinine Apical Transporters

P-glycoprotein, also called multidrug resistance protein 1; MDR1, is implicated to have a role in creatinine renal efflux, as single nucleotide polymorphisms of this transporter resulted in functional protein differences, with statistically significant differences in serum creatinine levels (Zhang *et al.*, 2007). MDR1 is encoded by ATP-binding cassette, sub-family B, member 1 (*ABCB1*) gene. It has a wide range of substrates that are usually bulky, hydrophobic organic ions. MDR1 is located apically in renal proximal tubule cells, where it effluxes its substrates to the urine at the expense of ATP.

Creatine transporter, encoded by *SLC6A8* gene, is also suggested to accept creatinine as a substrate with low affinity (Tachikawa *et al.*, 2008). It is subcellularly localized apically in the renal proximal tubule cells where it acts as Na^+/Cl^-/creatinine cotransporter (Garcia-Delgado *et al.*, 2007). Interestingly, the direction of transport of creatine transporter protein is supposed to be from urine back to the kidney proximal tubule cells by this transporter (Li *et al.*, 2010), conflicting with the net secretion and negligible reabsorption of creatinine. Thus, the role of this transporter in renal creatinine homeostasis is still to be elucidated.

Factors Affecting Active Creatinine Renal Secretion

Inter-individual differences in creatinine renal excretion may be attributed to environmental factors as age, muscular weight, gender and diet. Several transporter-related factors may modify creatinine renal secretion. These factors may be endogenous factors as naturally occurring genetic polymorphisms of transporter proteins or exogenous as drugs that may inhibit or simulate creatinine active transport. On the other hand, creatinine may act as a transport inhibitor of compounds competing with it for excretion by OCTs and/or MATEs. Furthermore, creatinine may inhibit other renal transporters not accepting it as a substrate. For example, in the unpublished data of Koepsell et al., creatinine acted as an inhibitor of OCT1 apical renal protein transport of 1-methyl-4-phenylpyridinium (Nies *et al.*, 2011). The implication of such inhibition is complex, knowing that OCT1 is not an apical efflux transporter, but rather an apical re-uptake protein of organic cations that, to date, was shown to be expressed in rodent kidney, but not in humans.

1. Gender-based Differences in Creatinine Transport

Gender-based differences in serum creatinine level have for long been well documented, varying significantly from 81 μM in men to 65 μM in women (Marescau *et al.*, 1997). This gender-based serum level variation is reflected on renal urinary excretion of creatinine, even in children (Mori *et al.*, 2006). The cause of such variation is still inconclusive, but may be strongly related to the significantly higher creatinine synthesis in males than females. It is possible that this variation may also be caused by inhibition of female sex hormones to creatinine renal transport.

Indeed, the anionic hormone, estrone sulphate; is a substrate for MATE1 and MATE2-k (Tanihara *et al.*, 2007). Another possibility is the regulation of transporters involved in creatinine renal secretion by sex hormones (Urakami *et al.*, 2000; Shu *et al.*, 2001; Asaka *et al.*, 2006).

2. Transporters Genetic Polymorphisms

Naturally occurring genetic variants have been identified in human OCTs and MATEs that lead to synthesis of functionally impaired transporters. This genetically-induced defect may cause impairment of creatinine secretion. Several genetic variants have been reported for OCT2 (Leabman *et al.*, 2003), eight of which caused amino acid changes, while one was a single-nucleotide insertion that lead to a premature stop codon (Fujita *et al.*, 2006). These variant transporters had diverse functional profiles that ranged from complete loss of transport activity to fully functional transport, with different ranges of kinetics and inhibition properties. Clinically, OCT2 protein-altered variants showed altered renal elimination of organic cations (Tzvetkov *et al.*, 2009). Some single nucleotide polymorphisms of MATE1 and MATE2-k (*SLC47A1* and *SLC47A2* genes, respectively) were also reported to completely abolish these proteins transport functionality (Yonezawa and Inui, 2011). Other mutations caused total lack of membrane expression of MATE1 and MATE2-k (Kajiwara *et al.*, 2009), thus affecting the pharmacokinetics of all their substrates, including creatinine.

3. Creatinine-Drug Interactions

Cationic drugs are pharmaceuticals whose molecules carry a net positive charge at physiological pH. These drugs comprise nearly 40% of all clinically prescribed medications (Neuhoff *et al.*, 2003). Creatinine is transported via organic cationic transporters that accept various cationic substrates. Such wide range of specificity of transporters involved in creatinine transport may anticipate several unwanted creatinine-drug interaction outcomes. One study showed the interaction of 59 structurally dissimilar compounds with MATE1 and MATE2-k transporters (Astorga *et al.*, 2012). OCT2 accepts drugs as metformin and cisplatin as substrates (Nies and Schwab, 2010). Still, it is not mandatory that all these substrates/inhibitors react with creatinine transport, due to possible multiple binding/inhibitory sites of these transporter proteins.

Cimetidine, quinidine and trimethoprim were shown to inhibit transcellular transport of creatinine in renal tubular epithelial cell line (Urakami *et al.*, 2005), probably through inhibition of OCT2-mediated creatinine transport. Fluoroquinolone and levofloxacin also inhibit creatinine transport via OCT2 (Okuda *et al.*, 2006), as well as procainamide, famotidine and ranitidine (Urakami *et al.*, 2004). A novel fluoroquinolone antibacterial agent, DX-619; at its therapeutic dose, was shown to inhibit not only OCT2, but also MATE1 and MATE2-k transporters, which probably leads to significant inhibition of renal tubular secretion of creatinine (Imamura *et al.*, 2011). Logically, administration of OCTs and/or MATEs substrates/inhibitors may impair the usefulness of creatinine as a marker of renal function.

4. Regulation of Creatinine Transporters

Up- or down-regulation of one or more transporters involved in creatinine active renal secretion may dramatically modulate serum creatinine levels. Up-regulation of transporters involved in both steps of creatinine renal uptake and efflux may aid in protecting the body from the hazards of high creatinine levels by promoting its renal excretion. On the other hand, down-regulation of such renal transporters, despite being considered nephro-protective as it decreases the accumulation of creatinine in the kidney, still may contribute to systemic increase in creatinine level. In this contest, fenofibrate (Asavapanumas *et al.*, 2012) and thymoquinone (Ulu *et al.*, 2012) are considered nephroprotective as they down-regulate OCT2. Nephrotoxic effects of cisplatin may be partially mediated by down-regulation of MATE1 (Morisaki *et al.*, 2008) involved in renal apical creatinine efflux. Disease conditions, as chronic renal failure, may also reduce OCT2 expression levels (Sun *et al.*, 2006), adding to the already existing creatinine retention. Similarly, ischemia/reperfusion-induced acute kidney injury causes down-regulation of both OCT2 and MATE1 (Matsuzaki *et al.*, 2008).

Extra-Renal Creatinine Transport

During renal impairment, pathologically high levels of creatinine are attained, which is associated with its accumulation as a uremic toxin in blood and tissues. This may amount to fatal conditions as uremic encephalopathy, where uremic toxins produce excitatory effects on the central nervous system especially at uremic concentrations similar to those producing convulsive effects, causing neurological complications seen in these patients (De Deyn *et al.*, 2009). Under normal conditions, serum creatinine concentration is 65-80 μM, whereas in non-dialyzed patients with renal insufficiency it may reach up to tenfold higher. Moreover, the blood-to-brain influx is much greater than the brain-to-blood efflux transport, which results in four- to fivefold higher brain creatinine concentration levels compared to that in serum (Tachikawa *et al.*, 2008). In such case, transporters at blood-brain barrier membrane may be the rate-limiting physiological determinant of the concentration of creatinine in brain. Cerebral clearance of creatinine occurs via OCT3 efflux protein in the blood-cerebrospinal fluid barrier (Hosoya and Tachikawa, 2011), expressed in hippocampal and cerebellar neurons and is localized in the brush-border membrane of choroid plexus epithelium. In addition creatine transporter may also comprise a central low affinity creatinine transporter (Tachikawa *et al.*, 2008).

Interspecies Variation in Creatinine Transport

The relatively recent availability of molecular biology techniques facilitated the identification of human proteins involved in creatinine transport. Still, the vast majority of available data related to creatinine excretion involve animal studies. For example, the first member of OCT family was isolated by expression cloning from rat kidney (Grundemann *et al.*, 1994). Unfortunately, creatinine excretion shows large inter-species variability that may present difficulty in interpretation of results from animal experiments in translational research. These differences are the reflection of tissue variability in expression levels of transporters involved in creatinine excretion among different species. One example is the contribution of OAT3 in creatinine renal proximal tubule uptake in mice (Vallon *et al.*, 2012), which is not reported for humans. It is possible that this species difference occurs so that mice oat3 take part in creatinine elimination to compensate for other transporter's low affinity for creatinine. Another example is OCT2, which is the main human renal uptake transporter protein of creatinine known so far, which is expressed in both rodent and human kidneys, but was shown not to participate in renal proximal basolateral uptake in oct2$^{-/-}$ mice (Eisner *et al.*, 2010). Furthermore, in rodent kidney, both OCT1 and OCT2 are expressed (Koepsell *et al.*, 2007), whereas OCT1 is not expressed in human renal tissue. Similarly, MATE2-k is not expressed in mice, although tissue distribution of MATE1 in mice is consistent with that in human (Yonezawa and Inui, 2011). This variability leads to the usage of OCT1/2 double knockout and MATE1 knockout mice to examine the roles of OCTs and MATE1/MATE2-K deficiency in humans, respectively.

Conclusion

A number of renal transporters contribute in creatinine renal active secretion, as well as other cationic compounds including drugs, toxins and endogenous metabolites. From these, OCT2, MATE1 and MATE2-k are the most prominent. Understanding creatinine renal transport pathways provides insight on potential drug interactions and may present the basis in prevention of drug toxic side effects. Despite of the difficulties facing translational research due to inter-species variations in creatinine transport, human molecular and pharmacogenomic studies can supply data concerning these transporters' substrate selectivity, transcriptional mechanisms, protein structure and genetic polymorphisms that can be employed to interpret *in-vivo* clinical outcomes.

References

Asaka J, Terada T, Okuda M, Katsura T and Inui K (2006) Androgen Receptor Is Responsible for Rat Organic Cation Transporter 2 Gene Regulation but Not for ROCT1 and ROCT3. *Pharm. Res.* 23:697-704.

Asavapanumas N, Kittayaruksakul S, Meetam P, Muanprasat C, Chatsudthipong V and Soodvilai S (2012) Fenofibrate Down-Regulates Renal OCT2-Mediated Organic Cation Transport Via PPARalpha-Independent Pathways. *Drug Metab. Pharmacokinet.* [Epub ahead of print; PMID: 22473497].

Astorga B, Ekins S, Morales M and Wright SH (2012) Molecular Determinants of Ligand Selectivity for the Human Multidrug And Toxin Extrusion Proteins, MATE1 and MATE-2K. *J. Pharmacol. Exp. Ther.* [Epub ahead of print; PMID: 22419765].

Barr DB, Wilder LC, Caudill SP, Gonzalez AJ, Needham LL and Pirkle JL (2005) Urinary Creatinine Concentrations in the U.S. Population: Implications for Urinary Biologic Monitoring Measurements. *Environ. Health Perspect.* 113:192-200.

BMJ Evidence Centre (2011). Assessment of elevated creatinine. Available from: URL: http://bestpractice.bmj.com/best-practice/monograph/935.html (accessed on 25th of April 2012).

Ciarimboli G, Lancaster CS, Schlatter E, Franke RM, Sprowl JA, Pavenstädt H, Massmann V, Guckel D, Mathijssen RH, Yang W, Pui CH, Relling MV, Herrmann E and Sparreboom A (2012) Proximal Tubular Secretion of Creatinine by Organic Cation Transporter OCT2 in Cancer Patients. *Clin. Cancer Res.* 18:1101-1108.

De Deyn PP, Vanholder R, Eloot S and Glorieux G (2009) Guanidino Compounds As Uremic (Neuro)Toxins. *Semin. Dial* 22:340-345.

Eisner C, Faulhaber-Walter R, Wang Y, Leelahavanichkul A, Yuen PS, Mizel D, Star RA, Briggs JP, Levine M and Schnermann J (2010) Major Contribution of Tubular Secretion to Creatinine Clearance in Mice. *Kidney Int.* 77:519-526.

Fujita T, Urban TJ, Leabman MK, Fujita K and Giacomini KM (2006) Transport of Drugs in the Kidney by the Human Organic Cation Transporter, OCT2 and Its Genetic Variants. *J. Pharm. Sci.* 95:25-36.

García-Delgado M, García-Miranda P, Peral MJ, Calonge ML and Ilundáin AA (2007) Ontogeny Up-Regulates Renal Na(+)/Cl(-)/Creatine Transporter in Rat. *Biochim. Biophys. Acta* 1768:2841-2848.

Glube N and Langguth P (2008) Caki-1 Cells As a Model System for the Interaction of Renally Secreted Drugs With OCT3. *Nephron. Physiol.* 108:18-28.

Gründemann D, Gorboulev V, Gambaryan S, Veyhl M and Koepsell H (1994) Drug Excretion Mediated by a New Prototype of Polyspecific Transporter. *Nature* 372: 549-552.

Hayer-Zillgen M, Brüss M and Bönisch H (2002) Expression and Pharmacological Profile of the Human Organic Cation Transporters HOCT1, HOCT2 and HOCT3. *Br. J. Pharmacol.* 136:829-836.

Holle SK, Ciarimboli G, Edemir B, Neugebauer U, Pavenstädt H and Schlatter E (2011) Properties and Regulation of Organic Cation Transport in Freshly Isolated Mouse Proximal Tubules Analyzed With a Fluorescence Reader-Based Method. *Pflugers Arch.* 462:359-369.

Hosoya K and Tachikawa M (2011) Roles of Organic Anion/Cation Transporters at the Blood-Brain and Blood-Cerebrospinal Fluid Barriers Involving Uremic Toxins. *Clin. Exp. Nephrol.* 15:478-485.

Huang DY, Boini K M, Lang P A, Grahammer F, Duszenko M, Heller-Stilb B, Warskulat U, Häussinger D, Lang F and Vallon V (2006) Impaired Ability to Increase Water Excretion in Mice Lacking the Taurine Transporter Gene TAUT. *Pflugers Arch.* 451:668-677.

Imamura Y, Murayama N, Okudaira N, Kurihara A, Okazaki O, Izumi T, Inoue K, Yuasa H, Kusuhara H and Sugiyama Y (2011) Prediction of Fluoroquinolone-Induced Elevation in Serum Creatinine Levels: a Case of Drug-Endogenous Substance Interaction Involving the Inhibition of Renal Secretion. *Clin. Pharmacol. Ther.* 89:81-88.

Kajiwara M, Terada T, Ogasawara K, Iwano J, Katsura T, Fukatsu A, Doi T and Inui K (2009) Identification of Multidrug and Toxin Extrusion (MATE1 and MATE2-K) Variants With Complete Loss of Transport Activity. *J. Hum. Genet.* 54:40-46.

Koepsell H, Lips K and Volk C (2007) Polyspecific Organic Cation Transporters: Structure, Function, Physiological Roles, and Biopharmaceutical Implications. *Pharm. Res.* 24: 1227-1251.

Leabman MK, Huang C C, Stryke D, Johns SJ, Kawamoto M, Ferrin TE, DeYoung J, Taylor TR, De La Cruz M, Herskowitz I and Giacomini KM (2003) PharmGKB Update: I. Genetic Variants of the Organic Cation Transporter 2 (OCT2, SLC22A2). *Pharmacol. Rev.* 55:399.

Li H, Thali RF, Smolak C, Gong F, Alzamora R, Wallimann T, Scholz R, Pastor-Soler NM, Neumann D and Hallows KR (2010) Regulation of the Creatine Transporter by AMP-Activated Protein Kinase in Kidney Epithelial Cells. *Am. J. Physiol. Renal Physiol.* 299:F167-F177.

Marescau B, Nagels G, Possemiers I, De Broe ME, Becaus I, Billiouw JM, Lornoy W and De Deyn PP (1997) Guanidino Compounds in Serum and Urine of Nondialyzed Patients With Chronic Renal Insufficiency. *Metabolism* 46:1024-1031.

Matsuzaki T, Morisaki T, Sugimoto W, Yokoo K, Sato D, Nonoguchi H, Tomita K, Terada T, Inui K, Hamada A and Saito H (2008) Altered Pharmacokinetics of Cationic Drugs Caused by Down-Regulation of Renal Rat Organic Cation Transporter 2 (Slc22a2) and Rat Multidrug and Toxin Extrusion 1 (Slc47a1) in Ischemia/Reperfusion-Induced Acute Kidney Injury. *Drug Metab. Dispos.* 36:649-654.

Mori Y, Hiraoka M, Suganuma N, Tsukahara H, Yoshida H and Mayumi M (2006) Urinary Creatinine Excretion and Protein/Creatinine Ratios Vary by Body Size and Gender in Children. *Pediatr. Nephrol.* 21:683-687.

Morisaki T, Matsuzaki T, Yokoo K, Kusumoto M, Iwata K, Hamada A and Saito H (2008) Regulation of Renal Organic Ion Transporters in Cisplatin-Induced Acute Kidney Injury and Uremia in Rats. *Pharm. Res.* 25:2526-2533.

Neuhoff S, Ungell AL, Zamora I and Artursson P (2003) PH-Dependent Bidirectional Transport of Weakly Basic Drugs Across Caco-2 Monolayers: Implications for Drug-Drug Interactions. *Pharm. Res.* 20:1141-1148.

Nies AT, Koepsell H, Damme K and Schwab M (2011) Organic Cation Transporters (OCTs, MATEs), in Vitro and in Vivo Evidence for the Importance in Drug Therapy. *Handb. Exp. Pharmacol.* 105-167.

Nies AT and Schwab M (2010) Organic Cation Transporter Pharmacogenomics and Drug-Drug Interaction. *Expert Rev. Clin. Pharmacol.* 3:707-711.

Okuda M, Kimura N and Inui K (2006) Interactions of Fluoroquinolone Antibacterials, DX-619 and Levofloxacin, With Creatinine Transport by Renal Organic Cation Transporter HOCT2. *Drug Metab. Pharmacokinet.* 21:432-436.

Rose BD, Post TW, Clinical Physiology of Acid-Base and Electrolyte Disorders, 5th ed, McGraw-Hill, New York, 2001, pp. 50-57.

Rosengart V (1944). Formation of Creatinine in the Animal Body. *Nature*, 154, 829. [DOI: 10.1038/154829a0].

Shemesh O, Golbetz H, Kriss JP and Myers BD (1985) Limitations of Creatinine As a Filtration Marker in Glomerulopathic Patients. *Kidney Int.* 28:830-838.

Shu Y, Bello CL, Mangravite LM, Feng B and Giacomini KM (2001) Functional Characteristics and Steroid Hormone-Mediated Regulation of an Organic Cation Transporter in Madin-Darby Canine Kidney Cells. *J. Pharmacol. Exp. Ther.* 299: 392-398.

Sun H, Frassetto L and Benet LZ (2006) Effects of Renal Failure on Drug Transport and Metabolism. *Pharmacol. Ther.* 109:1-11.

Tachikawa M, Kasai Y, Takahashi M, Fujinawa J, Kitaichi K, Terasaki T and Hosoya K (2008) The Blood-Cerebrospinal Fluid Barrier Is a Major Pathway of Cerebral Creatinine Clearance: Involvement of Transporter-Mediated Process. *J. Neurochem.* 107:432-442.

Tanihara Y, Masuda S, Sato T, Katsura T, Ogawa O and Inui K (2007) Substrate Specificity of MATE1 and MATE2-K, Human Multidrug and Toxin Extrusions/H(+)-Organic Cation Antiporters. *Biochem. Pharmacol.* 74:359-371.

Tzvetkov MV, Vormfelde SV, Balen D, Meineke I, Schmidt T, Sehrt D, Sabolic I, Koepsell H and Brockmöller J (2009) The Effects of Genetic Polymorphisms in the Organic Cation Transporters OCT1, OCT2, and OCT3 on the Renal Clearance of Metformin. *Clin. Pharmacol. Ther.* 86:299-306.

Ulu R, Dogukan A, Tuzcu M, Gencoglu H, Ulas M, Ilhan N, Muqbil I, Mohammad RM, Kucuk O and Sahin K (2012) Regulation of Renal Organic Anion and Cation Transporters by Thymoquinone in Cisplatin Induced Kidney Injury. *Food Chem. Toxicol.* 50:1675-1679.

Urakami Y, Kimura N, Okuda M and Inui K (2004) Creatinine Transport by Basolateral Organic Cation Transporter HOCT2 in the Human Kidney. *Pharm. Res.* 21:976-981.

Urakami Y, Kimura N, Okuda M, Masuda S, Katsura T and Inui K (2005) Transcellular Transport of Creatinine in Renal Tubular Epithelial Cell Line LLC-PK1. *Drug Metab. Pharmacokinet.* 20:200-205.

Urakami Y, Okuda M, Saito H and Inui K (2000) Hormonal Regulation of Organic Cation Transporter OCT2 Expression in Rat Kidney. *FEBS Lett.* 473:173-176.

Vallon V, Eraly SA, Ramachandra RS, Gerasimova M, Rose M, Nagle M, Anzai N, Smith T, Sharma K, Nigam SK and Rieg T (2012) A Role for the Organic Anion Transporter OAT3 in Renal Creatinine Secretion in Mice. *Am. J. Physiol. Renal. Physiol.* [Epub ahead of print; PMID: 22338083].

Yonezawa A and Inui K (2011) Importance of the Multidrug and Toxin Extrusion MATE/SLC47A Family to Pharmacokinetics, Pharmacodynamics/Toxicodynamics and Pharmacogenomics. *Br. J. Pharmacol.* 164:1817-1825.

Zhang WX, Chen B, Zhang W, Chen N, Yu ZC and Cai WM (2007) Effect of MDR1 Gene Polymorphism on Progression of End-Stage Renal Disease. *Acta Pharmacol. Sin.* 28: 579-583.

In: Creatinine
Editors: I. H. Perkins and C. M. Chapman

ISBN: 978-1-62257-475-9

Chapter XI

Acute Kidney Injury: Assessment of Kidney Function and Damage

Wonngarm Kittanamongkolchai**, *Napat Leeaphorn,
Pongsathorn Kue-A-Pai and Wisit Cheungpasitporn
Department of Internal Medicine, Bassett Medical Center,
Cooperstown, New York, US

Abstract

Acute kidney injury (AKI) is characterized by a rapid decline in glomerular filtration rate (GFR) over hours to days that results in the retention of urea and other nitrogenous waste products normally cleared by the kidneys. It is associated with a 25% to 80% risk of in-hospital death and has been rising in the incidence over the past several decades. The RIFLE and AKIN criteria have greatest utility in epidemiologic studies. However, these definitions may be problematic when applied to patients at bedside because the baseline creatinine may be unknown. The creatinine (Cr) level may not perfectly reflect the severity of kidney injury because serum Cr is altered by age, sex, muscle mass, nutritional status, and medications. The novel biomarkers, such as Kidney injury molecule-1 (KIM-1) and Neutrophil gelatinase associated lipocalin (NGAL), are promising in the diagnosis of intrinsic AKI and may permit development of a new paradigm for classifying AKI in the future.

Introduction

Acute kidney injury (AKI), previously known as acute renal failure is characterized by a rapid decline in glomerular filtration rate (GFR) over hours to days that results in the retention of urea and other nitrogenous waste products normally cleared by the kidneys. It is a common clinical event with fatal complications. Patients with AKI can present with a wide range of symptom severity from asymptomatic and transient changes in laboratory parameters

* Email: wonngarm.kittanamongkolchai@bassett.org.

of GFR, to rapidly fatal derangements in regulation of effective circulating volume, electrolytes and acid-base composition of the plasma.

In the United States, > 1 million hospitalized patients yearly receive a diagnosis of AKI, and recent studies showing a rising incidence over the past several decades estimated to have a yearly incidence of 500 per 100,000 populations [1–4]. AKI is associated with a 25% to 80% risk of in-hospital death, particularly in those admitted to the Intensive Care Units (ICU) where in-hospital mortality rates may exceed 50% [4–6]. AKI has also been implicated in the pathogenesis of chronic kidney disease (CKD) [7].

Causes of AKI are generally divided into three major categories: (1) prerenal AKI (~55%), caused by renal hypoperfusion and resulted in decreased function without frank parenchymal damage; (2) intrinsic AKI (~40%), caused by disease that directly involve the renal parenchyma; and (3) postrenal AKI (~5%), caused by urinary tract obstruction.

Diagnostic evaluations include history and physical examination, urine findings, laboratory findings, radiologic evaluation, renal failure indices, kidney biopsy and novel biomarkers. In this chapter, we would mainly focus on assessing kidney function in AKI and diagnosis of kidney damage by novel biomarkers.

Definition of Acute Kidney Injury (AKI)

The Acute Dialysis Quality Initiative (ADQI) was created by a group of expert intensivists and nephrologists to develop consensus and evidence based guidelines for the treatment and prevention of acute renal failure [8]. Recognizing the need for a uniform definition for ARF, the ADQI group proposed a consensus graded definition, called the RIFLE [9]. These criteria have their greatest utility in epidemiologic studies.

The RIFLE criteria consists of various graded levels of kidney injury based upon percent rise in serum creatinine (Cr), urine output and outcome measures [8].

- Risk: 1.5-fold increase in the serum creatinine or GFR decrease by 25 percent or urine output <0.5 mL/kg per hour for six hours
- Injury: Twofold increase in the serum creatinine or GFR decrease by 50 percent or urine output <0.5 mL/kg per hour for 12 hours \
- Failure: Threefold increase in the serum creatinine or GFR decrease by 75 percent or urine output of <0.5 mL/kg per hour for 24 hours, or anuria for 12 hours
- Loss: Complete loss of kidney function (eg, need for renal replacement therapy) for more than four weeks
- ESRD: Complete loss of kidney function (eg, need for renal replacement therapy) for more than three months

Compared to patients who did not have AKI, patients in the RIFLE stages of "risk," "injury," and "failure" had increased relative mortality risks of 2.4 (CI 1.94-2.97), 4.15 (CI 3.14-5.48), and 6.37 (CI 5.14-7.9) [10-16].

The AKIN (Acute Kidney Injury Network) criteria are a modification of the RIFLE criteria and include both diagnostic and staging system [17-19]. The AKIN proposed the term acute kidney injury (AKI) to represent the entire spectrum of acute renal failure. The proposed diagnostic criteria are an abrupt (within 48 hours) absolute increase in the serum Cr concentration of >/=0.3 mg/dL (26.4 micromol/L) from baseline, a percentage increase in the serum Cr concentration of >/=50 percent, or oliguria of less than 0.5 mL/kg per hour for more than six hours.

- Stage 1. Increase in serum creatinine 0.3 mg/dl or 1.5 to 2 fold increase from baseline or urine output less than 0.5 mL/kg per hour for more than 6 hours
- Stage 2. Increase in serum creatinine >2-3 folds from baseline or urine output less than 0.5 mL/kg per hour for more than 12 hours
- Stage 3. Increase in serum creatinine >3 fold from baseline or serum creatinine of 4.0 mg/dl with an acute rise of at least 0.5 mg/dl or urine output less than 0.3 mL/kg per hour for 24 hours or anuria for 12 hours.

These criteria have greatest utility in epidemiologic studies and in defining consistent inclusion criteria and/or endpoints for clinical studies. However, these definitions may be problematic when applied to patients at bedside because the baseline creatinine may be unknown, and placement of a urinary catheter may not be indicated [20].

Moreover, patients with subclinical AKI may not develop changes in creatinine level despite evidence of nephron damage [21]. Also, the serum Cr level may not perfectly reflect the severity of kidney injury because serum Cr kinetics are altered by age, sex, muscle mass, nutritional status, and medications [20]. These criteria will likely be revised, and possibly replaced, as biomarkers of tubular injury are developed.

Assessment of Glomerular Filtration Rate (GFR)

The most common method of assessing renal function is by estimation of the glomerular filtration rate (GFR). The glomerular filtration rate (GFR) represents the volume of water filtered from the plasma per unit of time. Estimation of this value is currently considered the best method of evaluating kidney function and ideally involves a substance that is freely filtered by the glomeruli. The normal value for GFR depends on age, sex, and body size, and is approximately 130 and 120 mL/min/1.73 m2 for men and women, respectively, with considerable variation even among normal individuals [22]. GFR is decreased in those with renal dysfunction, and is used to monitor renal function in those with chronic kidney disease.

The direct measurement involves administration of a radioactive isotope (such as inulin or iothalamate) that is filtered at the glomerulus but neither reabsorbed nor secreted throughout the tubule [23-25]. However, direct measurement of GFR is not available in most clinical circumstances, and the serum creatinine level is used as a surrogate to estimate GFR.

Serum Creatinine

Creatinine (Cr) is derived from the metabolism of creatine in skeletal muscle and from dietary meat intake. It is released into the circulation at a relatively constant rate and has a stable plasma concentration [26]. Creatinine is freely filtered in the glomeruli, excreted by the kidneys, and easily measured in the blood. Measurement of this value has historically been the study of choice to evaluate kidney function. However, approximately 10 to 40 percent of urinary creatinine is derived from tubular secretion by the organic cation secretory pathways in the proximal tubule [26]. Additionally, serum creatinine can only be used in patients with stable kidney function [27]. With severe acute kidney injury, the GFR is markedly reduced but there has not yet been time for creatinine to accumulate and for the serum creatinine to reflect the degree of renal dysfunction.

The serum creatinine level concurrently increases with decreased GFR in the setting of kidney injuries. For example, a 50% reduction in the GFR is associated with an increase in the serum creatinine level from 1.0 to 2.0 mg/dL (88.4 to 176.8 μmol/L). The serum creatinine level also generally increases by 1.0 to 1.5 mg/dL (88.4 to 132.6 μmol/L) daily in patients who develop anephric due to circumstances such as bilateral nephrectomy, end-stage kidney disease, or severe acute kidney injury.

Using the serum creatinine alone to estimate renal functioning is not an ideal measure of kidney function. As we mentioned earlier, a small amount of creatinine is normally secreted by the proximal tubules, and this amount tends to increase as progressive renal decline occurs, thereby overestimating the true GFR value [26]. Elderly patients, those with malnutrition, liver failure, amputees, as well as patients with spinal cord injury or disease tend to have less muscle mass; hence, lower serum creatinine values that results in overestimation of the GFR.

Conversely, there are factors that increase serum creatinine without truly affecting renal function, such as dietary meat (protein) intake, volume of muscle mass, and medications that interfere with tubular secretion of creatinine such as cimetidine, trimethoprim, and probenecid. This circumstance may result in an underestimation of the GFR, which may lead to misdiagnosis of acute kidney injury. In addition, it has been suggested that the serum creatinine rises more rapidly with rhabdomyolysis (up to 2.5 mg/dL or 220 μmol/L per day) than with other causes of acute kidney injury [28].

Estimation Equations

The NKF K/DOQI guidelines suggest the use of the Cockcroft-Gault and Modification of Diet in Renal Disease (MDRD) study equations as an alternative method of estimating kidney function in adults. The MDRD study equation is increasingly utilized in the United States. The CKD-EPI equation is a new equation that is more accurate than the MDRD Study equation has also been reported. As we mentioned earlier regarding serum creatinine interpretation, proper interpretation of the results from these equations also requires stable kidney function [27].

Cockcroft-Gault Equation [29]

Ccr (mL/min) = [(140 - age) × weight(Kg)]/72 × Cr (mg/dL) × 0.85 (if the patient is female).

Modification of Diet in Renal Disease Study Equation [30]

GFR = 186 × (Scr)-1.154 × (age)-0.203 × 0.742 (if the patient is female) or × 1.212 (if the patient is black).

Abbreviated Modification of Diet in Renal Disease Study Equation [31]

GFR = 175 × (Scr)-1.154 × (age)-0.203 × 0.742 (if the patient is female) or × 1.212 (if the patient is black)

The Cockcroft-Gault and MDRD equations were developed for patients with CKD and have not been shown to accurately estimate kidney function in healthy persons or in patients with AKI. Use of these equations should be limited to patients with stages 3 to 5 chronic kidney disease (CKD) or those with an eGFR of 59 mL/min/1.73 m2 or less [32-38].

Creatinine Clearance

The creatinine clearance is usually determined from a 24 hour urine collection from the following equation:

- Creatinine clearance (L/day) = Ucr (mg/dL) x V (L/day) /Serum Cr (mg/dL)

This value has to be multiplied by 1000 to convert into mL and then divided by 1440 (the number of minutes in a day) to convert into units of mL/min.

A 24-hour urine collection for creatinine clearance is needed in circumstances requiring a precise estimation of kidney function such as the evaluation of living donor kidney transplant candidates. Over- or undercollection of a sample obtained for 24-hour urine collection may result in an inaccurate estimation of the GFR.

The accuracy of 24-hour urine collection can be assessed by comparing the total urine creatinine excretion with the expected value of creatinine excretion (20 to 25 mg/kg/24 h [0.18 to 0.22 mmol/kg/d] in men, 15 to 20 mg/kg/24 h [0.13 to 0.18 mmol/kg/d] in women).

Radionuclide Kidney Clearance Scanning

Radionuclide kidney clearance scanning, also known as GFR scanning, is now considered the gold standard for measurement of the GFR in healthy persons and in those with AKI. It is also helpful in evaluation of renal infarcts and urinary tract obstruction. However, use of these studies is limited because of expense, lack of widespread accessibility, and operator technical difficulties.

Blood Urea Nitrogen

Blood urea nitrogen (BUN), formed in the liver by the deamination of amino acids, is derived from protein waste products and freely filtered in the glomeruli. The normal BUN/Cr ratio is 10:1 to 15:1.

Conditions that decrease kidney perfusion, such as dehydration or heart failure, are associated with increase in the BUN/Cr ratio, typically to 20:1 or higher. BUN is generally less useful than Cr because the BUN can change independent of the GFR. A high-protein diet, catabolic states, and gastrointestinal bleeding also may cause an increase in the BUN level.

Decreased urea production and inadequate protein intake associated with disease states such as liver failure and malnutrition may cause a decrease in the BUN level and a subsequent overestimation of kidney function. Thus, these conditions may be associated with near normal values for both the BUN (due to decreased urea production) and the SCr (due to muscle wasting) despite a relatively large reduction in GFR [39-40].

Serum Cystatin C

Cystatin C is a low molecular weight protein that is a member of the cystatin superfamily of cysteine protease inhibitors. It is filtered at the glomerulus and not reabsorbed. However, it is metabolized in the tubules.

Cystatin C is thought to be produced by all nucleated cells at relatively constant rate, and not affected by changes in diet, although this is not proven. Cystatin C levels increase with age.

Estimation equations based on serum cystatin C have also been formulated [41-43]. Cystatin C-based equations have been proposed to be more accurate in populations with lower creatinine production, such as the elderly, children, renal transplant recipients, or patients with cirrhosis [44-45].

Although cystatin C appears to be more accurate for the assessment of GFR than serum creatinine in certain populations, the clinical use of cystatin as an alternate marker for estimating GFR is still limited because of the absence of definitive cut-off values [46-47], conflicting results in clinical studies, the poor commutability of results, and no accurate examination of costs and of its routine use in a stat laboratory. In addition, testing for cystatin C is only available in a limited number of laboratories. Cystatin C may be useful in those cases where Cr measurement is not appropriate, particularly in patients with liver cirrhosis, obesity, or malnutrition.

Novel Biomarkers for the Diagnosis of Kidney Damage

As was mentioned earlier, serum Cr and GFR estimation equations can only be used in patients with stable kidney function. With acute kidney injury, for example, the GFR is initially markedly reduced but there has not yet been time for Cr to accumulate and for the Cr to reflect the degree of renal dysfunction. In addition, serum Cr level may not change until accumulating in the blood 24 to 48 hours after kidney damage. Thus, at-risk patients remain undetected.

Several novel kidney injury biomarkers have been investigated and show great promise for the early and precise diagnosis of AKI. Kidney injury molecule-1 (KIM-1) is a type 1 transmembrane glycoprotein that shows marked upregulation in the proximal tubule with AKI [48]. KIM-1 is not expressed in appreciable quantities in the absence of tubular injury or in extrarenal tissues. KIM-1 can be detected shortly after ischemic or nephrotoxic injury in the urine and, accordingly, may be an easily tested biomarker in the clinical setting.

Neutrophil gelatinase associated lipocalin (NGAL) is another leading novel biomarker of AKI. NGAL was first discovered as a protein in granules of human neutrophils. NGAL is markedly upregulated and abundantly expressed in the kidney after renal ischemia and can be detected in the plasma and urine within 2 hours of cardiopulmonary bypass–associated AKI [49]. Other injury markers including urinary tubular enzymes, urinary low-molecular-weight proteins, and urinary interleukin-18, are being studied in an attempt to increase the early recognition of injury and predict the outcome in AKI.

A large multicenter study significantly demonstrated the strength of association between NGAL and intrinsic AKI. Furthermore, the study also demonstrated that NGAL and KIM-1 predicted poor outcomes during hospitalization, even days after the initial measurements [20]. These biomarkers are promising and may permit development of a new paradigm for classifying AKI in the future.

References

[1] Chertow GM, Burdick E, Honour M, Bonventre JV, Bates DW. Acute kidney injury, mortality, length of stay, and costs in hospitalized patients. *J. Am. Soc. Nephrol.* 2005;6:3365–70.

[2] Hsu CY, McCulloch CE, Fan D, Ordonez JD, Chertow GM, Go AS. Community-based incidence of acute renal failure. *Kindey Int.* 207;72:208-12.

[3] Waikar SS, Curhan GC, Wald R, McCarthy EP, Chertow GM. Declining mortality in patients with acute renal failure, 1988 to 2002. *J. Am. Soc. Nephol.* 2006;17:1143-50.

[4] Xue JL, Daniels F, Star RA, et al. Incidence and mortality of acute renal failure in Medicare beneficiaries, 1992 to 2001. *J. Am. Soc. Nephol.* 2006;17:1135-42.

[5] Liano F. Pascual J. Epidemiology of acute renal failure: a prospective, multicenter, community-based study. Madrid Acute Renal Failure Study Group. *Kindey Int.* 1996;50:811-8.

[6] Nash K, Hafeez A, Hou S. Hospital-acquired renal insufficiency. *Am. J. Kidney Dis.* 2002;39:930-6.

[7] Venkatachalam MA, Griffin KA, Lan R, Geng H, Saikumar P, Bidani AK. Acute kidney injury: a springboard for progression in chronic kidney disease. *Am. J. Psysiol. Renal. Physiol.* 2010;298:F1078-94.

[8] Ronco C, Kellum JA, Mehta R. Acute dialysis quality initiative (ADQI). *Nephrol. Dial Transplant* 2001; 16:1555.

[9] Bellomo R, Ronco C, Kellum JA, et al. Acute renal failure - definition, outcome measures, animal models, fluid therapy and information technology needs: the Second International Consensus Conference of the Acute Dialysis Quality Initiative (ADQI) Group. *Crit. Care* 2004; 8:R204.

[10] Ali T, Khan I, Simpson W, et al. Incidence and outcomes in acute kidney injury: a comprehensive population-based study. *J. Am. Soc. Nephrol.* 2007; 18:1292.

[11] Uchino S, Bellomo R, Goldsmith D, et al. An assessment of the RIFLE criteria for acute renal failure in hospitalized patients. *Crit. Care Med.* 2006; 34:1913.

[12] Hoste EA, Clermont G, Kersten A, et al. RIFLE criteria for acute kidney injury are associated with hospital mortality in critically ill patients: a cohort analysis. *Crit. Care* 2006; 10:R73.

[13] Kuitunen A, Vento A, Suojaranta-Ylinen R, Pettilä V. Acute renal failure after cardiac surgery: evaluation of the RIFLE classification. *Ann. Thorac. Surg.* 2006; 81:542.

[14] Cruz DN, Bolgan I, Perazella MA, et al. North East Italian Prospective Hospital Renal Outcome Survey on Acute Kidney Injury (NEiPHROS-AKI): targeting the problem with the RIFLE Criteria. *Clin. J. Am. Soc. Nephrol.* 2007; 2:418.

[15] Ostermann M, Chang RW. Acute kidney injury in the intensive care unit according to RIFLE. *Crit. Care Med.* 2007; 35:1837. 16.Ricci Z, Cruz D, Ronco C. The RIFLE criteria and mortality in acute kidney injury: A systematic review. *Kidney Int.* 2008; 73:538.

[16] Mehta RL, Kellum JA, Shah SV, et al. Acute Kidney Injury Network: report of an initiative to improve outcomes in acute kidney injury. *Crit. Care* 2007; 11:R31.

[17] Levin A, Warnock DG, Mehta RL, et al. Improving outcomes from acute kidney injury: report of an initiative. *Am. J. Kidney Dis.* 2007; 50:1.

[18] Molitoris BA, Levin A, Warnock DG, et al. Improving outcomes from acute kidney injury. *J. Am. Soc. Nephrol.* 2007; 18:1992.

[19] Nickolas TL, Schmidt-Ott KM, Canetta P, et al. Diagnostic and prognostic stratification in the emergency department using urinary biomarkers of nephron damage a multicenter prospective cohort study. *J. Am. Coll. Cardiol.* 2012 Jan 17;59(3):246-55.

[20] Mishra J, Ma Q, Prada A, et al. Identidication of neutrophil gelatinaseassociated lipocalin as a novel early urinary biomarker for ischemic renal injury. *J. Am. Soc. Nephol.* 2003;14:2534-43.

[21] Stevens, LA, Levey, AS. Measurement of kidney function. In: Medical Clinics of North America, Singh, AK, (Ed), W.B. Saunders, Philadelphia 2005. p.457.

[22] Rahn KH, Heidenreich S, Brückner D. How to assess glomerular function and damage in humans. *J. Hypertens* 1999; 17:309.

[23] Levey AS. Measurement of renal function in chronic renal disease. *Kidney Int.* 1990; 38:167.

[24] Brändström E, Grzegorczyk A, Jacobsson L, et al. GFR measurement with iohexol and 51Cr-EDTA. A comparison of the two favoured GFR markers in Europe. *Nephrol. Dial Transplant* 1998; 13:1176.

[25] Shemesh O, Golbetz H, Kriss JP, Myers BD. Limitations of creatinine as a filtration marker in glomerulopathic patients. *Kidney Int.* 1985; 28:830.

[26] Rule AD, Bergstralh EJ, Slezak JM, et al. Glomerular filtration rate estimated by cystatin C among different clinical presentations. *Kidney Int.* 2006; 69:399.

[27] Grossman RA, Hamilton RW, Morse BM, et al. Nontraumatic rhabdomyolysis and acute renal failure. *N. Engl. J. Med.* 1974; 291:807.

[28] Cockcroft DW, Gault MH. Prediction of creatinine clearance from serum creatinine. *Nephron* 1976; 16:31.

[29] Levey AS, Bosch JP, Lewis JB, et al. A more accurate method to estimate glomerular filtration rate from serum creatinine: a new prediction equation. Modification of Diet in Renal Disease Study Group. *Ann. Intern. Med.* 1999; 130:461.

[30] National Kidney Foundation. K/DOQI clinical practice guidelines for chronic kidney disease: evaluation, classification, and stratification. *Am. J. Kidney Dis.* 2002; 39:S1.

[31] Poggio ED, Wang X, Greene T, et al. Performance of the modification of diet in renal disease and Cockcroft-Gault equations in the estimation of GFR in health and in chronic kidney disease. *J. Am. Soc. Nephrol.* 2005; 16:459.

[32] Rule AD, Larson TS, Bergstralh EJ, et al. Using serum creatinine to estimate glomerular filtration rate: accuracy in good health and in chronic kidney disease. *Ann. Intern. Med.* 2004; 141:929.

[33] Gonwa TA, Jennings L, Mai ML, et al. Estimation of glomerular filtration rates before and after orthotopic liver transplantation: evaluation of current equations. *Liver Transpl.* 2004; 10:301.

[34] Froissart M, Rossert J, Jacquot C, et al. Predictive performance of the modification of diet in renal disease and Cockcroft-Gault equations for estimating renal function. *J. Am. Soc. Nephrol.* 2005; 16:763.

[35] Lin J, Knight EL, Hogan ML, Singh AK. A comparison of prediction equations for estimating glomerular filtration rate in adults without kidney disease. *J. Am. Soc. Nephrol.* 2003; 14:2573.

[36] Ibrahim H, Mondress M, Tello A, et al. An alternative formula to the Cockcroft-Gault and the modification of diet in renal diseases formulas in predicting GFR in individuals with type 1 diabetes. *J. Am. Soc. Nephrol.* 2005; 16:1051.

[37] Botev R, Mallié JP, Couchoud C, et al. Estimating glomerular filtration rate: Cockcroft-Gault and Modification of Diet in Renal Disease formulas compared to renal inulin clearance. *Clin. J. Am. Soc. Nephrol.* 2009; 4:899.

[38] Papadakis MA, Arieff AI. Unpredictability of clinical evaluation of renal function in cirrhosis. Prospective study. *Am. J. Med.* 1987; 82:945.

[39] Sherman DS, Fish DN, Teitelbaum I. Assessing renal function in cirrhotic patients: problems and pitfalls. *Am. J. Kidney* Dis 2003; 41:269.

[40] Grubb A, Nyman U, Björk J, et al. Simple cystatin C-based prediction equations for glomerular filtration rate compared with the modification of diet in renal disease prediction equation for adults and the Schwartz and the Counahan-Barratt prediction equations for children. *Clin. Chem.* 2005; 51:1420.

[41] Sjöström P, Tidman M, Jones I. Determination of the production rate and non-renal clearance of cystatin C and estimation of the glomerular filtration rate from the serum concentration of cystatin C in humans. *Scand. J. Clin. Lab. Invest.* 2005; 65:111.

[42] Grubb A, Björk J, Lindström V, et al. A cystatin C-based formula without anthropometric variables estimates glomerular filtration rate better than creatinine clearance using the Cockcroft-Gault formula. *Scand. J. Clin. Lab. Invest.* 2005; 65:153.

[43] White C, Akbari A, Hussain N, et al. Estimating glomerular filtration rate in kidney transplantation: a comparison between serum creatinine and cystatin C-based methods. *J. Am. Soc. Nephrol.* 2005; 16:3763.

[44] Pöge U, Gerhardt T, Stoffel-Wagner B, et al. Calculation of glomerular filtration rate based on cystatin C in cirrhotic patients. *Nephrol. Dial Transplant* 2006; 21:660.

[45] Shlipak MG, Sarnak MJ, Katz R, et al. Cystatin C and the risk of death and cardiovascular events among elderly persons. *N. Engl. J. Med.* 2005; 352:2049.

[46] Mussap M, Plebani M. Biochemistry and clinical role of human cystatin C. *Crit. Rev. Clin. Lab. Sci.* 2004; 41:467.

[47] Vaidya VS, Ramirez V, Ichimura T, et al. Urinary kidney injury molecule-1: a sensitive quantitative biomarker for early detection of kidney tubular injury. *Am. J. Physiol. Renal. Physiol.* 2006; 290:F517.

[48] Herget-Rosenthal S. One step forward in the early detection of acute renal failure. *Lancet* 2005; 365:1205.

In: Creatinine
Editors: I. H. Perkins and C. M. Chapman
ISBN: 978-1-62257-475-9

Chapter XII

Retinol X Creatinine in Kidney Disease - A New Approach

***Miguel Roehrs*[1,3]**
***and José Antonio Mainardi de Carvalho*[2,3]**
[1]Post-graduate Program of Pharmacology, Center of Healthy Sciences, Brazil
[2]Post-graduate Program of Pharmaceutical Sciences,
Center of Healthy Sciences, Brazil
[3]Clinical Laboratory, University Hospital of Santa Maria,
Federal University of Santa Maria, Santa Maria, RS, Brazil

Abstract

Chronic kidney disease is renal injury in progressive and irreversible loss of renal glomerular, tubular and endocrine functions. Its most advanced stage is called chronic renal failure (CRF) and it is the final common pathway for a variety of renal disorders. According to a recent consensus of the National Kidney Foundation, the IRC is characterized by a glomerular filtration rate (GFR) below 60 ml/min/1, 73m2 body surface. The degree of CKD varies according to the glomerular filtration rate and values below 15 ml/min/1, 73 m2 already indicate kidney failure. In clinical practice, GFR is assessed by measuring creatinine in serum or plasma or by determining the creatinine clearance, being that the creatinine clearance remains one of markers most used in evaluation of renal function, despite of overestimating the GFR and depend on muscle mass. Retinol is the major circulating form of vitamin A and it plays an essential role in maintaining the health of mammals. After absorption, vitamin A is transported from the hepatic tissue to peripherals sites; for such transport to happen, retinol needs be connected to complex retinol-binding protein 4 (RBP4) - transthyretin. In order to allow excretion of retinol, catabolism of protein of the complex (RBP4) must occur, which takes place in the kidney, the main catabolic site of this protein; for this reason the homeostasis of circulating vitamin A depends on the renal function. Patients who have renal diseases present elevated levels of retinol because in this pathology the renal function decreases, as well as its catabolic activity will also be reduced, causing a reduction of the catabolism of RBP4 and consequently of excretion of retinol. In fact, there is a strong positive direct correlation between the concentrations of vitamin A and serum creatinine. Thus, according to the increase of the severity degree, chronic renal insufficiency suffers a decrease of renal function reflected by the augment of serum creatinine as well as of retinol levels. The determination of vitamin A in patients with renal disease has great importance because high concentrations of this vitamin have a pro-oxidant proven by the relation with biomarkers of oxidative stress such as malondialdehyde and antioxidant enzymes (glutathione peroxidase, catalase and superoxide dismutase). However, the determination of vitamin A in the laboratory routine has limitations mainly due to its high cost and for requiring more complex methodologies. Since there is a direct relation between serum retinol and creatinine, it can estimate the levels of retinol from the levels of creatinine. On the other hand, creatinine is considered a low cost methodology, standardized and accessible to all clinical laboratories, and the relation between retinol and creatinine consists an additional tool for clinical monitoring and treatment of patients with kidney disease.

Chronic Kidney Disease

Chronic kidney disease (CKD) is a serious public health problem which prevalence has increased in the last few years. Its progression is associated with high morbidity and mortality, especially with increasing overall prevalence of major causes of CKD as hypertension, diabetes *mellitus* (DM) and obesity, other risk factors for CKD include aging and family history [1]. According to data from the National Health and Nutrition Examination Surveys (NHANES), the prevalence CKD (excluding CKD terminal) in the United States was 13.1% in period 1999-2004. At the end of 2008, there were over 500 000 Americans living with end-stage renal disease (ESRD) [2]. Associated with this, the number of CKD terminal patients needing dialysis or transplantation of kidney has also increased significantly in developed and developing countries [3]. In CKD, the kidneys are damaged and/or cannot filter blood normally. However, CKD is usually asymptomatic until its most advanced state. CKD has been identified due to decreased kidney function and/or kidney damage persistent for at least three months. Kidney dysfunction is indicated by a glomerular filtration rate (GFR) of less than 60 mL/min/1.73 m^2, while kidney damage most frequently is manifested as increased urinary albumin excretion [4, 5].

Glomerular Filtration Rate and Creatinine

The endogenous creatinine is the most widely used marker to estimate GFR, endogenously produced and released in body fluids at a constant rate, creatinine has its plasma concentration maintained within a narrow limit [6]. As a marker of GFR, it is convenient and low cost. However, it is important to consider that plasma levels of creatinine may be affected by factors such as age, sex, exercise, use of certain medications, muscle mass and nutritional status of the individual [7].

The development of a formula based on calculation of estimated GFR (eGFR) has offered a very practical and easy approach for converting serum creatinine value into GFR result considering patient's age, sex, ethnicity and weight (depending on the equation type). The commonly used equations include Cockraft and Gault (1976), Modification of Diet in Renal Disease (MDRD) (1999) and Chronic Kidney Disease Epidemiology Collaboration (CKD-EPI) (2009). It is the implementation of these equations particularly the MDRD that has raised the medical awareness about diagnosis and management of CKD and its adoption by many guidelines in North America and Europe [8].

Retinol

Retinol, the major circulating form of vitamin A refers to a subclass of retinoic acids long understood to help regulate immune function and to reduce morbidity of infectious diseases. This vitamin is required for normal functioning of the visual system, maintenance of cell function for growth, epithelial integrity, production of red blood cells, immunity, and reproduction. Different forms of vitamin A include β carotene, which is found in plants, and preformed vitamin A, which is found in animal sources. Retinol is an essential nutrient that cannot be synthetized so it must be obtained through diet. Its deficiency increases vulnerability to a range of illnesses including diarrhea, measles, and respiratory infections. High intake of synthetic vitamin A over a prolonged period may lead to toxicity, though toxicity from natural food sources is rare. Periodic supplementation should not cause serious adverse effects [9]. Physiologically, retinol concentration is regulated by the hepatic synthesis of its specific carrier retinol-binding protein 4 (RBP4), a small visceral protein (21-kDa), which is catabolized by the kidney after delivering retinol to target tissues [10].

Retinol X Creatinine

Patients with renal failure on hemodialysis or peritoneal dialysis have high levels of retinol binding protein (RBP4) as well as retinol (vitamin A). The increases that are observed in both RBP4 and retinol occur due to metabolism, wich is greatly influenced by kidney function. It is known that vitamin A is transported from its hepatic stores to peripheral target sites in the form of retinol bound to its specific carrier protein, retinol-binding protein (RBP) and transthyretin (TTR). The retinol-binding protein 4 (RBP4) is a 21 kDa plasma protein that is mainly synthesized in the liver and adipose tissue and is known to transport retinol (ROH) in the blood. The binding of ROH to RBP4 guarantees the homeostatic regulation of plasma ROH levels, which is an essential aspect for a variety of physiological processes. In healthy individuals RBP4 is mainly synthesized in the liver and secreted into the circulation in a 1:1:1 complex with ROH and transthyretin (TTR). The binding with TTR increases the molecular weight of RBP4 and thus prevents its glomerular filtration and catabolism in the kidney. After releasing ROH into the target cells the remaining apo-RBP4 (unbound ROH) is rapidly filtered through the glomeruli and subsequently reabsorbed in the proximal tubular cells via the megalin–cubulin receptor complex and then catabolized. It was observed an increase in circulatory retinol in rats with experimental acute renal failure and have established that this increase is almost entirely due to retinol in the retinol–RBP–TTR complex. This retinol is derived from the hepatic pool of retinol newly acquired from the diet, suggesting that the kidney modulates its release [11].

In this manner, normal kidney function influences the release of hepatic retinol into circulation and contributes to circulatory vitamin A homeostasis. In this line, clearance and catabolism of retinol-binding protein depend on normal renal function. In fact, a correlation between plasma vitamin A and serum creatinine concentration has been observed, suggesting an association with increased severity of renal failure. In this way, it was demonstrated that the kidney, the main site of RBP4 catabolism, contributes to an elevation of RBP4 levels during chronic kidney disease (CKD) and regarding the kidney function, there was a strong correlation between serum creatinine and RBP4 levels [12]. Some studies have shown that levels of retinol in patients with kidney failure are increased, showing no damage to these patients. However, there is evidence that this increase can bring many consequences and may even in many cases have a toxic action. This discrepancy between results of different authors is due to differences in diet, wich varies from region region since vitamin A comes from animal sources. Thus, as there is a strong correlation demonstrated between retinol levels and creatinine. There is also a strong correlation between the retinol and creatinine levels with the malondialdehyde levels, classic marker of lipid peroxidation, wich shows that is occurring damage lipids, as well as antioxidant enzymes [13]. There are several methodologies for the determination of retinol and RBP4. These methods, besides being very sensitive and important for the diagnosis and maintenance of patients with renal failure are complex and costly, and for the normal routine of clinical laboratories these techniques have limitations. In addition, creatinine is still considered as a good marker of renal function, since the technique has a good sensitivity in the diagnosis and management of kidney disease, also having a low operating cost. This is very important for poor countries, where most advanced methodologies would be made impossible. Another aspect that emphasizes the use of creatinine is that it correlates strongly with other important markers in renal disease. Therefore, the simple determination of creatinine concentration can predict how much of retinol and RBP4 levels.

References

[1] Matsushita, K; Van der Velde, M; Astor, BC; et al. Association of estimated glomerular filtration rate and albuminuria with all-cause and cardiovascular mortality in general population cohorts: a collaborative metaanalysis. *Lancet* 2010, 375(9731), p: 2073-2081.

[2] United States Renal Data System. United States Renal Data System 2010 Annual Data Report: Atlas of Chronic Kidney Disease and End-Stage Renal Disease in the United States. National Institutes of Health, *National Institute of Diabetes and Digestive and Kidney Diseases*; 2010. www.usrds.org/adr.htm.

[3] Viana, HR; Soares, CMBM; Tavares, MS; et al. Inflammation in chronic kidney disease: the role of cytokines. *J. Bras. Nefrol.* 2011, 33(3), p: 351-364

[4] National Kidney Foundation. K/DOQI clinical practice guidelines for chronic kidney disease: evaluation, classification, and stratification. *Am. J. Kidney Dis.,* 2002, 39(2 Suppl 1), p: S1-266.

[5] Levey, SA; Eckardt, K; Tsukamoto, Y; et al. Definition and classification of chronic kidney disease: A position an statement from Kidney Disease: Improving Global Autocomes (KDIGO). *Kidney International* 2005, 67, p: 2089 -2100.

[6] Levey, AS; Bosch, JP; Lewis, JB; et al. A more accurate method to estimate glomerular filtration rate from serum creatinine. *Ann. Intern. Med.* 1999, 130, p: 461-470.

[7] Myers, GL; Miller, WG; Coresh, J; et al. Recommendations for improving serum creatinine measurement: a report from the laboratory working group of the National Kidney Disease Education Program. *Clin. Chem.* 2006, 52, p: 5-18.

[8] Mula-Abed, WA; Al Rasadi, K; Al-Riyami, D. Estimated Glomerular Filtration Rate (eGFR): A Serum Creatinine-Based Test for the Detection of Chronic Kidney Disease and its Impact on Clinical Practice. *Oman Med. J.* 2012, 27(2), p: 108-113.

[9] Mayo-Wilson, E; Imdad, A; Herzer, K; et al. Vitamin A supplements for preventing mortality, illness, and blindness in children aged under 5: systematic review and meta-analysis. *BMJ* 2011, 343, p: 1-19.

[10] Espe, KM; Raila, J; Henze, A. Impact of vitamin A on clinical outcomes in haemodialysis patients. *Nephrol. Dial. Transplant.* 2011, 26, p: 4054–4061.

[11] Frey, SK; Nagl, B; Henze, A; et al. Isoforms of retinol binding protein 4 (RBP4) are increased in chronic diseases of the kidney but not of the liver. *Lipid Healthy Dis.* 2008, 7, p: 29.

[12] Rock, CL; Jahnke, MG; Gorenflo, DW; et al. Antioxidant vitamins in hemodialysis. *Am. J. Clin. Nutr.* 1997, 65, p: 844–850.

[13] Roehrs, M; Valentini, J; Bulcão, R; et al. The plasma retinol levels as pro-oxidant/oxidant agents in haemodialysis patients. *Nephrol. Dial. Transpl.* 2009, 24, p: 2212-2218.

Index

B

C

D

E

F

G

H

I

J

K

L

M

N

O

P

Q

R

S

T

U

V

W

Y